Thomas Jefferson and Early American Health Care

Thomas Jefferson
and
Early American Health Care

Academic Medicine in the Nineteenth Century

Robert S. Gibson, M.D.

Frederic C. Beil
Savannah
2023

Frederic C. Beil
609 Whitaker Street
Savannah, Georgia 31401

Library of Congress Cataloging-in-Publication Data
Names: Gibson, Robert S., author
Description: First edition. | Savannah : Frederic C. Beil, 2023.
Includes bibliographical references and index.
"The story of Thomas Jefferson's belief in scientific advancement, especially in medicine and public health."
Identifiers: LCCN 2023025823 | 9781929490615
(cloth ; alk. paper)
Subjects: MESH: Jefferson, Thomas, 1743-1826. | University of Virginia. School of Medicine. | History of Medicine | Schools, Medical—history | Public Health—history | History, 19th Century | Virginia
Classification: LCC R747.U73 | NLM WZ WZ 70 AVB | DDC
610.71/1755—dc23/eng/20230703
LC record available at https://lccn.loc.gov/202302583

Printed in the United States of America

Design and composition by Isabella Sottile

Contents

Foreword

FOR THOSE WHO CHERISH (or condemn) our third president, *Thomas Jefferson and Early American Healthcare* is a revelation, combining a compelling series of stories with voluminous archive-based research to interpret little-known details about Jefferson that continue to be influential today. This book takes the reader into new territory by exploring Jefferson's roles in promoting science-based medicine and the educational prerequisites needed to foster it. The author, Dr. Robert Gibson, has more than compensated for his lack of formal historical training with decades of careful research in all pertinent primary and secondary sources, informed by his own background as a practicing physician and medical educator.

An unexpected portrait emerges. Jefferson exemplified and explored the science of health in its infancy, embracing principles espoused by Francis Bacon, Isaac Newton, Pierre Jean Georges Cabanis, and others. Indeed, one of the crucial points of the book is its demonstration that Jefferson prefigured and promoted scientific inquiry in general, and evidence-based medicine in particular. In an age in which bleeding, purging, and untested herbals were the norm of disease treatment, Jefferson, despite not being a physician, lived by the Hippocratic maxim that medicine should first do no harm and instead allow the body's defenses to work, in lieu of drastic or untested interventions. Far from advocating a simplistic trust in nature, Jefferson promoted a judicious restraint based on his assimilation of scientific and medical concepts drawn from Enlightenment thinkers. The careful analysis of how French *philosophes* helped fashion Jefferson's own scientific ideals is one of the many highlights of this volume.

The book is brilliant in presenting the often gory and ineffectual practices of medical treatment in colonial America. Against this historical backdrop Dr. Gibson analyzes the specifics of Jefferson's major contribution to scientific and pedagogical advance, grounded in in his painstaking planning of the University of Virginia. Particularly important is the author's exploration of the ways that the new university's curriculum, testing requirements, and faculty appointments, which Jefferson formulated and managed, led to higher and more rigorous academic training for medical students, establishing standards of scientific mastery that did not become widespread elsewhere until the beginning of the twentieth century. All this is enlivened by engaging descriptions of a library unique in scope, authority, and cost; a novel anatomy theater and teaching museum; treatment in a student infirmary; university clinics open to local residents; and innovative practice-based learning exercises in pharmacology and chemical experimentation. Jefferson's public-health contributions were by no means limited to the improved training of doctors. The book describes his numerous and often pioneering innovations in free vaccinations, hospitals for seafarers, hygiene-based architecture, drainage infrastructure, and the dissemination of health information to the general public. In one of his many foreshadowings of contemporary America, Jefferson subscribed to the belief that a prosperous republic required health consciousness in its citizenry.

Breaking new ground, the book shows that Jefferson's influence on medicine extended well past his death in 1826 by relating the achievements of his protégé and personal physician at the University of Virginia, Robley Dunglison, who later achieved prominence as an educator and author in Philadelphia, as well as the innovations of other prominent faculty members, especially James Lawrence Cabell, who remained in Charlottesville until his death in 1889. Through most of the nineteenth century, these men and their students propagated Jefferson's ideals nationwide via textbooks, academic journals, teaching technologies, and institutions such as the American Medical Association and what would become the United States Public Health Service. Their work ensured that the establishment of an American academic infrastructure in medicine, distinct from Europe's, would be informed by Jefferson's legacy.

In sum, the book demonstrates the lasting intellectual contribution that Thomas Jefferson made to American medicine when he founded the University of Virginia. Dr. Gibson's book deserves the attention of a wide range of readers ranging from individuals interested in American history, through health-care workers exploring the roots of their profession, to Jefferson researchers seeking to investigate links between the third president and the medical sciences.

Andrew J. O'Shaughnessy, *The Illimitable Freedom of the Human Mind: Thomas Jefferson's Idea of a University* (Charlottesville: University of Virginia Press, 2022).

Acknowledgments

THIS BOOK REPRESENTS years of research and writing, but it could not have succeeded without the assistance of many. First, I owe an enormous debt of gratitude to Andrew J. O'Shaughnessy, Vice President of the Thomas Jefferson Foundation at Monticello and Saunders Director of the Robert H. Smith International Center for Jefferson Studies (2004–2022). Andrew has been an unwavering source of support, encouragement, and inspiration. When others described my project as overly ambitious, especially for a non-historian, he convinced me that it was a worthy endeavor, and helped to enrich my ideas. Our many enlightening discussions and his amazing insights will forever be cherished.

J. Jefferson Looney, the Daniel P. Jordan Editor of *The Papers of Thomas Jefferson, Retirement Series*, twice read, corrected, and commented in detail on the final two drafts of the manuscript. His extensive editing resulted in essential improvements, and I am deeply grateful for his patience and expertise.

In this work extensive use has been made of quotations from Jefferson's writings, for good reason. Most often his own method of expression has proven superior to any possible paraphrasing or summarization, as his choice of word and phrase invariably revealed much about his complex persona and philosophy. The quotes used in this book are exact transcriptions that include Jefferson's idiosyncratic spellings and no capitals at the beginning of sentences, a point that Jeff Looney insisted upon.

I am especially grateful to Nicole Schroeder, a UVA graduate student in history, for her crucial research over four years, including a detailed investigation of book borrowing by students in the early years of the university. I'd also like to express an utmost appreciation to Joseph Eckenrode. He diligently read many drafts of the manuscript and astutely provided numerous suggestions for how to make my arguments more effective. Without his endless help, this manuscript would not be where it is today.

I am also beholden to those readers who graciously reviewed the manuscript at various stages, offering valuable feedback. These included: Robert M. Carey, W. Bernard Carlson, Robert L. Chevalier, Martin Clagett, Don Eugene Detmer, Michael A. Flannery, Arlene Keeling, Sylvia Kraemer, Vladimir Kryzhanovski, Lucia (Cinder) Stanton, Edward J. Stemmler, Keith Thomson, and Nadine Zimmerli. Others kindly answered questions, sent references, and/or shared unpublished manuscripts, including Robert Bloodgood, John Boles, Don Detmer, Jonathon Erlen, David Hudson, Joseph Kett, Richard M. Mikulski, Merrill D. Peterson, Curtis Tribble and Jennings L. Wagoner, Jr. Additional thanks go to Lynn A. Price, who provided much needed expertise in formatting endnotes and the bibliography.

All historical exploration depends enormously on the resources of libraries and their staff, so I am particularly grateful to Daniel Cavanaugh, Alvin B. and Nancy Baird Curator of Historical Collections, and his amazing associate Emily Bowden at the Claude Moore Health Sciences Library of the University of Virginia; the patience and always helpful staff at the University's Albert and Shirley Small Special Collections Library; to John McKee at the Thomas Jefferson Foundation at Monticello; Charles B. Greifenstein and Adrianna Link at the American Philosophical Society: Kelsey Duinkerken at Thomas Jefferson University Archives & Special Collections, Philadelphia; Jonathan Hoppe at the Philadelphia Museum of Art; Kenneth Johnson at the Library of Congress, Jessica Murphy at the Francis A. Countway Library of Medicine, Harvard University, and Kaitlyn Krieg at The Morgan Library and Museum New York.

My last thanks are reserved for my wife, Mary, of fifty years. She has been a quintessential support system, providing calm when I panicked and encouragement when I floundered. Moreover, she tolerated my interminable disappearances into my home office. For these and other reasons, I am forever grateful.

Finally, a number of concepts in this book are revised versions of previously published material by the author. This material appeared in *The Founding of Thomas Jefferson's University*, pp. 151–174, © 2019 by the Rector and Visitors of the University of Virginia.

Part I

JEFFERSON ON SCIENCE, HEALTH CARE, AND MEDICAL EDUCATION

The first wealth is health.

Ralph Waldo Emerson, 1860

Chapter 1

A STATESMAN OF SCIENCE AND FRIEND OF HUMANITY

Every discovery which multiplies the subsistence of men must be a matter of joy to every friend of humanity.

Thomas Jefferson to Jeudy de l'Hommande, 1787[1]

THOMAS JEFFERSON (1743–1826) was one of the great intellects of the eighteenth century. His genius had so many facets that in 1962, John F. Kennedy remarked at a White House dinner for all living American Nobel laureates his guests represented "the most extraordinary collection of talent, of human knowledge that has ever been gathered together at the White House, with the possible exception of when Thomas Jefferson dined alone."[2] In the letter in the chapter heading above and many others, Jefferson expressed his belief in scientific advancement, the idea that the diffusion of new useful knowledge was essential for a forward-looking young nation intent on establishing representative democracy, a way to lead it out of the colonial-era wilderness to a future promised land of egalitarian liberty, human prosperity and happiness.[3] More than most of his contemporaries, Jefferson recognized the transformative potential of scientific progress, and his personal commitment to it and its public dissemination was a lifelong pursuit.

Jefferson is acknowledged for his brilliance in many fields, but less well known is his great interest in the medical practices and customs of his time, and his contributions to the corpus of medical science, especially public health, and to the reform of medical education in America.[4] During his life, he became a crusading champion for all of the sciences, an avid student of medicine, a friend and colleague of many enlightened leaders in medicine, an advocate for the physical and mental well-being of the American citizenry, and the founding force behind two medical schools in America.[5] This chapter examines the influences that shaped Jefferson's intellectual development and fostered his lifelong interest in science, which subsequent chapters will show affected his personal and intellectual attitudes to the practice of medicine in the early nineteenth century.

Throughout this chapter, Jefferson's extraordinary esteem for knowledge and his unceasing dedication to the practical application of science are illustrated. It will present examples of his insatiable desire to learn and to discover new truths based upon "sober facts," and at the same time delve into the many factors that animated his lust for precision and logic in his quest for scientific progress and educational reform. This chapter will also introduce the thinkers who aroused Jefferson's passion for those characteristics that gave legitimacy and authority to science and show how Jefferson himself was a sophisticated practitioner in numerous scientific fields. It will be argued that insofar as Jefferson supported scientific endeavors through libraries, scholarly societies, voyages of discovery, high-level correspondence, and universities, as well as by government policies and monies, he was instrumental in establishing the infrastructure of scientific research in the United States and has been called aptly a "statesman of science."[6] These activities had a direct impact on Jefferson's vision for, and founding of, the University of Virginia and its medical department.

Jefferson's Interests in Science

Science and education were interests Jefferson pursued all of his life, notwithstanding his obligations as member of the Virginia House of Burgesses (1769–75); member of the Continental Congress (1775–76, during which he authored the Declaration of Independence, and 1783–84); member of the Virginia House of Delegates (1776–79); governor of Virginia (1779–81); minister plenipotentiary to France (1784–89);[7] secretary of state in President George Washington's cabinet (1790–93); vice president of the United States under John Adams (1797–1801); president of the United States (1801–09); and in his later years, venerable sage and founding father of the University of Virginia (1809–26). In 1791, Jefferson compared natural history [science] to politics and said that "the first in my passion, the last my duty," and in these few words he summarized a preoccupation which spanned more than five decades of public service, and a lifetime of scientific endeavor.[8]

Reflected in his papers, letters, and memoranda of his studies is the eternal mental struggle he endured, on the one hand to chase as a private citizen the scientific interests for which he felt he was destined, and on the other hand to fulfill the patriotic obligations to serve his state and the new republic of which he was an architect. As he was leaving the presidency, Jefferson wrote that "nature intended me for the tranquill pursuits of science, by rendering them my supreme delight. but the enormities of the times in which I have lived, have forced me to take a part in resisting them, and to commit myself on the boisterous ocean of political passions." Later he exulted "that I may at length be indulged in those studious pursuits, from which nothing but revolutionary duties would ever have called me."[9] Although Jefferson spent much of his life, however reluctantly and even complainingly, in the public service of his country, he preferred the pursuit of science to politics, because in his quest for scientific truth he had only to follow the evidence rather than bend to public opinion or the pressure of power groups.

More than any other of his contemporaries, with the possible exception of Benjamin Franklin, Jefferson displayed an extraordinarily wide range of scientific interests. Chief among these were agriculture, archaeology, astronomy, botany, chemistry, comparative anatomy and linguistics, cryptography, entomology, ethnology, geography and exploration, library science, mathematics, mechanical engineering, meteorology, medicine and surgery, paleontology, physics, public health, and zoology. Jefferson's interest in all of the sciences was not merely that of the dilettante, for he brought new knowledge to many different fields. More importantly, he came to view the nature of science as an endless frontier, rather than fixed and catechistic, and he used his accumulated knowledge and worldwide political status to enhance the reputation of science in his own country and at the same time to bring recognition of American science to the rest of the world.[10]

Early Influences

A combination of influences sparked Jefferson's passion for science. His early curiosity about the natural and physical sciences was likely kindled by posthumous accounts of his maternal grandfather, Isham Randolph (1684–1742), whose scientific interests and botanical expertise were widely recognized outside of colonial America; by his own father, Peter Jefferson, an accomplished explorer–surveyor and cartographer, who died in Jefferson's youth but left him with a fascination with western exploration; and by one of his early teachers, the Reverend James Maury, who went beyond providing a solid classical grounding by instilling a broad humanistic outlook and emphasis on service to society.[11] In his teachings, Maury argued that all ideas, including religious beliefs must pass the bar of reason; that is, a person should not accept any precept until he had "received rational satisfaction of [its] credibility."[12] During his time at Maury's school (1757–59), Jefferson was first introduced to the rudiments of natural history and possibly also to natural philosophy in the form of Isaac Newton's celestial mechanics.[13] Thus, as an adolescent, Jefferson was exposed to an ethos where beliefs, no matter the source, were required to be based on evidence, as well as the ideas of contemporary natural philosophers, the incubators of modern science.

From March 1760 to April 1762, Jefferson attended the College of William and Mary and came under the influence of William Small (1734–75), a graduate of Marischal College of the University of Aberdeen on Scotland's east coast.[14]

Small (see Figure 1), the only professor at the Williamsburg school to win Jefferson's admiration and affection, was also the only member of the faculty who was not an Anglican minister. Like most of its counterparts in the American colonies, the College of William and Mary had been founded as a seminary for educating young gentlemen and training others to become ministers of the gospel. One of Jefferson's objections to William and Mary, as he knew it from his student days, was the clerical control, exemplified by the requirement that professors subscribe to the Thirty–nine Articles of the Church of England. The board of visitors was appointed by the Anglican Church, and all students had to attend chapel twice daily and learn the catechism. Later, first in the Virginia legislature and then when he became the governor, Jefferson acted to secularize the school.[15]

Small was a delightful exception to his more strictly orthodox colleagues, a polymath who opposed all form of narrow dogmatism and exerted a decisive influence on Jefferson's intellectual development, including his thinking on what a university ought to be. In the time Small spent at the College of William and Mary (1758–64), he did more to modernize the institution than any man before him and his innovations had a powerful and enduring effect on his pupils, especially Jefferson's nascent passion for science. Not only did he bring new insights, based on the excellent schooling he had received in Scotland, to the teaching of natural philosophy and mathematics, he initiated a revolutionary pedagogical practice, the lecture–discussion–demonstration method whereby formal lectures were provided in the morning, followed by commentary and Socratic questioning, and a series of practical demonstrations in the afternoon. This mode of teaching broke completely with the traditional collegiate system in mid-eighteenth century colonial America; it constituted an outright abandonment of ancient, and all–together sterile, memory lessons and recitation exercises, and it proved to be more effective in engaging students and improving their critical thinking and reasoning skills. Small encouraged his pupils to undertake further private study. Under his influence, Jefferson's notion of a working day came to include independent reading and reflective learning. According to family members, he frequently spent fifteen hours a day in classroom work and his own study.[16]

Other weighty changes championed by Small at William and Mary included the teaching of belles-lettres, the introduction of the Scottish Common Sense School of Philosophy, and a rational and elevated course of study that systematically probed the latest developments in science, mathematics, moral philosophy (ethics, rhetoric, and logic) and natural law, and the avant–garde ideas of Enlightenment thinkers and empiricists such as Isaac Newton, Francis Bacon, John Locke, Francis Hutchinson, Lord Kames, David Hume, and Adam Smith.[17] Jefferson likened Small to "a father" to "whose enlightened & affectionate guidance of my studies while at College, I am indebted for every thing."[18] The influence of his tutelage is perhaps best captured in Jefferson's own words:

> it was my great good fortune, and what probably fixed the destinies of my life that Dr Wm Small of Scotland was then professor of Mathematics, a man profound in most of the useful branches of science, with a happy talent of communicn correct & gentlemanly manners, & an enlarged & liberal mind. he, most happily for me, became soon attached to me & made me his daily companion when not engaged in the school; and from his conversation I got my first views of the expansion of science & of the system of things in which we are placed.[19]

As a mature adult, Jefferson did not forget his beloved teacher, or the fact that Small's influence extended well beyond scientific and pedagogical enlightenment. In a letter to his grandson, then–president Jefferson paid further tribute to his college mentor, writing that, when confronted with "temptations & difficulties, I would ask myself what would Dr Small . . . do in this situation? What course in it will ensure me [his] approbation? I am certain that this mode of deciding on my conduct tended more to its correctness than any reasoning powers I possessed."[20]

Other "affectionate mentors" contributed greatly to Jefferson's intellectual development during his time in Williamsburg (1760–67). He became part of a "*partie quarrée*" (foursome) consisting of Small, Francis Fauquier (1703–68), George Wythe (1726–1806), and Peyton Randolph. From these "characters of very high standing," Jefferson wrote that he "heard more good sense, more rational & philosophical conversations than in all my life besides."[21] Fauquier served as the royal lieutenant governor of the Virginia colony from 1758 until his death. An energetic amateur scientist with a strong interest in natural philosophy and astronomy, his studies of weather and other subjects stimulated Jefferson's interest in scientific instrumentation that would last a lifetime. Wythe was an esteemed lawyer and judge who later joined Jefferson in signing the Declaration of Independence. As a law tutor from 1762 to 1768, he taught Jefferson the great principles of jurisprudence and much about the value of rigorous logic and precise rhetoric in argumentative dialogue.[22] Like Small, Wythe influenced Jefferson in ways more profound than mere intellectual attainments. Late in life, Jefferson wrote of Wythe in moving prose that went to the core of the man's character:

> No man ever left behind him a character more venerated than G. Wythe. his virtue was of the purest tint; his integrity inflexible, and his justice exact; of warm patriotism, and, devoted as he was to liberty, and the natural and equal rights of man, he might truly be called the Cato of his country, without the avarice of the Roman; for a more disinterested person never lived. temperance and regularity in all his habits gave him general good health, and his unaffected modesty and suavity of manners endeared him to every one. he was of easy elocution, his language chaste, methodical in the arrangement of his manner, learned and logical in the use of it, and of great urbanity in debate; not quick of apprehension, but with a little time profound in penetration and sound in conclusion. . . . In pleading [in court] he never indulged himself with an useless or declamatory thought or word; and became as distinguished by correctness and purity of conduct in his profession, as he was by his industry & fidelity to those who employed him.[23]

As a result of these early intellectual influences, Jefferson became an exceptionally tenacious lifelong learner, constantly endeavoring to absorb and understand the entire range of worldly wisdom, past and present, and to transmit his breadth of knowledge to others. Under the guidance and inspiration of William Small, Jefferson's innate curiosity for science was greatly enhanced and critically focused. His formal exposure to the writings of Francis Bacon and the mathematical demonstrations of Isaac Newton helped make clear to Jefferson the importance of reason and scientific method in man's attempt to understand the cosmos. And his introduction to the Scottish version of Enlightenment improvement, for both self and mankind, instilled in Jefferson a strong disposition to seek new knowledge rather than simply accepting handed-down dogma, codified his belief in the primacy of scientific investigation over intellectually nebulous oratory, and the need to combine scientific and humanistic inquiry with a degree of humility because human knowledge is always partial.[24] Moreover, his "benevolent mentors" sowed in Jefferson's mind the first seeds of what would become a rich harvest of revolutionary ideas concerning the purpose of higher education in America.

To Jefferson, school-based tutelage would never suffice in itself. From each and every stage, man must move forward in an unending process' of self–education. Never satisfied even with his own immense scientific learning, throughout his life Jefferson eagerly pursued knowledge with a steely resolve, a vigor and a steadfastness that set him apart from all of his contemporaries.[25]

Jefferson and His Private Libraries

Jefferson's education was continuous due to a lifelong love of books and reading that was evident by age five and a personal library to which he added throughout his life.[26] Jefferson's bibliophilic acquisitiveness complemented his scientific inquires and laid the foundation for the Library of Congress and the library of the University of Virginia. For the printed word, he had what he termed a "canine appetite for reading."[27] He became one of the best–read men of his day in America, and many of his philosophical arguments were inspired distillations of all the great works that he fed into his mind. Nobody knew better than he the cultural and scientific values that lay between the covers of a book or periodical. Indeed, he wrote that "I cannot live without books," which he regarded as "a necessary of life."[28] His literary interests were broad, as he avidly collected not only books but also newspapers, pamphlets, law manuscripts, Indian vocabularies, lectures, and scientific journals. Mere life experience, thought Jefferson, could not make a full man: "I know it is often said there have been shining examples of men of great abilities in all of the businesses of life, without any other science than what they had gathered from conversations, and intercourse with the world. but who can say what these men would not have been had they started in the science on the shoulders of a Demosthenes or Cicero, of a Locke, a Bacon, or a Newton?"[29] Clearly, Jefferson sought the wisdom of these great men and numerous other luminaries of classical scholarship from antiquity to his time, with indefatigable diligence, so that his mind would be properly prepared for a lifetime of scientific inquiry, discovery, and educational innovation. In his words, reading was the "lamp to lighten my path."[30]

Jefferson's compulsion to investigate all useful avenues of human knowledge had a strong and determining influence on what was and was not part of his library inventories. During his lifetime, he assembled at least five libraries: Shadwell (1757–1770), Monticello (1770–1815, his "great" library that was sold to the Library of Congress), his 1815–1826 "retirement library," the separate one he left at Poplar Forest, and the collection he planned for the University of Virginia.[31] Jefferson's choices were unusually purposeful, if not wholly utilitarian, pragmatic, and materialist.[32] Compared to other colonial libraries, especially those owned by New England book collectors, Jefferson's libraries contained a wider range of subject matter—a collection that revealed a more worldly or secular interest in subjects such as history and applied science and much less preoccupation with religious spiritualisms and metaphysical speculation.[33] Indeed, Jefferson's collection was not a mere retreat from the realities of present day existence. It showed him to be more concerned with learning how to live and create order in the present world than in speculating on how to prepare for an afterlife.[34]

In his lifetime Jefferson may have owned something like 10,000 books.[35] His first library of about 400 volumes, assembled during his formative years, was burned along with most of his papers when a fire destroyed his family home at Shadwell on February 1, 1770. He lamented at the time, "Would to god it had been the money [that the books cost rather than the books themselves]; then had it never cost me a sigh!"[36] Undeterred, Jefferson quickly began rebuilding his library. By 1773, he recorded a count of 1,276 books in his library at Monticello and by 1783 the number had doubled.[37] Jefferson further enlarged his library holdings by acquiring more than 2,000 volumes between 1784 and 1789, when he served as a diplomat in France. With him he brought his library catalogue, which served both as an inventory of books he already owned and a list of those he hoped to acquire, expanding the latter as he came into contact with the works of the French literati and the scientific community. Jefferson thus described his book–buying strategy long afterward: "While residing in Paris, I devoted every afternoon I was disengaged, for a summer or two, in examining all the principal bookstores, turning over every book with my own hands, and putting by every thing which related to America, and indeed whatever was rare & valuable in every science. besides this, I had standing orders during the whole time I was in Europe, in it's principal book–marts, particularly Amsterdam, Frankfort, Madrid and London, for such works relating to America as could not be found in Paris."[38] By the time he sold it to the nation to replace the one that was destroyed when the British burned the U.S. Capitol in 1814, Jefferson's library at Monticello had grown to more than 6,500 volumes, making it one of the largest and most expensive private collections of the time. Congress paid $23,950, which was probably well below market value, although the purchase still met with strident Federalist opposition.[39]

Jefferson organized his entire library according to a classification scheme based on Francis Bacon's *The Proficience and Advancement of Learning* (1605) and very likely also on an expanded taxonomic structure by Jean le Rond d'Alembert and Denis Diderot in the monumental *Encyclopédie* (1751). He divided human knowledge into three major categories: history, philosophy, and fine arts, which corresponded to Bacon's "faculties of the soul," namely memory (civil and moral history), reason (moral and mathematical philosophy), and imagination (the fine arts, comprising architecture, gardening, sculpture, painting, poetry, music) with forty–four sub–classifications. Individual titles within each sub–classification were listed according to an arrangement he referred to as "sometimes analytical, sometimes chronological, & sometimes a combination of both." This cataloguing system has been described as a "detailed and telling product of his distinctive imagination at work," one that offered great insight into the broad and systematic nature of his mind. Indeed Jefferson's taxonomic system was so advanced that the Library of Congress retained it into the twentieth century.[40]

The expansive scope of Jefferson's book collection has been called a "most perfect and general library," wherein could be found "whosoever the wit of man hath heretofore committed to books of worth," a collection that spanned nearly every subject from ancient history to zoology.[41] The largest proportion of titles in Jefferson great library—some 899, or nearly 27 percent of the total—was what we today recognize as science books.[42] Of these, medical subjects comprised the greatest quantity, followed in order by mathematics, botany and zoology, and agriculture. The next largest categories were ethics (which included law) and history.

As impressive as Jefferson's library was, it most certainly did not encompass the entire range of literary work. For example, there was no subdivision for metaphysics—a subject that Jefferson viewed as not worth reading because it considered questions "beyond our reach" and was replete with unprovable speculation around which one could not order the business of life.[43] In 1822, Jefferson explained implicitly the reason for his distaste of metaphysics: "I am myself an empiric in Natural philosophy, suffering my faith to go no further than my facts."[44] The one type of metaphysics, or rationalistic philosophy, which Jefferson did value, was what his friend, Antoine Louis Claude Destutt de Tracy called *idéologie* (English: "ideology"), a word that the Frenchman coined in 1796, meaning not a set of beliefs but a science of ideas aimed at the human mind of prejudices. Jefferson specifically included this subject, the "science of ideas," in his personal library and also in the curriculum of the University of Virginia. He praised Destutt de Tracy as "the ablest writer living on intellectual subjects," and described Tracy's Élémens d'Idéologie (1803) as "a production of the first order in the science of our thinking faculty." Jefferson was understandably attracted to this new discipline, for it was not a speculative system of thought, but rather a philosophical methodology for discovering new truths, based on experimentation and logical positivism, thus promising to purge philosophy of its rationalizations and spiritualisms and its abstractions from the material world and at the same time provide a more accurate means for arriving at evidenced truth.[45]

Besides texts on metaphysics, Jefferson also tended to eschew fiction—a genre that occupied an extraordinarily small portion of his library and the many syllabi of "required reading" he fashioned for his relatives and friends.[46] In a letter suggesting appropriate reading for women, Jefferson dismissed most novels and some poetry as leaving the mind in an unhealthy state of "bloated imagination, sickly judgment and disgust towards all the real businesses of life." Books that serve only to amuse, entertain, or gratify one's imagination were "A great obstacle to good education" and should be avoided. For women, Jefferson only approved of a handful of fictitious narratives "modeled on the incidents of real life," capable of being "useful vehicles of a sound morality," as well as some poetry for "forming style and taste."[47]

Proponent of Public Libraries, Newspapers, and Research Libraries

Jefferson's predilection for books was not just a private pursuit. He was the first Virginian to call for a state library accessible to the public and felt a responsibility to encourage reading through county libraries providing basic knowledge in six areas that would enhance one's navigation in the business of life and help citizens to know, respect, and safeguard their rights as free Americans. Unfortunately, Jefferson did not promote reading literacy for all of society. Most members of the enslaved communities at Monticello and Poplar Forest were barred from access to books. Jefferson did nothing to prevent them from learning how to read, but he also made no move to extend literacy to their communities at large. Thus, fundamentally, Monticello was an African American village, most of whose members lived at the foot of the continent's greatest library—and were effectively forbidden its use.[48] Even so, Jefferson laid out a vision for public libraries that was still quite progressive at the time, observing in 1809 that, "I have often thought that nothing would do more extensive good at small expence than the establishment of a small circulating library in every county, to consist of a few well chosen books, to be lent to the people of the county under such regulations as would secure their safe return in due time, these [chosen books] should be such as would give them [the people] a general view of other history & particular view of that of their own country, a tolerable knowledge of geography, the elements of Natural philosophy, of agriculture & mechanics."[49] The types of books that he favored included: Greek, Roman, and European history, for knowledge of global scale and the corrupting influences on past generations of ruling monarchies whose supreme authority was exercised without the consent of the people; American history, to illuminate the struggle for independence and the ensuing arduous work that was necessary for participatory democracy to succeed; basic geography, to show how the elements of the earth are represented; agriculture, from which citizens can learn how to feed and clothe themselves in the most efficient ways; and mechanics, which teaches people how things work. In addition, Jefferson attempted to foster the development of a free and truthful American press. At times he expressed serious concern about "the putrid state into which our newspapers have passed, and the malignity, the vulgarity & mendacious spirit of those who write for them; "complaining that "nothing can now be believed which is seen in a newspaper;" and suggesting that an editor intent on reform should "divide his paper into 4. chapters, heading the 1st Truths. 2d Probabilities.

3^d Possibilities. 4th Lies."[50] Nonetheless, he thought that perhaps the most important educative factor existent was dissemination of differing political ideas and opinions through a variety of newspapers.[51] "For god's sake," he said when an attempt was made to suppress an allegedly blasphemous book in 1814, "let us freely hear both sides, if we chuse."[52]

Jefferson's expansive thinking included a proposal for a publicly funded research library for the few who could benefit from it. Its real object was to provide scholars of superior talent with sufficiently specialized information to support projects that advance human knowledge, rather than to meet the basic reading requirement of an entire community from children to the elderly. In 1779, while a member of the Virginia House of Delegates, he urged the annual expenditure by the state of the rather large sum of two thousand pounds to procure, under the guidance of "three persons of learning and of attention to literary matters," such books and maps as would be useful to "the researches of the learned and curious."[53] Unfortunately, this legislative bill, the third pillar in Jefferson's comprehensive education plan for the new state of Virginia, was not approved.

Jefferson's conception of reading as a "lamp to lighten my path" was an attitude he hoped all of his free countrymen would embrace. Throughout his life, he advised dozens of friends and relatives on what books to read or what books they should ensure their children read, and in what order.[54] In the words of one historian, he ardently believed that an "informed citizenry was at the heart of a dynamic new democracy," and Jefferson underscored the importance of literacy when he wrote that "if a nation expects to be ignorant & free in a state of civilisation, it expects what never was & never will be."[55] The two aforementioned library proposals failed, as did suggestions to the U.S. Congress in 1791 that patent fees be used to start a public library and another in 1821 that all import duties on books be repealed as "detrimental to the progress of knowledge."[56] But Jefferson did succeed in founding one of the first truly academic libraries in America within a university environment by designing, supervising the construction, and choosing the books for the library at the University of Virginia. He was also a key figure in the reestablishment of the Library of Congress after the British burned it in 1814 by selling the nation his personal holding of 6,487 volumes so that Congress could "recommence" its own library. In honor of Jefferson's "visionary leadership in promoting an informed democracy," the Library of Congress renamed its main building of 1897 the Jefferson Building in 1980, and it initially christened its pioneering Open Multimedia Access System for federal legislative information THOMAS.gov.[57]

Republic of Letters and Scientific Societies

In Jefferson's era, the communication of scientific knowledge was more personal, comprising correspondence, conversation, and societies that were, in effect, intellectual clubs. Though Jefferson loved reading, it was an essentially one–sided act of intellectual exchange. Much of his influence, however, occurred through interaction with other people, either in correspondence or in public presentations, as well as, in his case, in legislative and scientific proposals. In his openness, Jefferson reinforced the emerging ideals of scientific transparency and the need for publication, which stood in contrast to authoritarian secrecy and individualistic mysticism. Like Benjamin Franklin, described by David Hume as "the first great man of letters, for whom we are beholden to America,"[58] and his coterie of correspondents, Jefferson enthusiastically participated in the transatlantic "republic of letters," which he described as "a great fraternity spreading over the whole world," emphasizing that "no republic is more real than that of letters," whose "correspondence is never interrupted by any civilized nation."[59] Members of his "republic" saw themselves as collaborating with each other on an intellectual level, and therefore, on equal terms without regard to politics, religion, or nationality. In hundreds upon hundreds of letters, if not thousands, correspondents tried out their ideas and new theories, critiqued those of others, relayed the newest gossip, and chronicled the mundane matters of life. Letters were in fact an important vehicle for spreading intellectual and scholarly developments throughout America and abroad. Through such connections, not one unified network but lots of little networks, Jefferson acquired an exceptional familiarity with an extraordinarily diverse range of "men of science" who both challenged and enlightened him. Among them was the great naturalist the comte de Buffon, who provoked and compelled Jefferson to conduct the most brilliant scientific survey of his time, *Notes on the State of Virginia*, and to break new ground in paleontological, anthropological, and ethnographic studies, as well as comparative linguistics.[60]

At the same time, albeit within a limited audience of high–level researchers, letters functioned as forerunners of scientific journals with their requirement that any idea should be public and open to criticism and possible refutation. The Republic of Letters was in effect a literary laboratory where concepts and descriptions of devices and experiments could be tested in the flames of epistolary give and take, with the unspoken rule that thoughts that could not pass muster in a public domain should be discarded.

In this Republic of Letters, ideas and technological innovations were shared not only between individual experimenters but also collectively through a number of "clearinghouses" of knowledge—the philosophical societies and various improvement clubs, such as the American Philosophical Society, founded in Philadelphia in 1743; the Aberdeen Philosophical Society of Scotland, founded in 1758; the Birmingham Lunar Society of England, founded in 1765; and the American Academy of Arts and Sciences, founded in 1780, located in Cambridge, Massachusetts.[61] During his life, Jefferson belonged to a great number of academic organizations in America and Europe and contributed many noteworthy publications.

In 1780, the American Philosophical Society (APS) elected Thomas Jefferson to its membership, thus beginning a relationship that would last until Jefferson's death in 1826. During his forty–six–year association with the APS, Jefferson served on many committees, was a member of the Society's Council (its governing board), and held the office of vice president from 1793–95, and president from 1797–1815.[62] The APS, probably more than any other learned institution, provided Jefferson with a great deal of intellectual sustenance, most importantly, access to the erudite world of ideas and cutting–edge research. It also afforded Jefferson ample opportunities to conduct his own research and to promote an agenda driven by the belief that American research was novel, unique, and worthy of consideration by scientists around the world.

But Jefferson did not only take from the APS's lode of scientific information. He gave back. Under his influence the tone of the APS became decidedly republican, deistic, and pro–French. Moreover, science came to be fully in service to the state. His numerous contributions included guiding the transformation of the fledgling Philadelphia institution into the nation's leading scientific organization and helping the APS become the preeminent collecting center for information and artifacts on North America's unique natural history and Native American past.[63] Jefferson promoted the concept that scientific endeavors could and should advance national interests. Examples include his work at the APS on the Hessian fly and on establishing uniform standards for coinage, weights and measures.[64] Using his network of associates to bolster APS membership by nominating those whose demonstrated learning impressed him the most, and raising funds to support ambitious scientists and their projects he leveraged his position as president to grow the society, to acquire books from Europe, and to establish the APS as the central node from which early American science could be conducted.[65] Carrying these initiatives into the area of publishing, he encouraged the dissemination of scholarly ideas and original research through the society's *Transactions*, in which 285 papers were published during Jefferson's APS presidency.[66]

The Perfecting of Man by Scientific Progress

Jefferson's scientific views were motivated by the Enlightenment ideals that reason could be cultivated and applied for the improvement of all mankind. Such a position was at once radical, heretical, and shared by few within the overall society of America at the turn of the nineteenth century. In its acceptance of the probability of scientific advancement based on human education and achievement, it was more optimistic than most popular philosophies founded on notions of essential human sinfulness and the need for supernatural incentives. Fault lines in the intellectual landscape of the early post–Revolutionary War period are partially revealed in the correspondence between Jefferson and John Adams. Several letters in particular suggest their wildly divergent views on the nature and limits of knowledge; on what was known and yet to be discovered; on the relative authority of scientific methodology, and on the improvability of the human mind.[67] Adams, who probably was the most pessimistic of the founding fathers, had serious doubts about the intellectual and moral capacities of the American people.[68] He had little patience with those who prated on about the reach of human imagination and the benefits of scientific advance, preferring only "to ascertain the limits of human knowledge already acquired." Jefferson went so far as to imply to a friend that Adams had rejected belief in scientific progress in favor of a reactionary "bigotry in Politics & Education."[69] In short, the philosophical bent of Adams looked backwards, not forward by testing the "evidentiary basis of our more comforting certainties."[70] Suspecting that "human Power, or human Wisdom, and human Virtue" were not only limited in fact but also in principle, Adams looked upon progress through critical inquiry as having built-in boundaries and utterly rejected the doctrine of human perfectibility.[71] In contrast, from his youth Jefferson held firm the precept that science required absolute freedom of inquiry and no ceiling to discovery. He fervently believed in and insisted upon freedom of the mind, in its right to inquire everywhere and to arrive at conclusions devoid of all partisan political and sectarian bias, in order to attain a greater certainty of scientific truth and progress.[72] As Jefferson's biographer, Dumas Malone, states: "To the venerable sage as to the bold Revolutionary patriot, freedom and knowledge were inseparable."[73]

Compared to Adams, Jefferson had great faith in people, progress, and the future of America and its institutions.[74] As a disciple of Newtonian science, Jefferson was hostile to setting boundaries on the nature and limits of knowledge, always questioning if it was appropriate to set any limits on the wisdom, power, or virtue of humans. He eschewed all theories based on "occult forces and invisible hands," meaning that religious authority and the superstitions of antiquity should be rejected, and empirically derived truth accepted as the only, certainly the most dependable form of knowledge. Unlike Adams, he dismissed scriptural accounts of miracles as primitive myths perpetuated by self–interested clergy seeking to maintain control.[75] Jefferson likened his sanguine belief in progress and the illimitable potential of the human mind to the similar ideas of the Marquis de Condorcet (1743–94). He agreed with Condorcet that man's "mind is perfectible to a degree of which we cannot as yet form any conception. it is impossible for a man who takes a survey of what is already known, not to see what an immensity in every branch of science yet remains to be discovered, & that too of articles to which our faculties seem adequate."[76] Adams and other Federalist leaders rejected this liberal view of a future rational society largely shaped by scientific progress, and fiercely attacked Condorcet and his fellow thinkers of the French Enlightenment, believing they were foolishly optimistic about human nature, government and new systems of education.[77] In 1813, Jefferson codified his thoughts on Adams and his political allies when he wrote that:

> one of the questions you know on which our parties took different sides, was on the improvability of the human mind, in science, in ethics, in government E^t^c. those who advocated reformation of institutions, pari passu, with the progress of science, maintained that no definite limits could be assigned to that progress. the enemies of reform on the other hand, denied improvement, & advocated steady adherence to the principles, practices, & institutions of our fathers, which they represented as the consummation of wisdom, & akmé of excellence, beyond which the human mind could never advance . . . you predict that [the freedom of enquiry] will produce nothing more worthy of transmission to posterity, than the principles, institutions, & systems of education recieved from their ancestors. I do not consider this as your deliberate opinion. you possess, yourself, too much science, not to see how much is still ahead of you, unexplained & unexplored … I consider it as an expression lent to the prejudices of your friends.[78]

Unlike Adams, Jefferson was an eternal optimist for the human species, believing man to be a highly sentient creature with the capacity to learn new truths and apply them for the benefit of mankind. He was keenly aware of the great progress that had been made during the scientific revolution of the seventeenth century, from René Descartes to Isaac Newton. Jefferson referred to Newton, Francis Bacon, and John Locke as "my trinity of the three greatest men the world had ever produced," because they "laid the foundation of those superstructures which have been raised in the Physical and Moral sciences." He clearly understood that allegiance to a more modern method of intellectual inquiry would result in an endless growth and development of human wisdom.[79]

Jefferson grounded his doctrine of human perfectibility in empirical scientific methodology that was itself rooted in tangible proof—an organized approach that emphasized objectivity, reason, and logic, and the accumulation of data from first–hand direct observation and experimentation. Concerning one question he remarked that "it is the actual experiment alone which can decide."[80] He also disapproved of speculative hypotheses that were destitute of direct evidence and which reason could not sanction. In such cases, the wisest philosophy was one of silence, or a truthful confession of ignorance, since "It is always better to have no ideas than false ones; to believe nothing, than to believe what is wrong." This principle, thought Jefferson, distinguished the true scientist from the charlatan who allowed his enterprising inclinations to carry him away into hazardous regions, and who vainly strived to support a fanciful theory through a shroud of heedless obfuscation. "The moment a person forms a theory, his imagination sees in every object only the traits which favors that theory; "all theory must yield to experience"; and "experience & frequent disappointment have taught me not to be over-confident in theories or calculations, until actual trial of the whole combination has stamped it with approbation."[81] Moreover, Jefferson showed remarkable insight when he argued that improvements in science could also inculcate virtue and enhance the morals of men. For Jefferson, education as the accretion of useful knowledge and the application of rational methods was in itself a moral activity, able "to develope the reasoning faculties of our youth, enlarge their minds, cultivate their morals, & instill into them the precepts of virtue and order." He saw learning and doing science as instances of ethical behavior.[82]

Jefferson's Personal and Political Efforts to Expand Scientific Knowledge

Jefferson was not only an inquirer into and communicator of scientific knowledge, he was himself a scientist. Throughout his adult life, he sought to enlarge the bounds of human knowledge by refining existing ideas and theories, inventing and/or improving technological devices, and making new discoveries in several different branches of science. Jefferson emphasized the importance of agricultural study: "It was among our wisest pursuits"; "a science of the very first order. it counts among it's handmaids, the most respectable sciences, such as chemistry, natural philosophy, mechanics, mathematics generally, natural history, and botany"; and, "Cultivators of the earth are the most valuable citizens. They are the most vigorous, the most independant, the most virtuous, and they are tied to their country and wedded to it's liberty and interests by the most lasting bands." As early as 1780, Jefferson and other progressive southern planters began formal experiments in agronomy designed to increase the crop productiveness of an increasingly exhausted land.[83] Operating largely by trial–and–error, Jefferson made several important new observations and advanced established techniques that helped lay the foundations for achievements associated with modern agricultural science. While he did not discover the techniques of plant breeding, contour plowing, and crop rotation, he promoted their advancement and played a major role in the improvement of the American rural economy. Examples include: field testing every variety of seed he could get his hands on by acquiring stock from purchase, gift, or exchange from other gardeners around the world; importing new crops (olive and caper trees, and a variety of fruits and vegetables) and livestock (Merino sheep and sheep dogs) from Europe to American farms; advocating for, and in some instances creating, inventions and innovations that would increase agricultural output and profits through reduced labor costs (for example, a more efficient threshing machine, the moldboard plow, and ha-ha fences); promoting the study and experimentation of techniques that would protect crops and livestock from destructive pests; and creating agricultural societies that would share discoveries and promote the best methods of land stewardship.[84] Jefferson was an early "environmentalist" intent on improving the American rural economy,[85] and his developed ideas were sufficiently important enough to gain this remark by Secretary of Agriculture Henry A. Wallace over a century later in 1937: "It was Jefferson more than any other man of his time who foresaw the fruitfulness of the application of science to agriculture, and through science, a smaller and smaller area of land will be able to produce commodities of greater value and wider enjoyment with less outlay."[86]

Jefferson was also an avid weather observer who went well beyond simple observation. He linked geography and meteorology analytically, which is to say, scientifically, and was among the first Americans to describe the phenomena of temperature inversion, foehn winds, and looming.[87] He also was a pioneer in advocating precise collection of climatological data every five to ten years, in every section of the country. To this end he established a network of fellow weather observers in Virginia and a few other states—choosing men who understood the need for care and attention to instrument calibration and placement. Moreover, Jefferson's written work between 1785 and 1824 detailing the results of his numerous meteorological studies, reveals his insightful commentary on the hazards of climate warming and the interplay among climate change, human agency, and health.[88]

Jefferson initiated the science of vertebrate paleontology in America with his erudite study of the megalonyx, a paper of February 10, 1797, with a March 10 postscript, published by the APS as "A Memoir on the Discovery of Certain Bones of a Quadruped of the Kind in the Western Parts of Virginia." Jefferson had secured the bones of this prehistoric animal from a cave in Greenbrier County, Virginia (now West Virginia), and sent them to Philadelphia where they were reconstructed. Eventually the skeleton was placed in the Academy of Natural Sciences in Philadelphia.[89] Jefferson's interest in paleontology continued well into his second presidential term. In 1807, he commissioned Captain William Clark to excavate fossilized bones from Big Bone Lick in northern Kentucky. Clark's work gave the world the first evidence of several mammalian species that lived during the Pleistocene Epoch, also known as the Ice Age. The explorations in Kentucky have been described as the beginning of American government work in paleontology and made Big Bone Lick the "first official paleontological collecting site in North America." At this time Jefferson's political opponents started mocking him with the name "Mr. Mammoth."[90]

Entomology was another scientific subject which engaged Jefferson's attention and his actions suggest it was far more than an idle interest. In 1791, he organized a committee of the APS to investigate the natural history and biological minutiae of the Hessian fly. So named because Americans suspected that German soldiers brought the insect to American shores during the revolution, it was wreaking havoc on American wheat crops, especially in New York and New England, and sparked a crisis when the British refused to accept imports of supposedly contaminated

American wheat.[91] Jefferson took detailed notes during a trip to New England in 1791 and dissected a specimen the following year, although he never reported his findings to the APS. His research remains valuable as an early and detailed account of the fly's migration patterns and a pioneering exercise in economic entomology.[92]

NOTES ON THE STATE OF VIRGINIA

Jefferson's most famous scientific endeavor, *Notes on the State of Virginia*, amply illustrates his immense erudition, his bent for experimentation, and belief in a "hierarchy of knowledge."[93] Originally drafted to answer a series of queries from the French government, the manuscript was expanded, revised, printed for private circulation in 1785, and then published by Jefferson two years later. Even after that he intended but did not complete a final major revision after retirement from public life.[94] The *Notes* gave Jefferson an important place among the pioneering scientific writers of the eighteenth century, and came to be regarded as "the first comprehensive treatise upon the topography, natural history, and natural science of the United States, the precursor of the great library of scientific reports which has since been issued by the States and Federal government."[95] Described by Gilbert Chinard as "one of the first masterpieces of American literature," it helped inspire other men of science to take up the task of describing all that was known and yet to be discovered in their respective states.[96] Moreover, the *Notes* reveal Jefferson's recognition that scientific information, far from being the pursuit of isolated scholars, has a direct bearing on issues of governance. In this sense, the *Notes* anticipate the support Jefferson, as a government official, was able to provide to science and exploration.

In his opus Jefferson documents his pioneering use of the principle of stratification in archeological excavation. He thus deserves the title of first scientific archeologist in America.[97] In addition, the *Notes* provide early evidence of Jefferson's skepticism about certain medicinal remedies. Of Virginia's mineral springs, he observed that, "There are several Medicinal springs, some of which are indubitably efficacious, while others seem to owe their reputation as much to fancy, and change of air and regimen, as to their real virtues. None of them having undergone a chemical analysis in skilful hands, nor been so far the subject of observations as to have produced a reduction into classes of the disorders which they relieve, it is in my power to give little more than an enumeration of them." This note of caution proved prophetic. While in France, Jefferson had a favorable experience with hot mineral baths, but similar treatment at the Warm

Springs of Virginia proved disastrous in 1818, leaving his health entirely prostrated by the use of the waters. they produced an imposthume [abscess] and eruption [boils]."[98]

In Jefferson's time, botanical medicine was a vital component of the healing arts, and his *Notes* show how well versed he was in this area. In Query VI, he lists one hundred and twenty-three plants, trees, fruits, and vegetables in four categories: the medicinal, of which there were twenty-one, the esculent, the ornamental, and those useful for fabrication. Jefferson grew and investigated many botanicals at Monticello, partly, to learn whether they had medicinal value, and he listed them with their scientific as well as their common names. Throughout his life, Jefferson was a patron of botany and undertook much work in that science. In 1792, in recognition of his contributions to the field, Professor Benjamin Smith Barton of the University of Pennsylvania named a plant *Jeffersonia diphylla* (commonly known as twinleaf or rheumatism root) in honor of Jefferson.[99]

Notes on the State of Virginia is much more than a dry collection of data. Its structure shifts—sometimes abruptly—from almost unreadable statistical compilations to impassioned argumentation, wrapped in a system of precise logic and rhetoric about the character of valid reasoning. Again and again, Jefferson goes out of his way to argue and propose, instead of merely describe.[100] The book moves from facts to judgment and then to reasoning and conviction based on empirically observed patterns. The structure of the book attempts to build agreement around "facts," in order to create a sound "starting point" for an effective argument, thus enabling Jefferson to refute more persuasively a number of incorrect assertions and slanderous statements of several prominent French naturalists, in particular, George Louis Leclerc, also known as the comte de Buffon (1707–88) and his associates, Louis Jean Marie Daubenton (1716–1800) and the Abbé Raynal (1713–96).[101] With a rush of patriotic fervor, Jefferson identified thirty-one false premises of the French naturalists and meticulously produced compelling evidence to discredit, if not completely annihilate, each one of their flawed theories about the "degeneracy" of animal species, including humans, in the United States.[102] The prodigious amount of knowledge that Jefferson accumulated in the *Notes* also served him well in his eloquent rebuttal to Raynal's contention "that America has not yet produced one good poet, one able mathematician, one man of genius, in a single art or in a single science."[103]

Jefferson's *Notes* contains a substantial body of facts, compiled with exactness and collated into well-reasoned and logical conclusions. It also includes controversial passages on philosophical topics that became the "subject of bitter partisan debate," including Jefferson's criticism of orthodoxy in general, and his pleas for freedom not only from religious dogma and superstition but from, as he memorably put it in 1800, "every form of tyranny over the mind of man." In one particularly provocative statement, in the *Notes* Jefferson asks," What has been the effect of religious coercion? it has made one half of the world fools, and the other half hypocrites."[104] He attacks the assumption and usurpation of power by the rich and well born, the laws of entail and primogeniture in his own state, the enslavement of man by man and the injustice of racial superiority. He also argues for the need to educate all who have the capacity to learn, regardless of their social or economic status, and for the right of the individual to freedom and happiness under just and equitable laws.[105]

For his devotion to the cause of the common man, Jefferson was labeled an "apostate and traitor to his class"; for his interest in science without boundaries, a "howling atheist" and a "confirmed infidel;" for his sympathy for an Indian victim of the white man's cruelty, he was called a "liar" and "hypocrite"; and, for some of his scientific assertions, he was deemed "impetuous," "too visionary" and "hallucinatory."[106] After his retirement from politics, Jefferson offered one of his very rare responses to his critics: "of all of the charges brought against me by my political adversaries," he commented, "that of possessing some science has probably done them the least credit. Our countrymen are too enlightened themselves to believe that ignorance is the best qualification for their service." Later he complained of those who thought, "even science itself as well as my affection for it, a fit object of ridicule and a disqualification for the affairs of government."[107] Jefferson's enlightened philosophy regarding science–based medicine and his blueprint for reforming medical education in America aroused criticism that plagued him regularly.[108]

In the *Notes* Jefferson does sometimes opine on subjects without any credible empirical evidence. One of the most regrettable passages is found in Query XIV, where he accepts and discusses the supposed inferiority of Blacks. In Query XI, he extolled the virtues of America's native people, but here Jefferson theorizes that the physiological functions and aesthetic characteristics of persons of African descent are distinctly different, and that their faculties of comprehension, reason, and imagination are far less developed than those of Whites or Indians.[109] He goes on to suggest that in their present state, Blacks are unfit to possess all of the rights of full citizenship. Jefferson believed slavery violated the natural rights of man. But he merely hoped for its "conditional" abolition and was equally convinced that Blacks and Whites could not peacefully coexist in freedom because of hostility due to their previous relationship and their differences in color, temperament, and above all, intellectual ability. In his words, White Americans and enslaved Blacks constituted two "separate nations." Jefferson therefore argued that emancipation must be accompanied by colonization of the freed slaves beyond the limits of the United States, preferably Africa or the West Indies, with due compensation to the masters. He was never able to imagine America as a multiracial country. His vision of a racially pure American devoid of free Blacks was tantamount to apartheid. Admittedly many other prominent Americans and cognoscenti supported emancipation followed by colonization and feared a biracial America.[110] The nonegalitarian view of race was soon enshrined in the fractional mode by which slaves were counted in the Constitution.[111]

Jefferson's belief in the eventual necessity of ending slavery never changed. To his credit, he proposed antislavery legislation both before and after he wrote *Notes.* Between the early 1770s and his death, he proposed a number of steps that might facilitate his plan for gradual emancipation, and he tried without success to include an antislavery clause in the Declaration of Independence. Some proslavery groups later denounced him for his abolitionist views.[112] Nonetheless, his denigration of Blacks in *Notes* in chillingly harsh terms has earned him enduring, and richly deserved criticism. From a twenty–first–century perspective, "the contradiction between his republican ideas of freedom and equality," and his complicit lifelong entanglement with race–based chattel slavery, "is quaintly described by some as a paradox and by others as rank hypocrisy in what has been called America's tragic original sin."[113] In this case, Jefferson was not ahead of his time; he was at best a product of a time when a sizable body of European literature undoubtedly familiar to Jefferson, authored by such prominent philosophers and men of science as David Hume, Adam Smith, Oliver Goldsmith, C. F. Volney, Carl von Linné (Linnaeus), and Georges Cuvier, viewed Blacks and Native Americans as inferior to whites.[114]

Jefferson held complex and contradictory views on slavery and Blacks. He recognized the evils of slavery and acknowledged the contradiction with his professed beliefs in personal liberty. Throughout his life he never wavered from his view that slavery was morally wrong and should ultimately be abolished. However, he freed only seven of his slaves in his lifetime and in his will. In his final year, he wrote about the "deplorable entanglement" of slavery and reiterated his belief that it was unlawful for "one man to appropriate to himself the faculties of another without his consent."[115] At one time, he thought Blacks were naturally inferior, that their ineptitude was innate, indelible, and unchangeable. At other times, he conceded that the despotic regime of forced servitude, reinforced by dehumanizing social practices, may have had a damaging impact on Blacks' capacities, and that, given opportunity, they might achieve equality with whites.

Beginning in the 1990s, some authors have called Jefferson a "proto–hereditarian," alleging that he believed nature was the dominant determinant in human behavior, intelligence, and other characteristics, and that Blacks would always be inferior to Whites because their destiny was genetically fixed at birth. The weight of the evidence, however, suggests otherwise. Jefferson espoused the importance of nurture, that man's destiny is largely shaped by one's surroundings (environment), or opportunities for improvement. In 1785 he wrote that "I believe the Indian to be in body and mind equal to the whiteman. I have supposed the blackman, in his present state, might not be so, but it would be hazardous to affirm that, equally cultivated for a few generations, he would not become so."[116] In the end, Jefferson left it to science to determine whether nature (heredity) or nurture (the cruelly oppressive social structure of enslavement) was responsible for what he perceived to be a distressing absence of intellectual accomplishment among Blacks, especially in the arts and sciences. "I advance it therefore as a suspicion only," he concluded, "that the blacks whether originally a distinct race, or made distinct by time and circumstance, are inferior to the whites in the endowments of both body and mind."[117] In chapter 6, we will see that the issue of enslaved people being inferior in some sense as human beings was still being examined in the hotbed of the pre–Civil War era by one of Jefferson's intellectual descendants at the University of Virginia.

International Statesman of Science

Jefferson was unceasingly dedicated to the practical application of Enlightenment science in its most general meaning, as the most certain means of advancing progress and human happiness in the new republic. As an example of his "zeal to promote the general good of mankind by an interchange of useful things," Jefferson devoted much of his time while in France between 1785 and 1789 to seeking out the best achievements of the Old World to report them to the New. He assiduously studied the recent advances in the useful arts and sciences, particularly agriculture, chemistry, astronomy, natural history, and such inventions as the steam engine; kept four major American colleges—Harvard, Yale, the University of the State of Pennsylvania (after 1791 the University of Pennsylvania) and the College of William and Mary—informed of scientific activities in

Europe; and supplied the American Philosophical Society with many European inventions and artifacts that intrigued him and that he considered useful to American enterprise. Jefferson also endeavored to provide the French with correct information about the United States, its geography, natural history, socially responsible political principles, and the worthy accomplishments of its people. In this manner he served both continents as an international statesman of science, doing so mindful of the writings of Francis Bacon, who perhaps was the "first statesman of science"[118]

Jefferson did not shy away from calling out European falsehoods, even if it might cost him a valued friendship. In 1784 he learned about the new European health craze, animal magnetism, popularized by Franz Anton Mesmer (1734–1815), a Viennese healer, hypnotist, and flamboyant showman. When he heard that the Marquis de Lafayette, America's heroic ally during its war for independence, planned to promote the therapeutic power of mesmerism while on a U.S. tour, Jefferson did his part to keep what he called the "hocus pocus theory" from starting up in America.[119] While in Paris, he sent copies of the highly critical investigative report of a commission headed by Benjamin Franklin to members of Congress and six of his other American correspondents to alert them to what he regarded as mesmeric fraud, and he continued to attack Mesmer as a charlatan thereafter.[120]

Inventions, Patent Law, and Intellectual Property Rights

Jefferson was fascinated by mechanical inventions. While not himself a prolific inventor, Jefferson was an innovator who improved on items already in existence. His reputation was derived primarily from his consuming interest in time- and labor-saving devices, and his compulsion to modify and attempt to improve existing utilitarian devices to meet his own needs. He recognized the transformative potential of truly novel inventions that had a beneficial impact on society. "Although Jefferson greatly admired the ingenuity of inventors, he was also critical of them when, in his view, they attempted to restrict access to their inventions." He was not opposed to inventors seeking legitimate "economic compensation for use of their genuine creations;" however, he opposed patent and other intellectual property rights that granted exclusive control over right of use for an indefinite or extensive period of time. Jefferson was also "skeptical of the ability of a single inventor, acting in isolation, to create true advances over all prior work, believing instead that [most] invention was a collaborative act involving many connections with colleagues, present and past."[121]

Whatever his reservations about the extent and exclusiveness of intellectual property claims, Jefferson was an influential pioneer in the early development of American patent law, beginning when the United States Constitution, Article 1, Section 8, clause 8, gave Congress exclusive jurisdiction over patents and copyrights. As secretary of state when Congress passed the first Patent Act on April 10, 1790 (see Figure 2), Jefferson became the "guiding spirit" of a three-member board responsible for examining and approving (or denying) patent applications. Before he became overwhelmed by the number of applications and guided the transition to a simple registry procedure, Jefferson took great pride in this work, examining every invention brought forward, but approving few.[122]

He never took out a patent on his own mechanical inventions, among which were the moldboard plow of least resistance, which won him a gold medal from the *Societe d'Agriculture de Paris* in 1807; a machine to break up hemp fibers; a swivel chair; and a cryptographic device he called his "wheel cipher" for secret diplomatic communication. His ideas for improvements on or innovations to existing technology included a dry dock, a folding stool, a portable lap desk or "writing box," a dumb waiter, a window designed to admit air but not rain, an improved cistern design, various devices that facilitated meteorological observations, and improvements in fireproofing ceilings. Jefferson even bought and made improvements in the copying press and the polygraph, two forerunners of the photocopier, and used them to keep a complete record of his correspondence.[123]

Despite being chronically in debt, Jefferson showed no interest in advantaging himself financially by securing exclusive privilege for any idea expressed in his *Notes on the State of Virginia* or his voluminous correspondence, which was allowed and even encouraged by the Copyright Law of 1790. In speaking of his own discoveries and inventions, and why he never patented one, Jefferson wrote that he "never thought of monopolising by patent any useful idea which happens to offer itself to me." When he imagined one useful improvement, he stated that "as soon as I can speak of it's effect with certainty, I shall probably describe it anonymously in the public papers, in order to forestall the prevention of it's use by some interloping patentee."[124] Clearly, Jefferson had little or no taste for money made from any form of monopoly, including ones resulting from exclusive rights to intellectual property. And when the new Constitution of the United States was being drafted, both Jefferson and Franklin, perhaps even Madison, initially seemed to agree that monopolies "are justly classed as among the greatest nuisances in government," and that a list of inalienable rights should include a "restriction against monopolies," even limited ones for intellectual property, the benefit of which was "too doubtful to be opposed to that of their general suppression." Before Jefferson left Paris, however, he had concluded that the progress of science and the arts would be promoted by the granting of patents, if the rules for doing so were based on sound principles.[125]

Jefferson maintained that all products of the human mind—every idea arising from "the fugitive fermentation of an individual brain" should be freely and readily available to the general public, and he feared that patents, as temporary monopolies, would delay the transfer of new advances to citizens and put them in the hands of greedy businessmen. In his lengthiest and cleanest statement on the subject, he argued in 1813 that patentability should be based on the novelty in usefulness and importance, and on social benefit (i.e. social contract doctrine). New inventions were to be encouraged without being made inaccessible to the general public.[126] A decade later he described "multiplied testimony" as a necessary condition to establish truth, since "much is known to one which is not known to another, and no one knows everything. it is the sum of individual knoleges which is to make up the whole truth, and to give it's correct current thro' future time." Jefferson admitted no natural, or a priori, property right in a new invention because many inventions are based on preceding ideas and thus few individuals can assert exclusivity to an idea. "The fact is," he commented, "that one idea leads to another, that to a 3^d^ and so on thro' a course of time, until some one, with whom no one of these ideas was original, combines all together, and produces what is justly called a new invention." At the same time he recognized the need to give effective encouragement regarding the introduction of new and useful inventions from abroad as well as to the exertions of skill and genius in producing them at home.[127]

Despite his misgivings, Jefferson promulgated the concept that the interposition of government policy in matters of invention, if sensibly administered, was necessary for science to advance and improve American prosperity. He soon admitted the patent law "has given a spring to invention beyond my conception."[128] In his deliberations leading to approval of sixty–seven patent applications, Jefferson took full advantage of a provision in the patent law that required inventors to demonstrate not only the usefulness but also the novelty of their devices, and to provide precise, publishable specifications with drawings, as well as a miniature working model.[129] This provision was intended to preserve the public's right to know in the face of an inventor's right to exploit. In 1791 Jefferson had unsuccessfully proposed a revision of the original Patent Act of 1790 that would have required petitioners to prove that their inventions were sufficiently "new and useful" to merit patenting, and to file and publish a record of them in every United States' district court.[130] Historians have suggested that Jefferson's "rationale for requiring filing and publication of the patent certificate in every judicial district was to give the public notice of the thing invented . . . in terms sufficient to point out the general nature thereof, and to warn others against an interference therewith."[131]

As head of the three–man patent board, Jefferson occasionally found it necessary to test a proposed new invention personally. In 1791, for example, at the request of Congress, he was called upon to investigate a claim made by Jacob Isaacks of Rhode Island that he had developed a new method for distilling potable water from salt water by means of "the common iron Cabouse." Such a process, if successful, would be invaluable for ships at sea and castaway seamen. Jefferson performed many experiments with and without the apparatus that Isaacs had erected (the latter intended to be "a controlled distillation") and sought counsel from several fellow members of the APS. His scholarly *Report on Desalination of Sea Water* of November 21, 1791, was published and distributed by the House of Representatives, which may make it the first American scientific paper to be published under governmental auspices. As a result of these experiments Jefferson advised Congress that a patent should not be granted. While Isaac's distillation system was shown to be somewhat effective, it was judged to be no more effective than various other desalination systems that preceded it.[132] This conclusion reflected Jefferson's standard that "only true novelty of invention should be rewarded, and that public dissemination of different systems, methods, and practices, past and present, should be widely promoted." His operating rules have been summarized thus: "patents should be given to particular machines, not to all possible applications or uses of them; that mere changes in materials, or form gave no claim; and that exclusive rights of an invention must always be considered in terms of the invention's social benefits."[133] Jefferson reached a similar conclusion after examining the work of other inventors. When Oliver Evans (1755–1819) claimed to have discovered an improvement in milling, Jefferson demonstrated that the Egyptians and the Persians, among others, had long used similar systems.[134]

Purpose-driven Exploration and Discovery

Jefferson's greatest contribution to scientific exploration and the mapping of the western half of the continent was his promotion of four military expeditions to the South and West between 1803 and 1807, of which the best known is the "Corps of Discovery" led by Meriwether Lewis and William Clark.[135] This multiyear venture was the culmination of a dream that Jefferson had nurtured for more than two decades. After three failures involving George Rogers Clark (1752–1818), John Ledyard (1751–1789), and André Michaux (1746–1802), Jefferson's dream of a geographic exploration of the western half of the continent became a reality when his election to the presidency gave him access to greatly enhanced resources with which to investigate, characterize, and occupy the vast wilderness of the continental west in a manner that would extend scientific frontiers while helping to secure the geopolitical and commercial future of an expanding empire of liberty stretching from "sea to shining sea."[136]

During his presidency, Jefferson invested his time, energy, political capital, and knowledge of Enlightenment science in the Lewis and Clark Expedition. He obtained the necessary money from Congress, in what was likely the first, precedent–setting, sponsorship of science by the federal government. Then he selected Meriwether Lewis (1774–1809), a captain in the U.S. Army and his private secretary, to command the expedition and personally prepared his instructions, which advised that all observations were "to be taken with great pains & accuracy, to be entered distinctly & intelligibly, for others, as well as yourself, to comprehend all the elements necessary, with the aid of the usual tables, to fix the latitude and longitude of the places at which they were taken."[137] Because Lewis had no technical background in science or diplomacy, Jefferson dispatched him to Philadelphia, where fellow APS members, leading figures in the American Enlightenment, provided tutoring in botany, zoology, geography, astronomy and instrumentation, surveying and mapping, Indian ethnology and linguistics, and medical science before starting on the expedition.[138] Later, when Lewis, disappointed and depressed, committed suicide on October 11, 1809 in an obscure frontier tavern in Tennessee before publishing any of his findings, Jefferson assumed responsibility for disseminating the discoveries to the public. Clark was given the task of writing the history of the expedition. Not comfortable as an author, he delegated the work to others, including Nicholas Biddle, and a two–volume book was published in 1814 with an introductory sketch of Lewis supplied by Jefferson.[139] More than any other man, Jefferson inspired and sustained the enterprise, determined its course, and secured its benefits for his countrymen. Although his instructions to Lewis were so extensive as to be almost impossible to fulfill and the expedition far exceeded its original budget, Jefferson viewed the expedition as a tremendous success. During its twenty–eight months the expedition traveled nearly eight thousand miles, learned much about the continent's geography and native inhabitants, and discovered more than three hundred plant and animal species, as well as many diseases not previously known to science. The revelations proved so valuable that this voyage of discovery became one of Jefferson's most enduring legacies. The three other exploratory expeditions that were sanctioned during Jefferson's presidency were the Ouachita River Expedition of 1804–05, which explored early southern Arkansas and northern Louisiana, the Red River Expedition in 1806, which ventured to the Southwest, including land that was under Spanish control, and the Zebulon Pike Expedition of 1806–07, which went to the western Great Plains and the Rocky Mountains and discovered El Capitan, later renamed Pike's Peak. Additional geographical and geological expeditions followed in fairly rapid succession, leading first to the creation of an army unit in 1812 that would eventually become the Corps of Topographical Engineers. Ultimately, the United States Geological Survey was formed in 1879.

During Jefferson's second term as president, he persuaded Congress to create the U.S. Coast Survey, America's first federally funded scientific agency. While the bill's objective was specific – to conduct surveys of the entire Atlantic seaboard plus portions of the Gulf coast and produce nautical maps – it reflected larger issues of great concern to the new nation, namely national boundaries, commerce, and defense.[140] After signing the bill on February 10, 1807, President Jefferson turned immediately to men of science, most of whom had provided counsel on previous explorations, for their ideas and recommendations on such matters as organizational structure, instrumentation and other material resources, capital requirements, and who had the expertise to lead the project.

Jefferson as Vaccination Advocate and Empirical Investigator

Jefferson had a "consuming interest in all fields of education and science, including the practice of medicine and public health. . . . Although a close friend of eminent physicians, his rationalism and scientific method placed him ahead of many practitioners of his time."[141] He frequently disparaged contemporary medical practice, believing it was more often ruinous than restorative of health, and instead actively promoted personal and public preventative health measures that careful observation and empirical evidence had proven to be both safe and effective.

One of Jefferson's greatest contributions to medical science, and the one in which he acted the part of medical researcher and provider, was the integral role he played in the advancement and distribution of the smallpox vaccine in early nineteenth–century America.[142] Smallpox was arguably the most feared and destructive scourge of that time. The single greatest cause of death in America, its worldwide case fatality rate hovered around 25 percent for adults, was even higher for infants, and left most survivors with severe disfiguring scars. As many as one–third became incurably blind.[143] Jefferson was well aware that smallpox epidemics had bedeviled humankind for many centuries, engendering panic and fear among all levels of society and ethnic groups, devastating commerce, disrupting government, and causing legislators to enact laws intended to halt its importation and spread, usually without much success. In his own time, smallpox wiped out slave populations, eradicated Indian tribes, and debilitated large armies. During the Revolutionary War, for example, the British general Charles Cornwallis captured Jefferson's Elk Hill farm on the James River and took those enslaved there to Yorktown, where almost all died from smallpox.[144]

During Jefferson's youth, the only known method of acquiring immunity against smallpox (*Variola* virus) was a form of inoculation known as variolation. Referring solely to inoculation with the live, pathogenic smallpox virus by nasal insufflation or subcutaneous ingrafting, it is not to be confused with vaccination.[145] First practiced in China by the sixteenth century, variolation then spread to the Middle East where the Turks altered the technical aspects of the procedure and touted it as an effective preventative throughout the latter half of the seventeenth century. Early in the eighteenth century, it was introduced to Europeans by Lady Mary Wortley Montagu, the wife of the British ambassador to the Ottoman Empire, who observed its success among the Turkish people and elected to have her own children variolated. The procedure soon gained significant popularity in England, but not in all European countries, and some influential institutions like the Sorbonne condemned the procedure.[146]

During a severe outbreak of smallpox in Boston in 1721 that affected more than six thousand people, almost half of the city's population, the procedure was introduced to America by two fellows of the Royal Society, the Reverend Cotton Mather (1679–1728), a Harvard College graduate with a keen interest in science and medicine, and Dr. Zabdiel Boylston

(1679–1766).[147] Although their inoculation program was entirely voluntary and highly successful, both men were widely criticized, threatened, and even attacked. Boylston was threatened with hanging for his efforts and bombs were thrown into the homes of both men in protest of their advocacy of variolation.[148] This opposition did not abate even after many additional reports of success, one of the most famous being Daniel Bernoulli's mathematical demonstration that widespread use of variolation to control smallpox epidemics would benefit not only individuals, but also the state and society at large.[149] During the next five decades, the promotion of variolation in America proved exceedingly controversial for a variety of reasons, some of which were legitimate. Because the procedure involved an arm–to–arm (direct) transfer of the *live virus* from the "fermenting pus" of an infected patient, the very real possibility existed that it could spread rather than prevent smallpox. An inoculated individual could start an epidemic of natural smallpox among friends and neighbors if he or she was not quarantined for at least three weeks after the procedure. Only those who could afford long convalescences (at times two to three months) were realistic candidates. Furthermore, if not done properly, especially before germ theory and antiseptic methods were understood, it might expose recipients to cross–contamination with other diseases, later identified as erysipelas, septicemia, syphilis, and tuberculosis. However, many who opposed variolation did so without bothering to examine the evident proof, safety, and success of the procedure. Some physicians, even at least one with European medical training, decried the dangerous "infatuation" with smallpox inoculation, believing it to be tantamount to poisoning, a "criminal act comparable to murder, and grounds for a felony indictment."[150] Others rejected the practice because it was "a thing learnt from Heathens and it is unlawful for Christians to learn the way of the Heathen." Defenders countered that the procedure was a divine gift, the abstention from which would itself be sinful.[151] The fiercest objection against variolation, however, came from clergy who railed incessantly about attempts to interfere with God's almighty plan regarding when and how people should die, preaching from the pulpit and in printed pamphlets that variolation should be condemned since it was never mentioned in the Bible.[152] These concerns collectively led many colonies including Virginia to adopt laws prohibiting the practice of variolation.

In May of 1766, aged twenty-three, Jefferson traveled a distance of nearly three hundred miles to be inoculated. Jefferson was encouraged to undergo the variolation procedure by Dr. George Gilmer, his friend and former classmate at the College of William and Mary. Because inoculation was illegal in Virginia, he went to Philadelphia, where William Shippen (1736–1808) was performing this procedure without fear of retaliation.[153] The young Jefferson suffered no ill effects. By undergoing the arduous and risky variolation procedure, he demonstrated his familiarity with emerging medical knowledge about infectious diseases and also signaled what would become a lifelong progressive commitment to personal and public preventive health.[154] Jefferson clearly recognized the risks of the procedure, but he was sufficiently convinced of its prophylactic efficacy that he had seven family members and at least five of his slaves inoculated between 1775 and 1782.[155] And as a lawyer, he willingly agreed to defend Dr. Archibald Campbell, a physician who practiced the procedure in 1768 and 1769 in Norfolk County, Virginia, and had his house burned down in an ensuing riot. Jefferson gave up his law practice before the case was resolved, but he later served on a legislative committee that recommended that the Virginia General Assembly ease the 1769 restrictions on smallpox inoculation.[156]

Jefferson eventually learned of the British physician Edward Jenner's successful experiments with the much milder and safer cowpox vaccine.[157] In contrast to variolation, vaccination was based on the use of a mild attenuated virus (cowpox virus) that produced a local, not systemic, infection at the site of inoculation yet led to a high level of immunity without need for post-procedure isolation. The procedure was called "vaccination" because the material came from cows (Latin *vacca*, cow). Jenner's work is widely regarded as the foundation of immunology. While he was neither the first to suggest that infection with cowpox conferred specific immunity to smallpox nor the first to attempt cowpox vaccination for this purpose, in 1798 he became the first to publish experimental evidence that cowpox elicited immunity, and to distribute the vaccine freely. Jefferson became an advocate for a national immunization program, promoting it as a social good rather than simply a strategy to protect individuals. He viewed Jenner's work as a revolutionary scientific advance[158] and optimistically embraced the possibility that the devouring monster of smallpox might be more successfully controlled, perhaps even exterminated, in his lifetime. He wrote: "Every friend of humanity must look with pleasure on this discovery, by which one evil the more is withdrawn from the condition of man; and contemplating the possibility that future improvements & discoveries, may still more & more lessen the catalogue of evils."[159]

Shortly after Jefferson assumed the presidency in 1801, he helped initiate generalized vaccination in the southern states and beyond.[160] But Jefferson did much more than promote its popular acceptance and dissemination; the many letters between him and allies like Dr. Benjamin Waterhouse

(1754–1846) of Harvard (see Figure 3), show that Jefferson brought his own ingenuity, patronage, and personal scientific experimentation to this seminal public health procedure. For his part Waterhouse is appropriately credited with the introduction of Jenner's vaccine to America in 1799. He was the first physician to test the cowpox vaccine there, and in September 1800, he sent a copy of his newspaper article favorably reviewing Jenner's work to then-president John Adams, his former roommate, with an appeal for help in introducing vaccination throughout the United States. When he found Adams unresponsive, Waterhouse turned to Vice President Thomas Jefferson for support, which was promptly given.[161]

The correspondence carried on between Jefferson and his medical friends illustrates the unique situation of a president of the United States cast into the unfamiliar roles of administrator of a vaccination clinic within his own and several other plantation households, as an innovative, problem-solving scientist, and as a capable clinical investigator. In his own neighborhood Jefferson took the lead in about two hundred vaccination cases. First he forwarded some vaccine with carefully detailed instructions for its use by his family's physician, Dr. William Wardlaw, in Albemarle County. Wardlaw was the first Virginia doctor to use Jenner's method, but he inoculated only about six members of Jefferson's household, before stopping because his medical practice proved too demanding for him to continue. Thereupon, Jefferson and his two sons–in–law, Thomas Mann Randolph and John Wayles Eppes, assumed responsibility and became temporary medical practitioners in their own right. Later in 1801 Jefferson reported: "In the course of July and August, I inoculated about 70. or 80. of my family; my sons in law about as many in theirs, and including our neighbors who wished to avail themselves of the opportunity our whole experiment extended to about 200 persons." In his "family" Jefferson included enslaved individuals.[162]

This exercise amply illustrates how Jefferson applied the scientific method of observation and experimentation to his extensive technical knowledge, including adherence to Jenner's two–part "Golden Rule," that vaccine fluid be harvested early, before the appearance of the areola, and that there be no interruption in the stages of pustule formation. Jefferson personally conducted several studies to determine whether or not the procedure was safe and effective.[163] His observational work included meticulous recordings of the temporal course of the immune reaction in each case, and it allowed him to determine the exact time when it was best to harvest immunologically active material from his patients' infection-induced vesicles, in order to prepare new vaccine. The optimal time turned out to be the eighth day.[164] He even asked for, and received, from Dr, John Redman Coxe in Philadelphia, active smallpox-infected material (which contained variola, the live virus), and used it to test the immunity of subjects he had previously vaccinated, thus producing what would now be called "protection trials" of the validity of the method as practiced in his part of Virginia.[165] And Jefferson freely shared his experimental findings, procedural instructions, and the genuine vaccine (his "Virginia strain") with many influential physicians in America so that they might inaugurate safe and effective vaccination programs in their local communities.[166] In an 1802 letter to Dr. Coxe, who had been the first to introduce the Jenner vaccine in Philadelphia, Jefferson wrote, "I think it an important object in such a work to bring the practice of the [smallpox] inoculation to the level of common capacities; for to give to this discovery the whole of it's value, we should enable the great mass of the people to practise it in their own families & without an expence, which they cannot meet."[167]

In addition to manufacturing and distributing vaccine, Jefferson also devised a method for preserving and transporting effective vaccine material. In the early days of cowpox vaccination in America, all of the material came from England to Boston. Jefferson was aware of the many failures that ensued, and he himself experienced disappointment when the first three batches of vaccine that Waterhouse sent him proved unsuccessful in producing immunity against smallpox. At this point Jefferson made a helpful observation. Consulting his weather charts, he noted that those days on which the vaccine had been in transit had been excessively hot, and hypothesized that heat might have destroyed the effectiveness of the virus. Jefferson then proposed that the vaccine material be placed in a special double–chamber container, in which the vaccine was first enclosed in a small glass vial, "well corked" and then the latter was immersed in a larger one partially filled with water and also corked. Jefferson reasoned that "it would be effectively preserved against the air, and I doubt whether the water would permit so great a degree of heat to penetrate to the inner phial, as does when it is in the open air. it would get cool every night, and shaded every day under the cover of the stage, it might perhaps succeed." His hypothesis that cooling could prevent degradation of cowpox vaccine was soon verified. Vaccine sent in this way proved effective in conferring immunity.[168]

Waterhouse, in one of his most important publications in 1802 (see Figure 4), credited Jefferson with "forwarding the practice of vaccination . . . by at least two years," noting that Jefferson was entirely responsible for distribution of effective inoculation samples throughout Virginia,

Pennsylvania, Delaware, Maryland, and North Carolina. An early medical historian maintained that "Thomas Jefferson was not only a patron and student of vaccination but an active practical disciple of Jenner and the direct introducer of vaccination into Pennsylvania and the whole south . . . Waterhouse and Jefferson were the two men to whom the introduction of vaccination in America was wholly due." Indeed, the meticulous research done by Jefferson and Waterhouse, including a "decisive" experiment by the latter at Noddle's Island in Boston harbor in November 1802 in which Waterhouse vaccinated nineteen volunteers with cowpox, exposed them to smallpox, and none fell ill, were brilliant demonstrations of methodologically sound, controlled clinical trials.[169]

Jefferson's interest in vaccination did not stop with the completion of his neighborhood project. During his retirement he continued to perform vaccinations at Monticello, and he worked with Waterhouse to educate the public and the profession.[170] Jefferson had a strong belief in the intelligence of the common man. If Americans could be educated about the increased effectiveness and safety of the Jenner vaccine, Jefferson believed that most people would take advantage of it to protect themselves and their families, and ultimately would strengthen the vitality of the nation. He sought to refute false statements, especially those from anti–vaccination groups. Many of the same criticisms leveled against practitioners of variolation were used to denounce cowpox vaccination. Some practitioners also claimed that the introduction of an "animal disease" into the human body was dangerously unethical, and that it might bring about a "metamorphosis into horned beasts" (see Figure 5).

As late as the turn of the twentieth century, anti-vaccination hostility resurfaced in the face of the call for compulsory vaccination during the smallpox epidemic of 1898–1903. Even today, despite overwhelming evidence of safe and effective preventative technologies, the scourge of vaccine misinformation, unrelated to the insular preferences of some ultra–orthodox religious groups, has made a sizable proportion of Americans fear vaccines more than the diseases they prevent. This "plague of science denial" represents a serious challenge for medical practitioners and public health officials, as it did in Jefferson's time.[171]

Mindful of the epidemics that had decimated Indian populations, during his first term as president, Jefferson engaged in what might be termed vaccine diplomacy.[172] Between December 1801 and February 1802, when several groups of Native Americans arrived in Washington to meet with Congress, Jefferson invited an Indian chieftain to the White House, stating that he had a message to convey to him of grave importance to the entire

Indian nation.[173] As later recounted by Waterhouse, Jefferson informed the warrior leader "that the Great Spirit had lately made a precious donation to the enlightened white men," and he then proceeded to explain the history of vaccination, which was "a gift from heaven" that would protect them from smallpox. The chieftain, who had been listening with close attention, then requested to be the first of his tribe to receive the benefits of vaccination, whereupon Jefferson arranged for Dr. Edward Gantt to inoculate the chieftain and many of his warriors in his entourage. Before the tribe departed Washington, Jefferson provided them with instructions and an amount of vaccine to use after arriving home. Another example of Jefferson's desire to see vaccination more widely disseminated among Native Americans came in his instructions for the Lewis and Clark Expedition to "carry with you some matter of kine–pox [another name for cowpox]; inform those of them with whom you may be, of it's efficacy as a preventative from the small pox; and instruct & encourage them in the use of it. this may especially be done wherever you winter." Both Jefferson and Waterhouse were pleased that the "salutiferous powers" of the cowpox vaccine would be carried "into the wilderness of the new World." Unfortunately, by the time the Lewis and Clark Expedition reached its winter encampment in today's North Dakota, the vaccine had become inert. Thus Jefferson's philanthropic initiative to vaccinate the indigenous people in the American West was stillborn. Still, by testing and publicizing Jenner's technique, with the care of a scientist and the authority of the presidency, Jefferson hastened its popular acceptance and thus indirectly helped to reduce the mortality from this dread disease.[174]

Views on Health, Education, and Scientific Literacy

Jefferson framed his philosophy on health and healing as a matter of correct political principles and polices that advanced human prosperity and happiness through universal, state–supported education. He spelled out his educational views clearly in seven legislative proposals that he drafted between 1779 and 1818. These included four bills he submitted to the General Assembly of Virginia in 1779: A Bill for the More General Diffusion of Knowledge (Bill 79); A Bill for Amending the Constitution of the College of William and Mary (Bill 80); A Bill for Establishing a Public Library (Bill 81); A Bill for Establishing Religious Freedom (Bill 82); his 1817 Bill for Establishing a System of Public Education; the Rockfish Gap Report of the University of Virginia Commissioners, August 4, 1818;

and his Bill for Establishing Elementary Schools, September 9, 1817.[175] For Jefferson, education was the only corrective of societal abuses and the chief instrument whereby the condition of man is to be progressively ameliorated. He expected broad social and economic benefits to flow from universal public education and regarded it as necessary to secure the legacy of the American Revolution.[176] The health of a nation and its individual members hinged on education. Collectively, a sound body politic depended on the sound mind of those constituting it. His crusade against ignorance recognized the hazards of false beliefs based on scientific illiteracy, which in turn could lead to destructive health behaviors, whether at the individual or population level. To guard against this, functionaries of the government needed to play a role in enriching public understanding of useful scientific knowledge, including what kinds of knowledge ought to be promoted and how they ought to be legitimized. In contrast to many of his contemporaries, Jefferson fervently believed scientific literacy would help citizens make informed decisions about medical care and healthy lifestyles, environmental issues, and the expanding array of technological choices that were coming into play. Learning about science would not only allow citizens of the new republic to share in the joy of humanity's great ongoing adventure of discovery and exploration, but it would also encourage an interactive dialogue between healers and patients by locating sources of power on both sides of the sickbed. Throughout his life, Jefferson was never a passive recipient of authoritarian, paternalistic medicine. He made his own informed choices, usually rejecting heroic interventions, and promoted empowerment among consumers. He similarly encouraged the citizens of the new republic to acquire sufficient medical knowledge so that they might take charge of their own destiny by using their minds as an important health asset. Late in life Jefferson wryly observed that in promoting scientific literacy through public education, he had been "discharging the odious function of a physician pouring medecine down the throat of a patient insensible of needing it."[177] He obviously hoped that an educated public would no longer need such interventions, medically or otherwise. Although his vision evidently did not extend beyond free inhabitants, Jefferson intended his system of universal education to reach "every description of citizens, from the richest to the poorest," and thereby to benefit those of all ages.[178] His conception of America was predicated on a philosophical purpose that mirrored the functions of biomedical research as we know it today: scientific study leading to the mastery of nature, to health, to a better quality of life, and to greater human dignity. Jefferson wrote that "the main objects of all science" are "the freedom & happiness of man," "that knolege is power, that knolege is safety, and that knolege is happiness," and that freedom is "the firstborn daughter of science."[179] The connection in his day between an informed citizenry and healthcare will be further explored in the next chapter.

Throughout much of his adult life, Jefferson promoted a strongly held notion that more science should be taught in American colleges and universities. For example, in 1789 he urged the president of Harvard University to cultivate among his students research in biological science,[180] and a decade earlier, while a member of the Virginia General Assembly, he proposed a radical piece of legislation to amend the constitution and curriculum of the College of William and Mary so as "to enlarge the sphere of science, and make it in fact a University." This reform bill, which dealt with all aspects of the college, from governance and salaries to the curriculum and the library, was Jefferson's first effort to legislate his vision of a university and anticipated many features of the future University of Virginia. The plan was partially implemented on December 4, 1779, and included provisions to abolish the schools of grammar and divinity, drop the teaching of Latin and Greek, and reorganize the college into six schools: Moral Philosophy and the Fine Arts; Mathematics, Natural Philosophy and Natural History; Anatomy, Medicine and Chemistry; Law and Police; Modern Languages; and the Brafferton Indian School.[181] The Schools of Law and Modern Languages were the first in America, and the School of Medicine became the third, although its existence was short–lived.[182] In creating the faculties of law, medicine, other sciences, and fine arts, the College of William and Mary arguably became the first to attain the character of a genuine university, a name used in the faculty records in 1781.[183] Partially influenced by the revolutionary plan that Jefferson executed at the College of William and Mary, the curricula of other American colleges were later remodeled, though with some modification. Chapter 3 will show how Jefferson infused science into the curriculum, including the medical curriculum, of the University of Virginia, which is thus the second university-based program he helped organize.

Jefferson's promotion of science in higher education was further realized in the founding of the U.S. Military Academy at West Point as an engineering school, when he signed into law the Military Peace Establishment Act on March 16, 1802. The statute, which outlined in twenty–nine sections a new set of laws and limits for the U.S. military, specified in sections 26–28 that the academy's primary function was training a "Corps of Engineers" loyal to the United States. This action thus created the first scientific school in America. Its curriculum was modeled, in part, on French precedents that combined engineering with a military education, and on English "popular science" precedents. The program of technical education at West Point influenced future scientific schools founded in 1846 as part of Yale and later named the Sheffield Scientific School, and in 1847 at Harvard with the Lawrence Scientific School. The Military Academy supplied the first engineering professors at these and other schools and graduates who played an outsized role nationwide in exploration, in cartography, and in building canals, bridges, roads and railways.[184] In his efforts to increase and improve the teaching of science in America, Jefferson hoped to import some of the best professors in Europe, particularly those from Edinburgh and Geneva, which he called "the two eyes of Europe in matters of science."[185] At one time he entertained hopes, which never materialized, of bringing to Virginia the entire scientific faculty of Geneva "where the sciences are there more modernized than anywhere else."[186] Recruiting European professors, especially from English–speaking nations, was critical, as will be seen, for populating the faculty of the University of Virginia.

Government and Science and Government as Science

Jefferson was among a small vanguard of political leaders who perceived the mutual advantages of a reciprocal relationship between science and government. He was preceded by George Washington, who, on January 8, 1790, in his first regular annual message to Congress, advised it "that there is nothing, which can better deserve your patrionage, than the promotion of Science."[187] Jefferson also believed that government should be made useful to science and science should be made useful to government.[188] In turn, through governmental support—that is, intelligent public policy decisions—science would be beneficial for society. Late in life Jefferson proclaimed his "conviction that Science is important to the preservation of our republican government, and that it is also essential to it's protection against foreign power." He understood the advantages of science and democracy working together, and that their effective interplay could help individuals and prosper the nation. Admittedly, Jefferson was philosophically committed to having a smaller rather than a larger national government, famously remarking to James Madison that "I am not a friend to a very energetic government." Despite his strong advocacy for applied (practical) science, Jefferson did not endorse direct federal funding in the sciences. The APS in Philadelphia and its sister organizations in New York and Cambridge were the leading promoters of science in Jefferson's time, and the only focused source for scientific advice to the government until the founding of the National Academy of Science in 1863.[189]

Jefferson exemplified a kind of bold American pragmatism that placed problem solving above partisanship and sought to base government policies on the best available data and most up–to–date understanding of the world. The government was not only to be a supporter of science but was itself to be operated scientifically. Both the government and the scientific community would be held to a common set of precepts that fostered a transparency of methodology in all decision-making processes. The testing and retesting of hypotheses, rigorous examination of ideas, review and critique by technically qualified peers, free speech and open exchange, and protection against retaliation for one's beliefs or findings were all healthy best practices in both science and government.[190] This gave credence to a view of government as a kind of laboratory whose leaders were willing to adjust public policy to accord with emerging data and critical review, which implied that such policies, including the constitution of the United States, would be adaptable and open to revision. Jefferson wrote "that the earth belongs in usufruct to the living: that the dead have neither powers nor rights over it." Usufruct means a form of stewardship, in which the living generation has a responsibility to maintain and improve the family, community, and societal welfare for the next generation—to make it better, more expansive.[191] Through vigorous debate, informed by the best-available scientific and technological understanding, Jefferson surmised that the functionaries of the new republic would find the most promising approaches for many of the most pressing problems of the day.

We can conclude that Jefferson's appetite for useful knowledge about scientific developments was insatiable, and he eagerly seized all means of obtaining it.[192] Because of his wide range of knowledge, he was ahead of his time in several lines of inquiry and in advance of contemporary scientists. He believed all knowledge should serve some practical purpose and that the study of science was the most certain means of advancing social progress, and human prosperity and happiness.

Jefferson brought to science a philosophical interpretation founded on French and Scottish Enlightenment thinkers, while always maintaining a broader view in contrast to the views held by most of his contemporaries. To him, good science was a central element in overcoming targeted social problems in the early national period of America. He was stalwart in his promotion of those characteristics that gave legitimacy and authority to science, namely objectivity, freedom of inquiry, an arduous disciplining of the mind (including avoidance of bias), and techniques crucial to new discovery. He preferred rationalistic thinking in contrast to metaphysical or moralistic thinking, and specific problem solving by proof-oriented investigation. Jefferson's philosophy was a blend of Isaac Newton's search for *omniscience* (grounded in basic science) and Francis Bacon's quest for *omnipotence* (applied science).[193] Jefferson saw two intertwined goals for science: a fuller, more complete understanding of nature and its judicious application to improve and sustain the liberty, health, and happiness of man,[194] as well as the success of a new form of republican government that was dependent on the sovereignty of an educated citizenry. Indeed, his many scientific endeavors illustrate his uniquely purposeful ideology: to inquiry into a narrowly defined area of scientific ignorance that was at the heart of a social problem, or one of persistent national or global interest.[195] In his lifetime crusade against ignorance, Jefferson's words and actions were concentrated in favor of omnipotence, or as Bacon had put it, "our aim is the knowledge of causes, and . . . on "the enlarging of the Human Empire, to the effecting of all things possible." Given enough scientific information, Jefferson believed that all human ills would yield to serious application of human intelligence," and he seemed to anticipate many of the predicates for establishing an effective argument for causation (for example, Bradford Hill criteria).[196]

Jefferson was not a pure scientist, nor was he simply "a great man of science." He was a statesman in the service of science, just as he was a statesman in his country's diplomatic service. His portfolio and power were sufficiently broad to enable him to weave scientific principles and practice into many fields not normally associated with pure science, including government policy, agricultural technologies, territorial expansion, and public health. At the same time, the questions of whether or how science informed his positions on the nature of man and race remains problematic.

Jefferson's lifelong preoccupation with science and his confidence in the future were succinctly stated in his comment to Dr. Benjamin Waterhouse in 1818: "when I contemplate the immense advances in science, and discoveries in the arts which have been made within the period of my life, I look forward with confidence to equal advances by the present generation; and have no doubt they will consequently be as much wiser than we have been, as we than our fathers were, and they than the burners of witches."[197]

This passage reveals Jefferson's confidence as he projects the causes of current breakthroughs into the future and sees greatness in those who would follow him. Western thinking, he perceived, was moving forward, at home and abroad, and Jefferson took great pleasure in the tangible strides it made, always encouraging those who labored to advance the cause of science.[198] But one scientific discipline disappointed him—medicine. The next chapter examines the reasons for Jefferson's largely negative attitudes toward medical theory and practice, a position that he counterbalanced by efforts to apply scientific thinking to personal and public health and to medical education.

Chapter 2

JEFFERSON'S IDEAS ON HEALTH AND THE STATE OF MEDICINE

He remarked, that whenever he saw three physicians together he looked up to discover whether there was not a turkey buzzard in the neighborhood.

Thomas Jefferson to Dr. Charles D. Everette, as reported to Dr. Robley Dunglison[1]

THIS CHAPTER will examine Jefferson's ideas on health, both theoretical and personal, and the state of medicine in the early 1800s. Among the domains to be explored are: his holistic philosophy of physical health and mental well–being; his habits of healthy living; his promotion of public and preventive health, including precepts of "prophylactic" architecture for hospitals and other built environments; the reason for and origins of his criticism of medical practice and institutional care; and, his conception of the scientifically minded physician intent on serving the public in a morally honest and humane fashion. Throughout, Jefferson's notions of health and medical treatment will be seen as closely tied to his concepts of science and epistemology presented in Chapter 1, where public evidence or the lack thereof was the criterion regulative of what deserved to be accepted as true belief. These criteria, as applied to medical concepts and practice, were influenced by Jefferson's contact with French thinkers, especially Pierre Jean Georges Cabanis (1757–1808). What Jefferson counted (and discounted) as medical science came to dictate his ideas of medical education and the professoriate and curriculum of the medical school he founded.

Attitudes Towards Medicine as Practiced

Like Moliere and Voltaire in preceding centuries, Jefferson railed against physicians with the same sarcasm and skepticism that Cicero heaped on the profession of augurs.[2] He did so because of his belief that medical science was the most important since in the final analysis, health, happiness, and life itself depend on it, and because medicine, when practiced as a scientific discipline, affords the greatest opportunity and widest scope for the exercise of humanity.[3] Jefferson also saw that of all the sciences, medicine was the one most in need of reform. In a lengthy letter to his good friend, Dr. Caspar Wistar of the University of Pennsylvania, Jefferson showed an amazing grasp of the state of medicine in late eighteenth and early nineteenth century America, including its deficiencies and the possibilities of future improvement.[4] In this writing and others, he admonished physicians for their allegiance to an unscientific assemblage of overly simplistic theories about the cause, seat and cure of disease, for their puerile observations and deceptive remedies that were often shrouded in a language of concealment and obfuscation, and for promoting a degree of heroic intervention that was often more ruinous of health than restorative.[5]

Jefferson firmly believed in the classical doctrine of "*Vis medicatrix naturae*" (the healing power of nature), the belief that, if left alone, nature would restore the balance that had been undone by disease. Doctors, he believed, interfered with this restorative process, with slavish devotion to purging, harsh emetics, and bleeding serving only to torment the patient. Jefferson made this precept a foundational element of his thinking about medicine.[6] In his letter to Wistar, he contended that because little was known about many morbid conditions physicians could rarely establish a definite cause of disease, and "to an unknown disease there cannot be a known remedy." Jefferson urged therefore that, "having been so often a witness to the salutary efforts which nature makes to reestablish the disordered functions, he [the physician] should rather trust to their action than hazard the interruption of that, and a greater derangement of the system, by conjectural experiments on a machine so complicated, & so unknown, as the human body, & a subject so sacred as human life. or, if the appearance of doing something be necessary to keep alive the hope & spirits of the patient, it should be of the most innocent character."[7] In this letter, which can be seen as a synopsis of his views on clinical medicine, Jefferson deftly applies his ethical conception of empirical science, implying that the absence of proven etiology is tantamount to ignorance, which cannot and ought not to be the basis of therapeutic interventions.

Absent experience–based cures, he notes that many diseases will resolve on the basis of natural causes. That is, observation shows that nature can be construed as a healer and, indeed, one more rooted in reliable experience than most interventions of a "trained" physician. Finally, Jefferson adds that if a physician must appear to be active, his ministrations should be innocuous. In effect, Jefferson recommended that a physician, aware of the dearth of scientific fact underlying his treatment, undertake minimal steps, which turns out to be to imitate nature.

Being a staunch supporter of the scientific method, Jefferson was particularly opposed to physicians who allowed their "fanciful theories" to outrun their facts. He distrusted orthodox medical practice, which he considered woefully medieval and subject to whim, and preferred a simple statement of ignorance when facts were insufficient. This is well illustrated in his *Notes*, where he wrote that "Ignorance is preferable to error; and he is less remote from the truth who believes nothing, than he who believes what is wrong."[8] In his admonition, Jefferson goes on to say,

> I have lived myself to see the disciples of Hoffman, Boerhave, Staalh [presumably Georg Ernst Stahl (1659–1734)], Cullen, [and] Brown, succeed one another like the shifting figures of a magic lanthern, & their fancies, like the dresses of the annual Doll–babies from Paris becoming, from their novelty, the vogue of the day, and yielding to the next novelty their ephemeral favor. the patient treated on the fashionable theory sometimes gets well in spite of the medicine ... it is in this part of medecine that I wish to see a reform, an abandonment of hypothesis for sober facts, the first degree of value set on clinical observation, and the lowest on visionary theories ... the only sure foundations of medecine are an intimate knolege of the human body, and observation on the effects of medicinal substances on that.[9]

Jefferson was aware that improper treatment could produce iatrogenic problems and believed that overly aggressive physicians often produced more harm than good. Moreover, he seemed convinced that had physicians left their patients to nature, instead of bleeding them and prescribing excessive doses of drugs of unproven benefit, more lives would have been saved. He expressed this by saying:

> the adventurous physician goes on, & substitutes presumption for knolege. from the scanty field of what is known, he launches

> into the boundless region of what is unknown. ... I believe we may safely affirm that the inexperienced & presumptuous band of Medical tyros let loose upon the world, destroys more of human life in one year, than all the Robin hoods, Cartouches, & Macheaths do in a century ... I would wish the young practitioner especially to have deeply impressed on his mind the real limits of his art, & that when the state of his patient gets beyond these, his office is to be a watchful, but quiet spectator of the operations of nature, giving them fair play by a well–regulated regimen, & by all the aid they can derive from the excitement of good spirits & hope in the patient.[10]

Jefferson expressed strong antagonism to any instruction in unproven medical theory, which he characterized as "the charlatanrie of the body," as theology was that "of the mind."[11] Believing that facts must displace theory, he argued that in the absence of scientifically documented observations, "the judicious, the moral, the humane physician should stop."[12] This last admonition reveals Jefferson's belief in one of the most enduring principles of Hippocratic medicine – that of *Primum non nocere,* or "First, do no harm."[13] To this, however, Jefferson added the importance of affectionate optimism. Indeed, the state of medicine in his time and beyond was such that the best medicine available was often the healer's sustained empathetic vigilance and spiritual solace, and his hopeful reliance on the recuperative power of nature (see Figure 6).

During Jefferson's lifetime and well into the nineteenth century, doctors emphasized the primacy of intrusive medical treatment, often to the exclusion or subordination of scientifically obtained findings.[14] Most orthodox physicians feared being branded an "inert" practitioner; the imperative to intervene, usually aggressively, was crucial to their professional image, standing, and income. Such physicians held inflated beliefs about the efficacy of their remedies, ignoring the healing powers of nature. They denounced "expectant methods of treatment," implicitly equating non-intervention with an immoral abrogation of professional responsibility. Many physicians feared that a "scientific emphasis," understood as a desire to locate the cause and seat of disease, rather than singularly combatting its systemic manifestations, could "corrupt" the practitioner's duty to "cure" the patient. Above all else, prescribing "active and intrusive measures" (e.g., blistering, copious bloodletting, and use of toxic emetics and purgatives) to "subdue" all symptoms was fundamental to "proper" medical practice. To Jefferson, treating symptoms without some understanding of their origins was malpractice.

The 1799 death of George Washington is one of the best-known examples of a patient finished off by the misguided heroics of eighteenth-century medicine.[15] During his final twelve hours of life, three physicians engaged in an unrelenting battle to subdue his "septic throat" without ever acting to relieve his obstructed windpipe.[16] They bled him four times, removing more than 80 ounces of blood (2.4 liters or 40 percent of his total blood volume), "painfully blistered" his throat, feet, legs and arms with a "Spanish fly," and administered three powerful evacuates that induced severe vomiting with a combination of mercurous chloride (calomel) and antimony tartrate. These indiscriminate interventions only worsened Washington's excruciating sense of suffocation due to the ever advancing throat and laryngeal edema, which was readily apparent by his stridorous breathing and the cyanotic hue of lips.[17] A sedating dose of opium would have been a more humane treatment, and if combined with a surgical procedure to open his airway, far more effective. Had the treatment been less debilitating, the normally healthy Washington might well have survived the illness.[18] His death calls to mind Moliere's statement in *Le Madade Imaginaire,* (1673) that "nearly all men die of their remedies, and not their illness."[19]

Holistic Philosophy of Health

Jefferson was a medical practitioner in his own right, serving himself, his immediate and extended family, and the broader community that included the enslaved persons of his estate, friends, and neighbors.[20] Unlike that of most of his contemporaries, he acknowledged many different and intertwined dimensions of human life that were all very relevant to health and happiness.[21] Jefferson saw the human condition in its fullness, not just as a physical body, and understood the disease implications of individual and societal behavior, especially when wrapped in "disordered thinking" and fueled by unhealthy emotions, attitudes or beliefs.

Jefferson's view of health and healing, and the world of medicine to which he subscribed, stemmed in part from his belief in the ancient wisdom, "mens sana in corpore sano" (a "sound mind in a sound body").[22] This conceptual framework influenced his personal health habits and the actions he took on behalf of the public he served. His philosophy called attention to the fact that sickness, like aging and death, is inevitable, and it promoted a psychosomatic notion that the body reflected the state of one's mind. He emphasized the importance of mind cultivation for the betterment of self and others and suggested a more modern-day definition of health—rather than simply the absence of pain and illness, he may have intuited it as the presence of physical, mental, and socioeconomic well–being.[23] To Jefferson, the body possessed incredible potential for innate healing, for repair and regeneration, if the mind and body were in a state of "tranquil permanent felicity."[24]

Jefferson clearly understood the connection between human disposition and bodily function—that a runaway or "disordered imagination" could produce ill health.[25] As early as 1787, he warned his daughter, Martha Jefferson (Randolph), "Idleness begets ennui, ennui the hypochondria, and that a diseased body. . . . If at any moment, my dear, you catch yourself in idleness, start from it as you would from the precipice of a gulph."[26] In 1816, when Jefferson's thought that his physical health was already beginning to deteriorate, he wrote to John Adams that "there are indeed . . . gloomy & hypocondriac minds, inhabitants of diseased bodies, disgusted with the present, & despairing of the future; always counting that the worst will happen, because it may happen. to these I say How much pain have cost us the evils which have never happened!"[27] Jefferson was enough of a realist to know that aging and death belonged to the lawful processes of nature, but he was still a sturdy optimist when he said it did not follow that the soul ought to wallow in anxious anticipation of what might occur. Happiness can derive as easily from the life of the body as the mind, as long as there is "a just equilibrium of all the passions."[28] Rather than hold onto the false notion that preservation of a youthful body will help achieve some sense of spiritual balance or well–being, aging people should rejoice that they have lived long enough to choose not only the right causes but to have had the opportunity to create more good than turmoil.[29] Through the power of positive thinking and intense intellectualism, Jefferson in his retirement years (1809–1826) extracted more from life than most do in a lifetime. He invested passion and considerable mental toil during his final seventeen years to the construction of the University of Virginia, in his own neighborhood.[30] And he lived to see it open in 1825 and was greeted with near awe whenever he descended from his mountaintop home of Monticello and paid the school a visit. Though his physical infirmity was certainly real and pronounced at the close of life, Jefferson died possessing far more felicitous thoughts than solemn regrets. He died worn down in body but as vigorous intellectually as he was in his prime.[31] By striving for a realistic balance of physical and mental pursuits in his later years, Jefferson sustained a very sound mind even in a body that was less so.

Personal Health Habits

Jefferson's interest in health included habits intended to preserve his own health, and it can be surmised that the implementation of his regimen functioned as a one–person clinical trial, in which he retained strategies that worked while discarding those that failed.

Jefferson embraced several strict habits. His personal regimen suggests that he was ahead of his time in appreciating the value of moderation, discipline and order in one's daily affairs, healthy eating habits and regular exercise. Unlike many of his contemporaries, he was scrupulous in his diet. Vegetables, rather than meat, made up the bulk of his meals. In a letter to Dr. Vine Utley, Jefferson stated he was in the habit of "eating little animal food, & that, not as an aliment so much as a condiment for the vegetables, which constitute my principle diet."[32] He did not use tobacco or "ardent spirits in any form."[33] Wine, however, was his favorite beverage and his wine cellar probably contained the finest selection of European wines in the United States.[34] He preferred only the "weak" varieties and consumed several glasses at dinner, sometimes more.[35] And, Jefferson may have discouraged visitors to Monticello from giving toasts after dinner because it encouraged them to drink more than they should.[36] He had observed in France that, unlike in America, dinner guests refrained from excessive drinking that could "terminate the most sociable meals" by "transforming themselves into brutes."[37]

Regular physical exercise was also important to Jefferson, who thought that "the time necessary to secure it [i.e., health] by active exercises, should be devoted to it in preference to every other pursuit."[38] Both as a college student at William and Mary and as an adult, he dedicated a couple of hours in the afternoon to walking, explaining that "The sovereign invigorator of the body is exercise, and of all the exercises walking is best," that "It is of little consequence to store the mind with science if the body is permitted to be debilitated. If the body be feeble, the mind will not be strong," and that "exercise and application produce order in our affairs, health of body, chearfulness of mind, and these make us precious to our friends."[39] Later in life, when he described himself as "too feeble indeed to walk much," Jefferson began riding a horse from three to four hours a day. As late as 1819 he could still ride "without fatigue 6. or 8. miles a day, and sometimes 30. or 40."[40] Jefferson enjoyed riding horseback through the final days of his life. Thomas Jefferson Randolph, his oldest grandson, recalled that "He retained to the last his fondness for riding on horseback; he rode within three weeks of his death, when, from disease, disability, and age, he mounted with difficulty."[41]

Jefferson avoided the health hazards of idleness himself and his correspondence reveals his disdain for indolence and wasting time.[42] He was a "miser of his time" who unerringly structured it according to "regular and systematic" habits, a man who kept a timepiece in nearly every room of his house and gave gold or silver watches to his grandchildren. During the day, he was always busy.[43] When not writing, he was reading,[44] exercising, working on some new invention or experiment, developing his interest in herbal medicines, cultivating his "garden pharmacy" at Monticello, or communicating with men of science.[45] James Holmes, a medical historian, said of his interest in plant pharmacy that "the level of Jefferson's interest in self–prepared medicine was heightened by the fact that no doctor was involved in the treatment'," and "that he most certainly viewed self–treatment as a safer method of health care."[46]

Jefferson had similarly disciplined sleeping habits. He would "rise with the sun" every morning and slept "from 5. to 8. hours, according as my company or the book I am reading interests me."[47] Before giving himself up to sleep, he read to fill his mind with felicitous thoughts, saying, "I never go to bed without an hour, or half hour's previous reading of something moral, whereon to ruminate in the intervals of sleep."[48]

Jefferson's personal regimen and his musings suggest that to progress in mind cultivation, one must maintain a healthy body and a productive daily routine, without becoming fanatical about it. Although Jefferson placed much value on learning, he held firm a belief that "health must not be sacrificed to learning," because "A strong body makes the mind strong" and "the most uninformed mind with a healthy body, is happier that the wisest valetudinarian."[49]

Among the founding fathers, Jefferson was arguably the strongest proponent of disease prevention.[50] He practiced and promoted a "surprisingly modern" philosophy of health preservation to avoid the more difficult task of health restoration.[51] Safeguarding one's health, including dental hygiene,[52] by incorporating sensible health measures into one's daily routine was a responsibility Jefferson took seriously, and he hoped his countrymen would do the same. Staying healthy and fit might provide citizens with the possibility of living longer and reducing the risk of disease, of having greater vitality and independence in one's twilight years and lessen the likelihood of overly intrusive responses of physicians who had little or no chance of restoring health should a person lose it.

In contrast to many of his blood relatives and friends, who died early, Jefferson lived to the age of eighty–three, nearly twice the life expectancy of the time.[53] His longevity and oft–stated freedom from serious illness[54] can be attributed to his philosophy of temperate living and his forward–looking ideas on health and preventive medicine, as well as his skepticism about physicians and the unscientific, often harmful medicine they practiced.[55]

Throughout his life, Jefferson was never a passive recipient of authoritarian, paternalistic medicine. Taught to be self–reliant from youth, he made his own informed choices, usually rejecting all forms of heroic intervention, and promoted empowerment among consumers. He encouraged the citizens of the new republic to acquire medical knowledge sufficient to take charge of their own destiny by using their mind as a health asset. This view of locating power through knowledge on both sides of the sickbed was consistent with his philosophy of republican democracy that emphasized collective decision making.[56]

According to Holmes and other historians, not all of Jefferson's peers shared his prejudices against physicians, heroic medicine, or even tobacco.[57] Benjamin Franklin, George Washington, John Marshall and John Adams all left correspondence indicating their willingness to seek the services of doctors, and usually early in the course of illness. For Washington in particular, the use of intrusive medical treatment was readily accepted; he was an insistent advocate and recipient of both bloodletting and purging, sincerely believing that "poisonous" matter in the body had to be evacuated to allow healing and "that a few days neglect, or want of bleeding, might render the ailment incurable."[58] At times, he performed the procedure himself on his slaves. As previously noted, his faith in heroic medical measures very likely contributed directly to his own death. Adams recorded his own early introduction to tobacco and his continued use for almost sixty years.[59] Ironically, as pointed out by Holmes, "Adams, the tobacco user, outlived Jefferson, who shunned it, by eight years," dying at the age of nearly ninety–one.[60]

Promotion of Public Health, Salutogenic Architecture, and Sensible Urban Design

Throughout his life Jefferson relished the sensation that rendered human beings capable of unselfish commitment to one another. In 1796, he wrote of "a debt of service due from every man to his country, proportioned to the bounties which nature and fortune have measured to him," and his actions as a staunch proponent of public health and social legislation show that he conscientiously responded to this call of duty.[61] During his five years in Paris, from 1784 to 1789, he worked with a committee to reform the city's ailing public-health system.[62] As governor of Virginia (1779–81) and later when he was president of the United States (1801–09), Jefferson voiced concerns about local domestic conditions within the environment, such as poor sanitation, noxious air, inadequate ventilation and polluted water supplies, overcrowded city conditions and warm climates in the transmission of disease.[63] He argued that the proper role of local, state and federal agencies in protecting public health and commerce through a clear–sighted use of practical quarantines based on sound knowledge and scientific methodology.[64]

In 1802, two years after the federal government officially moved to Washington, the city enacted its first public–health ordinance, "An Act to Establish and Regulate Public Markets," which forbade the sale of "unsound, blown or unwholesome meat."[65] That same year a law providing for an overseer of the poor required the mayor to contract a physician to administer medical care for the poor, and to make provisions for promptly burying the deceased poor.[66] In 1803, the presence of yellow fever in neighboring Alexandria led to the creation of a superintendent of police for Washington, whose "chief duty was to protect the public health by preventing the accumulation of stagnant water and other nuisances such as dead animals."[67] According to John Duffy, a medical historian, "President Thomas Jefferson was a firm exponent of the miasmatic [pollution] theory, and his influence undoubtedly helps to explain the Washington City Council's willingness to vote money in these years to eliminate stagnant pools, swampy areas and decaying animal debris."[68] It is also noteworthy that Jefferson's prior advocacy and continuing prestige after leaving office undoubtedly contributed to the passage on February 27, 1813, of a federal law encouraging vaccination.[69] This statute sought to regulate the purity of the Jenner vaccine in order to protect Americans from unscrupulous purveyors who offered adulterated versions,[70] sometimes with "contaminants" that produced iatrogenic illnesses. It authorized the president to appoint an official vaccine "agent to preserve the genuine vaccine matter" and send it through the post office to any American who requested it. Soon thereafter, the government was providing free vaccine for tens of thousands of people each year, an action that can be viewed as the first health-care entitlement for the general population, and the first federal law to oversee drug purity with an eye towards consumer protection.[71] However, the repeal of this law on May 4, 1822[72] reflected the prevailing view that the federal government should intervene in health concerns only in times of national emergency.[73]

Jefferson also showed his commitment to public health by advancing both statewide and federally funded health-care programs for "the relief and maintenance of ill and disabled seamen." In October 1780, when Jefferson was governor, the Commonwealth of Virginia enacted a law mandating the collection of nine pence per month from each mariner to fund a "hospital for the relief of sick and disabled seamen."[74] A subsequent act (December 20, 1787) funded the first hospital in America dedicated to caring for men who made their living at sea.[75] This state-sponsored hospital in the port of Norfolk was sold to the Federal government in 1801, three years after President John Adams signed into law a congressional act creating the Marine Hospital Service, which eventually morphed into the US Public Health Service.[76] Of note, Jefferson presided over the Senate when the Fifth Congress approved the act that authorized the Marine Hospital Fund and specified that its revenue would come from a payroll tax levied on merchant seaman.[77] During Jefferson's presidency, the fund was used to establish federally run treatment facilities in Norfolk, New Orleans, and Boston.[78] Jefferson also named his friend and political ally, Benjamin Waterhouse to be the third director of the Boston Marine Hospital.[79] Although Waterhouse was a controversial character whose appointment excited considerable criticism from professional rivals and political opponents,[80] Jefferson made sure that he was suitably qualified and ready to assume the position.[81] As the new head of the hospital, Waterhouse was quick to channel his impressive energy and intellect, and set one precedent after another.[82] According to Surgeon General C. Everett Koop, Waterhouse established "the first out–patient service for merchant seaman who didn't need to be hospitalized, and thus radically expanded the range of federal medical care," and "he wrote the first regulations governing the way federal medicine would be dispensed, who would dispense it and who would be eligible to receive it."[83] After Jefferson retired from the presidency, partisan politics resulted in the dismissal of Waterhouse from his hospital post amid charges of nepotism and corruption that were probably fabricated.[84]

In his annual message to Congress in 1805, Jefferson clearly articulated the interconnected responsibilities of local, state and federal officials, stating that "I have strictly enjoined of the officers at the head of the customs to certify, with exact truth, for every vessel sailing from a foreign port, the state of health respecting this fever which prevails at the place from which she sails. Under every motive from character and duty to certify the truth, I have no doubt they have faithfully executed this injunction." Jefferson went on to issue a challenge imbued with a degree of cautious optimism, saying that

> Much real injury has however been sustained from a propensity to identify with this endemic, and to call by the same name, fevers

> of very different kinds, which have been known at all times and all countries, and never have been placed among those deemed contagious. As we advance in our knowledge of this disease, as facts develope the source from which individuals receive it, state authorities charged with the care of the public health, and Congress with that of the general commerce will become able to regulate with effect their respective functions in these departments. The burthen of quarantines is felt at home as well as abroad; their efficacy merits examination. Although the health laws of the states should be found to need no present revisal by Congress, yet commence claims that their attention be ever awake to them.[85]

In exhorting the cities and states to work with Congress, Jefferson was calling for collaboration so that a more effective, practical and judicious use of quarantine for yellow fever might occur, along with an improved methodology for distinguishing the dangerous yellow fever from other more benign illnesses. If this happened, there surely would be better protection of the public as well as the nation's commercial interests.

Jefferson was in Philadelphia during the height of the 1793 yellow–fever epidemic, and he then took a different position on its cause. Some Federalists, led by Alexander Hamilton, claimed that yellow fever was an imported contagion that had arrived in Philadelphia through French citizens fleeing the slave rebellion in Haiti (then Saint-Domingue), and that the solution was quarantine and a limitation, if not an outright ban of immigration. Jefferson assigned more blame to local domestic conditions. His insightful commentary on the health crisis included its adverse effect on government and a belief that a warm climate, lack of sanitation, and crowded living conditions played at least some role in spreading the disease.[86]

A concern for community health led Jefferson to set up a student health service and establish a free clinic at the University of Virginia;[87] to study housing, urban planning, and hospital and prison design as public health problems; to propose new building rules for the prevention of diseases and to insure the most healthful climates in architectural designs for human habitation, including those associated with colleges and universities.[88] Many of the principles that guided Jefferson's conception of socially responsible environmental design, including public architecture surrounded by open space, might today be considered *salutogenic* because they focused on the positive impact of structural design on human health, safety, and emotional well–being, and avoided the pathogenic factors that contributed to the destruction or debilitation of the body, mind and morals of American citizens.[89] Examples include natural lighting, planned air circulation, and pleasing sightlines, which will be discussed below in Jefferson's plans for the buildings of the University of Virginia.

Jefferson also warned people about the hazards of tobacco cultivation and was troubled that Virginia was "an agent for the dissemination of this injurious agent," as one of the great tobacco–growing states. As he wrote in his *Notes*, tobacco was "a culture productive of infinite wretchedness."[90] Jefferson also spoke out in favor of child welfare, women's hygiene, the importance of choosing a spouse based on virtue rather than physical beauty, the health advantages of breastfeeding for mother and child,[91] and even the right to die by assisted suicide.

Like many of his ideas, Jefferson's views on euthanasia were ahead of their times. In a letter to Dr. Samuel Brown, Jefferson addressed the use of the plant *Datura stramonium* or jimsonweed.[92] He suggested to Brown that a lethal drug produced from the plant, if "restrained to self-administration," could be a "rational relief" to individuals with terminal afflictions such as "the inveterate cancer." The plant, wrote Jefferson, "brings on the sleep of death as quietly as fatigue does the ordinary sleep."[93] Despite his general dedication to preserving life, Jefferson was at ease with the moral and ethical conundrum associated with his proposal, perhaps because he saw the value of alleviating unrequited agony by granting patients the liberty of compassionate choices.[94] The first legal sanction for physician–assisted suicide only came in 1994 with passage of an Oregon referendum.[95]

Jefferson promoted concepts that are now recognized as essential protective measures for individual and community health – notably, immunization and control of the environment, which included sanitary reform, salutogenic architecture and sensible urban design. Moreover, he seemed to understand that such measures can have maximum value only when those for whom they are intended cooperate intelligently in their use.

Criticism of Medical Practice

This chapter opened with Jefferson's scientifically based criticism of contemporary medical practice. While it was not an obsession, references to the "reform" of medicine occur frequently in his writings.[96] His encyclopedic knowledge and reputation as a man of science helped him influence contemporary medical practice. Jefferson received all sorts of inquiries about human health and was often asked about the qualifications of certain physicians.[97] Some wished to know his views on the causes of certain diseases. Young physicians sent him copies of their inaugural dissertations, and medical professors presented him with copies of their medical lectures and essays—including Dr. David Ramsey of South Carolina, one of the first significant American historians;[98] Dr. Daniel Drake of Cincinnati, Ohio; Drs. Benjamin Waterhouse, George C. Shattuck, Jacob Bigelow and John Collins Warren from Boston and Cambridge; Drs. James Woodhouse, Benjamin Barton Smith, John Redman Coxe and Benjamin Rush from Philadelphia; and Drs. John Bard, David Hosack, William James Macneven, Alire Raffeneau-Delile, Edward Miller and Samuel Latham Mitchill from New York CIty.[99] Each sought Jefferson's opinion, and he responded freely, sometimes drawing from his personal experience or reading and sometimes relying on his conversations with leading American medical figures. These interactions with young physicians and established medical educators, and the public at large, enhanced Jefferson's knowledge of medicine and its most popular theories, as well as its serious limitations in late 18th and early 19th–century America. In the following sections, we will sketch a number of Jefferson's critiques of the theory and practice of medicine in his era and then clarify the intellectual influences that governed his objections.

Far into the nineteenth century, the medical profession in America lacked any semblance of a unified culture that promoted scientific investigation and application to public health or personalized medical care. The field of medicine was cluttered with many unsubstantiated theories, the most popular of which were of European origin, namely, those of Thomas Sydenham (1624–1689), Hermann Boerhaave (1668–1738), William Cullen (1710–1790), John Brown (1735–1788), and François–Joseph–Victor Broussais (1772–1838).[100] The predilection of this period for reductive theorizing was not confined to Europe. The colonies showed the same fondness for speculation about the cause and mechanisms of disease and their therapy, all based on hypothesis rather than empirical evidence. Many of these theories were "wild and irresponsible generalizations," typically grounded in an overly simplified theory of pathology and therapeutics.[101] During the latter part of the eighteenth century in America, it seemed natural to compliment an "important medical system builder" as an individual who, "to avoid the contagion of opinion… had read no medical book for five whole years." Such was the dubious praise that Samuel Latham Mitchill (1764–1831), a professor of chemistry and natural history at Columbia College, accorded the work of John Brown and the Brunonian system of medicine which he founded.[102]

Many equally benighted examples of medical theorizing surfaced in America.[103] None received more acclaim than the "single–entity theory of disease", espoused by Dr. Benjamin Rush (1745–1813) of the University of Pennsylvania. In 1789, Rush boldly proclaimed that all previous schemes of physic were faulty and that he was formulating "a more simple and consistent system of medicine" than the world had yet seen.[104] By 1796, he had amplified his unitary principle of fever into a unitary principle of disease, when he said to a class of medical students, "I have formerly said there is but one fever in the world. Be not startled, Gentlemen, follow me and I will say there is but one disease in the world. The proximate cause of disease is irregular, convulsive or wrong action in the (vascular) system affected."[105] Although Rush was perhaps America's best–known physician at the time and widely praised there and abroad,[106] his scheme was little more than a revival of the ancient tension theory that ascribed all illness to "excessive action" within the walls of blood vessels.[107] From this monistic pathology, he deduced a monistic depletion therapy.[108] Every condition could be treated by bleeding, or purging, to relieve tension and restore the patient to healthy balance. If a patient were bled long enough he would – sooner or later – relax.[109] This simple approach was precisely what some patients and busy practitioners desired. If the one cause and the one remedy were known, what need was there for unpleasant and difficult research such as autopsies? Further investigation was simply unnecessary.[110] Like other "system–makers" in Europe and America, Rush never recanted his doctrine of "one proximate cause." Instead, he presented it as a final truth with no expectation of revision.[111]

During the massive yellow-fever epidemic of 1793 in Philadelphia, Rush promoted his doctrine with religious zeal and eventually carried his practice of bleeding to extremes.[112] In an early account he wrote that "I preferred frequent and small, to large bleedings, in the beginning of September; but towards the height and close of the epidemic, I saw no inconvenience from the loss of a pint, and even twenty ounces of blood at a time. I drew from many persons seventy and eighty ounces in five days; and from a few, a much larger quantity."[113] Rush boldly and widely proclaimed the success of his method to the public and his medical colleagues without offering any scientific evidence.[114] He even declared that his doctrine of one disease had done for medicine what a belief in one God had achieved in religion![115] Being proud of his potent art, Rush not only eschewed the healing power of nature, he banished it from the sick room "as one would a stray dog or cat."[116]

A few prominent members of the medical community rejected Rush's unitary doctrine of disease and his claims of cure, surmising that his reliance on heroic bleeding did nothing to stem the devastation brought on by yellow fever.[117] But he dismissed such caution and criticism from the more conservative practitioners in Philadelphia as arising from their own self–interest, arguing to his wife in September of 1793 that, "Hundreds have been sacrificed by this mistake. We have but *one*, we cannot have but *one* fever in this town. The contagion of the yellow fever like Aaron's rod swallows up the seeds of all other diseases. We might as well talk of two suns or two moons shining upon our globe as of two different kinds of fever now in our city."[118] Furthermore, Rush stated of "the multiplication of diseases" that "It is as repugnant to truth in medicine, as polytheism is to truth in religion. The physician who considers every different affection of the different systems in the body, or every affection of different parts of the same system, as distinct diseases, when they arise from one cause, resembles the Indian or African savage, who considers water, dew, ice, frost, and snow as distinct essences."[119] Several historians have pointed out that Rush was at least partially triumphant in fighting the "false temerity" in the streets, the press, the medical societies and even the courts, as he successfully sued William Cobbett for his impolite observation that "the good doctor's claim of a sure cure was one of those great discoveries which are made from time to time for the depopulation of the earth."[120]

Rush can be celebrated as well as criticized. His laudatory accomplishments include: staying and fighting the outbreak when most physicians fled the city; his promotion of prison reform, education of women, free public schooling, veterinary medicine, abolition of slavery and capital punishment; establishing the Philadelphia Dispensary to provide medical care for the poor (1786); and advocating changes to humanize psychiatric treatment. He was also an early and active patriot who signed the Declaration of Independence, and he helped to found Dickinson College in 1783 and Franklin and Marshall College in 1787.

But with the benefit of modern understanding of medicine, Rush's veneration of venesection certainly clouds his legacy. Furthermore, he and through him many of the roughly three thousand student disciples he trained during a thirty–year career at the University of Pennsylvania promoted the practice of extreme purging.[121] To Jefferson and many others he recommended his "thunderbolt," an explosive laxative made up of the purgatives jalap and calomel (mercurous chloride) for the treatment of just about everything.[122] Several of Rush's colleagues renounced his large purgative doses as hurtful, even murderous.[123] Another American systematizer, Dr. John Esten Cooke (1783–1853), carried purging with calomel to amazing extremes in the South and Midwest. He prescribed as much as an ounce of calomel and repeated it at frequent intervals. Households sometimes harbored a pound or more of this mercurial.[124] Not until the middle-third of the nineteenth century did patients begin to protest against excessive purging with poisonous and sometimes fatal doses of calomel.[125] One writer expressed his opposition to the "abuse" of calomel by physicians with a poem that appeared in the *Richmond Enquirer* in 1825:[126]

Calomel: An Old Song, Altered and Enlarged

Physicians of the highest rank
To pay their bills we need a bank:
Not talents bright, nor art, nor skill,
Preserve us safe from *Calomel.*

Howe'er their patients do complain
Of head, or heart, or nerve, or vein,
Of fever, thirst, or temper fell,
The Medicine still, is *Calomel*

Since Calomel's become their boast
How many patients have they lost?
How many thousands they make ill,
Of poison, with their *Calomel?*

The writer then proceeded to relate the details of a patient's last illness, due entirely to mercury poisoning, and concluded with the following peroration:

Physicians, hear a friendly voice
Receive my counsel, take advice,
Be not offended, tho' I tell,
The dire effects of *Calomel.*

And when I do resign my breath,
Pray let me die a natural death,
And bid you all a long farewell,
Without one dose of *Calomel.*

In addition, the prevailing wisdom of contemporary medical practice, combined with an element of nationalism, asserted that the "idiosyncratic harshness of American disease" demanded more "heroic" measures than the diseases of Europe.[127] The idea that American disease was singularly vigorous was a widely held notion. Because of this, Rush and his contemporaries insisted that the citizens of the United States required more "copious depletion" than effete Europeans.[128]

A Commitment to Intelligent Empiricism and its Practical Application

To Jefferson, the therapeutic methods practiced by the medical fraternity of his day were irrational, entirely unscientific, and promoted complacency in the face of what really was a vast and appalling ignorance.[129] His criticism of medicine grew out of his long–standing acceptance of the maxim that beliefs had to be verified over time by intelligent observation and experiment.[130] Moreover, this true disciple of the Enlightenment in America promoted the body's natural defenses, good hygiene and healthy living, while advocating therapeutic restraint when evidence of benefit was lacking.[131] He was openly critical of physicians who routinely bled or prescribed as a matter of course excessive amounts of medicaments, such as calomel or opium.[132] Jefferson firmly believed that morbid conditions about which little was known did not require such fashionable, and at times painful, remedies. Instead, "honest and humane physicians" should place more reliance on innate restorative power of nature, without the aid of which all efforts would be in vain. The physician might do more harm than good by interfering with Nature's propensity to heal itself. Jefferson implored America to be distrustful of unsubstantiated theory and orthodoxy, which he considered subject to change at whim, advising an honest confession of ignorance from healers when understanding was insufficient. Speaking of theological issues, but with more general applicability, Jefferson said that "when I meet with a proposition beyond finite comprehension, I abandon it as I as do a weight which human strength cannot lift:, and I think ignorance, in these cases, is truly the softest pillow on which I can lay my head."[133]

Jefferson promoted and sought to establish a more rational basis for medical therapeutics, one rooted in the "certainty" of good science.[134] During his ninth and last decade of life, Jefferson did not believe that certainty in medicine was imminent, but he did argue that a commitment to intelligent empiricism would in time bring something authentic and lasting. According to historian Courtney B. Hall, two characteristics of Jefferson's thinking led him to make some rather sharp criticisms of the medical customs and practices of his time.[135] The first of these mental traits was his firm belief in observation, quantitative measurement likely fueled by his interest in mathematics, and experiment as *sine qua non* conditions for any scientific inquiry. Jefferson seemingly recognized two paths to knowledge of nature's secrets: keen observation of natural events as they occur, and experimentation in which the effect of a controlled intervention is scrupulously examined to determine whether it had a beneficial, neutral, or harmful effect.[136] This was illustrated in his many careful agricultural and mechanical experiments, his fieldwork in paleontology and archaeology, his elaborate arrangement of tabular data regarding weather and climate, his own experimentation with the smallpox vaccine, and with his personal habits of diet and exercise. The second trait reflected his utilitarian attitude. Jefferson was a pragmatist whose chief interest was in adapting the revelations of science to human need. To be worthy of man's consideration, Jefferson believed that science in all of its branches should contribute positively to human welfare, and he demonstrated this in action.

These basic criteria, the first a description of his scientific method, and the second a definition of what was to him the true objective of all science, suggest his remarkable insight as a scientist and free–thinking secular humanist. Jefferson assumed that to be helpful medical therapeutics must square with his basic criteria. He discounted "visionary theories" or empty hypotheses in the absence of "sober facts"— facts derived from a systematic investigation of phenomena intended to add to the sum total of verifiable knowledge through observation, experiment and clear reasoning. He approved heartily of remedial activities that medical experience had proven beneficial. He never tired of praising the work of John Coakley Lettsom, Edward Jenner, Benjamin Waterhouse and others who had taken part in the international vaccination effort, and he was quite proud of his own part in the American phase of smallpox vaccination. To Dr. Jenner, Jefferson wrote in 1806, with characteristic sweep, "Medecine has never before produced any single improvement of such Utility … you have erased from the Calendar of human afflictions one of it's greatest. yours is the comfortable reflection that mankind can never forget that you have lived. future nations will know by history only that the loathsome small pox has existed & by you has been extirpated." In another passage in this letter that further illustrates Jefferson's belief in the importance of bringing new knowledge to the bedside, he wrote that, "Harvey's discovery of the circulation of the blood was a beautiful addition to our knowledge of the animal economy. but on a review of the practice of medecine before & since that epoch, I do not see any great amelioration which has been derived from that discovery."[137] To Jefferson, Harvey's discovery, while potentially important,[138] paled in comparison to Jenner's vaccine since it had no discernable payoff as yet in terms of therapeutic advance.[139]

Many examples illustrate Jefferson's strident opposition to medical practice based solely on speculative schemes for healthful living and disease management.[140] One such writing was directed at Rush's followers and recalled the way Rush had treated many hundreds of patients during the yellow-fever epidemic in Philadelphia in 1793, with a variety of depletion techniques mostly bleeding and purging with mercury. Jefferson regarded this approach as harsh and harmful, probably killing more patients than it helped, when he said that, "I have in absolute abhorrence the fanciful and ephemeral theories under which dashing practitioners are so wantonly sporting with human life. our country is overrun with young lads from the Philadelphia school, who with their mercury & lancet in hand are vying with the sword of Bonaparte which shall have shed most human blood."[141] To William G. Munford in 1799, Jefferson wrote:

> from Hippocrates to Brown we have had nothing but a succession of hypothetical systems each having it's day of vogue, like the fashions & fancies of caps & gowns, & yielding in turn to the next caprice. yet the human frame, which is to be the subject of suffering & torture under these learned modes, does not change. we have a few medecines, as the bark, opium, mercury, which in a few well defined diseases are of unquestionable virtue, but the residuary list of the materia medica, long as it is, contains but the charlataneries of the art; and of the diseases of doubtful form, physicians have ever had a false knowlege, worse than ignorance.[142]

And in 1812 to Dr. John Crawford, he said, "for some forms of disease well known and well defined, she [i.e., medicine, as opposed to surgery] has found substances which will restore order to the human system; & it is to be hoped that observation & experience will add to their number. but a great mass of diseases remains undistinguished, & unknown, exposed to the random shot of the day. if on this chaos you can throw such a beam of light … you will … render great service to mankind."[143]

Unlike other founders, Jefferson strongly opposed just about every intrusive intervention, whether it be heroic depletive or stimulant treatment, and he himself avoided almost all forms of it throughout his life. As the letter to Munford reveals, he also was skeptical of pharmaceutical treatments available in his era. His disdain for indiscriminate, and often violent bleeding and purging extended not only to all of his family members but he forbade his plantation overseers from having it performed on slaves.[144] In 1773, Jefferson made an entry in his Garden Book under the title "articles for contracts with overseers," which expressed his antipathy towards venesection.[145] It read "never bleed a negro."[146] Many years later he informed another overseer that Dr. William Steptoe should only be called in sparingly for sick slaves. For "pleurisies, or other highly inflammatory fevers, intermitting fevers, dysenteries & Venereal cases, the doctors can give certain relief; and the sooner called to them the easier & more certain the cure. but in most other cases they oftener do more harm than good." Reflecting his belief in the healing powers of nature and limited intervention, in most cases he recommended treating the ill with "a lighter diet and kind attention" and to administer "a dose of salts," which "is salutary in almost all cases, & hurtful in none."[147]

Jefferson's rhetoric and actions both show that he firmly believed that the empirical pursuit of truth—knowledge to be gained and verified by direct observation, experimentation and careful reasoning—was the essence of scientific medicine.[148] He longed for the day when practitioners and medical educators would disavow the baggage of the past (e.g., repudiation of therapeutic specificity leading to indiscriminant treatment) and shift their service of the sick to a more enlightened approach to healing with an emphasis on biomedical research and the principle of specificity (i.e., creating a science of disease biology that includes knowledge of what works and why in specific cases), institutions of higher education with an unwavering public purpose (i.e., educating students as skeptics of reductive theories and inquisitors of facts), and specialization (fostering deeper, more specific, investigation) so that treatment can be matched to the differentiating features of the individual and their physical and social environment. Jefferson seemingly recognized the principle of specificity in medical therapeutics when he wrote a friend in 1815 that "Your practice of the cold bath thrice a week during the winter, and at the age of 70. is a bold one, which I should not, a priori, have pronounced salutary. but all theory must yield to experience, and every constitution has it's own laws."[149]

Intellectual Origins of Jefferson's Criticism of Medicine

Jefferson's criticism of his era's medical practices derived from his experience jin Paris, between 1784 and 1789, with a group of enlightened intellectuals called the *Idéologues*.[150] Initially through the good offices of Benjamin Franklin, Jefferson came to know and revere Anne-Catherine de Ligneville Helvétius (1720–1800). At her "delicious village" of Auteuil, he exchanged ideas with the leading Idéologues, many of whom he befriended, among them Abbé André Morellet (1727–1819), who was later to translate his *Notes on the State of Virginia*; the economist Jean Baptiste Say (1776–1832); the historian Constantin François Chasseboeuf Volney (1757–1820); the political theorist Antoine Louis Claude Destutt de Tracy (1754–1836); and physician-philosopher Pierre Jean Georges Cabanis (see Figure 7).[151] All of these men promoted empirical "substantiation of a philosophic position." They rejected fanciful literary arguments in the absence of "meaningful knowledge that entered the mind through the organs of the senses," evidence which was to be buttressed by experience and reason, and grounded in the laws of nature.[152] "By all accounts, Jefferson was an apostle of the Enlightenment. He fervently believed that a rational, evidence-based explanation existed for all medical phenomena and clearly felt that the healing profession was still in that long night of superstition, intolerance and misery.

While Jefferson was in France, in the middle- to late 1780s, many of the Idéologues undertook an elaborate revamping of traditional beliefs in religion, politics, economics, and medical science. Cabanis promoted a sweeping reorganization of medical education and practice and worked to reform hospital care and public-assistance programs; Philippe Pinel (1745 –1826) laid the foundations of modern psychiatry; and Marie François Xavier Bichat (1771-1802) made impressive contributions to organ-specific pathological anatomy.[153] After his return to the United States, Jefferson carried on considerable correspondence with several of the Idéologues, notably Cabanis, Destutt de Tracy, and Volney. And he helped to translate and facilitate publication of several of their original works, including Volney's *Les Ruines des Empires* (*The Ruins: or A Survey of the Revolutions of Empires*) and Destutt de Tracy's *Commentaire sur l'Esprit des Lois de Montesquieu* (*Commentary and Review of Montesquieu's Spirit of Laws*) and his *A Treatise on Political Economy.* Jefferson wanted these works placed in the hands of every reader in America. His editions were completed in 1801, 1811, and 1818, respectively, with his translation of Volney's work published anonymously due to the book's highly controversial religious content.[154]

Cabanis was one of the more vocal members of this group, and Jefferson respected him. An eminent neuroscientist, medical philosopher, and one of the founders of modern psychophysiology, Cabanis was a harsh critic of unsubstantiated medical theorization, and a pivotal player in the transcontinental promotion of intelligent empiricism.[155] In his book, *A Sketch of the Revolutions of Medical Science, and Views relating to its Reform*, he repeatedly emphasized the importance of observation, examination, and experimentation, and clear reasoning.[156] Cabanis sought to debunk all unproved medical theories prevalent at the end of the eighteenth century by correlating disease states with factual knowledge. Informed by the writings of Étienne Bonnet de Condillac (1715–80) and others, Cabanis urged practitioners to observe and not invent truth, arguing that in medicine, every thing, or nearly so, depended on *Coup d-oeil*, the acuteness of perception, and on an happy instinct—certainties are found to exist, in the sensations of the artist himself, rather than in the principles of the art. In another work he commented that "For studying the phenomena, which living bodies exhibit to our view, and for tracing their history with accuracy ... Observation, experience, and reasoning are sufficient for our purpose — We require nothing more."[157]

Cabanis believed that only a carefully performed empirical study of the physical aspects of man would allow an understanding of health and sickness, including the intertwined connection between flesh and spirit. Such research would also make it unnecessary to refer to revelation or ecclesiastical authority to explain medical phenomena.[158] Jefferson's interest in Cabanis's medical writings may have been aroused by his respect for scientific medical studies; their shared belief that a liberal political system probably ensured a high level of public health; a mutual interest in exploring the connections between health, disease and the sociopolitical environment of nations; and a desire to reform an anachronistic system of medical education.[159] Other Americans were to follow Jefferson's lead in adopting Cabanis' ideas and rhetoric and inveighing against the established medical profession. Most prominent in the mid-nineteenth century were Drs.Elisha Bartlett (dubbed the "Rhode Island Philosopher" by William Osler) and Jacob Bigelow of Harvard college.[160] For example, in 1844, when reviewing Rush's essays on the theory and practice of medicine, Bartlett wrote that "It may be safely said, I think, that in the whole vast compass of medical literature, there cannot be found an equal number of pages containing a greater amount and variety of utter nonsense and unqualified absurdity."[161] By the late 19th century, the condemnation of Rush was widely endorsed.[162]

Communication between Jefferson and Cabanis is well documented. They spoke frequently during their years together in Paris when Jefferson was the minister to France. They resumed their interactions beginning in 1802 and subsequently exchanged a number of letters and books.[163] Among the 6,500 books in Jefferson's private library, two noteworthy readings were by Cabanis—*Du Degré de Certitude de la Médecine* ("On the Degrees of Certainty in Medicine", 1803) and *Coup d'Oeil Révolutions et sur la Réforme de la Médecine* ("A Sketch of the Revolutions and Reform of Medicine", 1804).[164] These books and other writings by Cabanis combined a history of medicine with satirical attacks on the successive schemes proposed and implemented by most contemporary doctors. Cabanis ridiculed their theories and flawed hypotheses and laid out his own ideas emphasizing research and logic as the only way to improve the practice of medicine. Jefferson heartily approved, writing that "I am glad that M. Cabanis is engaged in writing on the reformation of medecine. it needs the hands of a reformer, and cannot be in better hands than his."[165] Both men genuinely respected the positive benefits of medicine while keenly appreciating its serious limitations. A comparison of the writings of Cabanis and Jefferson reveal a remarkable similarity in thought about the medical science of their time and the possibilities for future improvement.[166]

Views on Institutional Care and the "Echo of Inspiration"

Jefferson's criticism of medicine, as known and practiced in his time, extended to institutional care. In 1800, there were only two general hospitals in the United States—one in Philadelphia and another in New York—and these "novel institutions played only a minor role in the provision of medical care."[167] The great majority of inpatient beds were provided in almshouses, which also served as workhouses. Jefferson considered these institutions to be instruments of human degradation and indignity, altogether lacking in the ability to deliver individualized care.[168] Rather than being a place of healing, he viewed as a death trap "a general hospital, where the sick, the dying, and the dead are crammed together, in the same rooms, and often in the same beds."[169] Over the course of almost forty years, Jefferson was consistent in his criticism of hospital care, observing as late as 1824 that "It is poverty alone which peoples hospitals," and asking, "how many families in Richmond would send their husbands, wives, or children to a hospital, in sickness? to be attended by nurses hardened by habit against the feelings of pity, to lie in public rooms, harrassed by the cries and sufferings of disease under every form, alarmed by the groans of the dying, exposed as a corpse, to be lectured over by a clinical professor, to be crowded and handled by his students, to hear their case learnedly explained to them, its threatening symptoms developed, and its probable termination foreboded?"[170]

Like his friend of more than thirty years, Pierre Samuel Du Pont de Nemours, Jefferson favored dehospitalization of disease and poverty.[171]

In his *Notes on the State of Virginia*, he described the parish-relief system of his native state as the most effective, inexpensive, and compassionate scheme of self-help and medical assistance at home, and one that probably promised greater therapeutic success free from cross-infection. Both men believed that a natural environment combining domesticity with kind nursing not only fortified familial and social relationships, but also saved a much greater proportion of citizens from abuse. Removal of the sick or downtrodden to a hospital deprived the sick of a better chance of recovery through therapeutic ministrations of family and neighbors, while the vastly greater mortality of almshouse wards threatened permanent loss of income and the viability of the family itself.[172]

Jefferson's critical attitude towards hospital-based care in eighteenth-century America may have been partially shaped by his experience in Paris while serving as minister to France from 1785 to 1789. [H] He gained firsthand knowledge of the Hôtel-Dieu in Paris, an ancient municipal hospital with a deplorably high mortality rate—so high that it was known as "the gateway to death," "antechamber to the mortuary," and even as a "septic tank."[173] The care of the sick was simply appalling. The hospital held a crowded mass of 3,000 patients—four to six per bed—and mixed diseases in the same wards and even in the same beds.[174] Additionally, the unsafe environment—located in the most densely populated part of the city and a potential firetrap—provided insufficient and contaminated water to its unlucky inmates. The French Académie des Sciences recognized the Hôtel–Dieu as a source of contagion with its vitiated air and polluted city water, and took the lead in bringing about much-needed hospital reform. Owing largely to the efforts of three academy members—the Marquis de Condorcet, Pierre Samuel Du Pont de Nemours, and Pierre Jean Georges Cabanis,[175] all close friends of Jefferson—Louis XVI ordered the construction of four new hospitals—all of pavilion, or isolated ward, design, where patients could be segregated by disease and placed in separate beds,[176] and situated outside the city limits where there was less crowding, more healthy air and fresh water. Each held 1,200 patient beds organized in twelve symmetrically parallel pavilions aligned along a main axis—six on either side of an open garden, with a central chapel building at its head—connected by covered walkways for convalescing patients (see Figure 8).[177]

This new design promised superior ventilation, economy and efficiency of space, as well as cleanliness, privacy, and safety, while cutting down the risk of fire and contagion and reducing noise.[178] The pavilion design would become one of the Enlightenment's most important medical legacies and became the model for hospitals built all over Europe and America during the course of the nineteenth century.[179]

Many years later, when Jefferson began to sketch the buildings of his new university, he remembered the pavilion design of the Paris hospitals. As early as 1805, he had ruled out a single large building (like the old Hôtel-Dieu or the College of William and Mary) because such a design is "always ugly" and "exposed to the accident of fire, and bad in cases of infection."[180] In 1810, he termed his university design an "academical village"—referring to the healthiness of the countryside, free from the noise, disease and vice of large cities,[181] a design that "would afford that quiet retirement so friendly to study, and lessen dangers of fire, infection & tumult."[182] He envisaged an intergenerational community dispersed among many buildings, with separate "lodges" to house classrooms and professors, dormitory rooms for students, hotels for communal dining and a covered walkway "to give dry communications between all schools." All of the buildings would face onto a central grassy lawn, at the head of which would be the Rotunda that would serve as the library—the repository of wisdom, knowledge of the past, and ideas for the future.[183] In contrast to almost all colleges and universities of the time, Jefferson insisted that a library, not a church or chapel, be the focal point of the University of Virginia.[184]

As Figure 9, in the illustration galley shows, Jefferson's eventual architectural plan for the grounds of the University of Virginia is strikingly similar to the pavilion hospital design of the French Académie des Sciences in the 1780s, having not only the same symmetrical placement of neoclassical buildings, but also five symmetrical pavilions situated on either side of an open lawn, communicating by covered porches, with a dominating building (the Rotunda) at the central axis.[185] For a man so concerned with public health and enlightened thinking,– "what better health–inducing plan could Jefferson have come up with for his university than that of a modern, carefully planned hospital?"[186] Although the ground plan of Jefferson's academical village may have reflected "an echo of inspiration" from French hospital planning, as noted by Louis S. Greenbaum, the design of the individual structures that formed Jefferson's University of Virginia campus had very different origins.[187]

The Morally Honest and Humane Physician-Scientist

In his criticisms of the medical profession, Jefferson expressed a belief that physicians needed to move upwards on the scale of good. On a personal level, the medical practitioner had to be a moral individual, and on a theoretical level ethics had to govern medical epistemology. In Jefferson's view, a belief that know-how ought to be restrained by evidence was itself an ethical principle, a kind of ethics of knowledge.

In advocating for change in the behavior of those who were called to serve the sick and afflicted, he recognized that any beneficial transformation would depend, first and foremost, on the steadfast character and virtue of physicians, individually and collectively. His conception of a morally honest and humane healer included both cardinal and transcendent virtues. He commended the doctrines of Epicurus and his four cardinal virtues of prudence, temperance, fortitude (to meet and surmount difficulty, not to fly from them like cowards), and justice. In his correspondence, Jefferson developed a rhetoric of virtue that includes: honesty, truth telling, integrity, sincerity (avoiding harmful deceit and duplicity, thinking innocently and justly), authenticity, charity to and for all, benevolence, compassion, vigilance, perseverance, probity, gratitude, sound judgment, acting on principle, generosity and humility.[188] By steadfast character, Jefferson did not mean mere reputation or position that birth, wealth or "any adventitious aid from external circumstances" might give an individual, but the great aggregate of life, based upon fixed and conscientious principles and made up of deliberations that directed all "passions towards noble ends" and the steady pursuit "of what is right, turning neither to right nor left for the intrigues or popular delusions of the day."[189]

To Jefferson, medicine could be elevated to a rank amongst the exact sciences only by demonstrating to the public a willingness to change through a repudiation of speculation and hypothesis in favor of empirical evidence. This essential condition, if widely adopted in America, would advance medical science and practice, especially physiology and therapeutics, to a position of increased certainty, completeness, and consequent usefulness to society. Of all the branches of medical science, Jefferson seemed most interested in human physiology in health and disease, and a more rational basis for therapeutic action.[190] The novelty of the Parisian reform movement and its break with the norms of the ancient régime, especially intellectual despotism, captivated Jefferson. He was eager to help establish a new cultural ethos within the medical profession of the United States, believing that in a country forging a new social and political order, the symbolic value of the French medical revolution would serve a useful purpose. In the New World environment where principles of free thought and free speech were beginning to take hold, Jefferson hoped that medical men of courage would speak out against baseless theories and denounce Syndenhamism,

Boerhaavism, Cullenism, Brownism, and even Rushism. Jefferson seemed confident in the ability of American physicians to try new ideas, rejecting those that experience proved worthless or useless. He challenged them to assume an advocacy position on the science of medicine, calling for an improved epistemology grounded in experience and good judgment, one that was comprehensible and accessible to all citizens, including the common farmer, merchant, and others of modest or meager means. To accomplish this, physicians needed to free themselves of imprecise, confusing, or ambiguous language so that patients could more easily understand the scientific basis for all medical ministrations, and thus be in a better position to make informed choices about health care. Moreover, he sought from leaders in medicine an emphasis on preventive health measures, which to Jefferson offered far more reward than efforts to restore health when it was lost. He believed that all of these steps would improve health care, banish the evils of heroic drugging and bloodletting, and foster a healthier, more democratic and more authentically American society.

In pushing for reform, Jefferson suggested steps that pertained to the training and publicly accessible qualifications of those who presumed to cure the sick. The profession needed to rid itself of the common herd of charlatans and quacks and change a climate where mental cultivation, scientific evidence, and philanthropy weighed not a feather in the scale of reputation. It needed to create a self–regulating tradition based on a meritocracy and promote the idea that specialized knowledge, grounded in evidence and dispensed for the benefit of mankind, constituted a valid basis for professional distinction in American society. Long before the term was coined, and unlike most of his contemporaries, Jefferson favored a meritocracy or natural aristocracy based on talent, virtue, competence and commitment to public service rather than birth or wealth.[191] Indeed, Jefferson's philosophy worked to prod medical practitioners to adopt basic science, in anatomy, physiology, pathology and chemistry, and applied learning from real-world experience as the dominant forms of knowledge, and to administer social justice in healing tactics based on reason rather than faith and revealed religion. Such standards, moreover, were not to be limited to a hermetic order of medical specialists but were to be visible to the lay public, so that they could know and trust the qualifications of those presuming to treat them.

Jefferson sought to reshape therapeutic thought and practice in America. Most physicians, regardless of their educational backgrounds or professional reputation, were ignorant of the modus operandi of drug actions.[192] Jefferson, however, did not accept the prevailing notion that observation of the effect of various remedies on symptoms was, by itself, a sufficient and proper guide to therapeutic action. More was required. Medical therapeutics, like every other useful science, must rest on three pillars: expert knowledge, scientific proof and ethics. The first pillar required an intimate knowledge of human physiology in health and disease, and, when a physiological process became disordered, an understanding of what was likely to occur if recovery was left to nature alone. By knowing the physiognomy of a disease when allowed to run its own course, the scientifically minded physician can, without risk of error, begin to estimate the value of different medications which have been employed, whether, for example, the remedy caused no harm, reversed the deviant physiology and cutshort the duration of the disease.

The second pillar required extensive observations of the effect of a specific intervention on the natural course of disease. The research had to be exacting and include a numerical method that was untainted by prejudices, grounded in the rules of experimentation and valid reasoning, and informed by knowledge of discoveries already made. In 1823, he postulated as a necessary condition to establish truth that individual findings must be examined "seriatim and publically" in light of the totality of knowledge, which requires patience and one's "own judgement" that are "unbiased by party views and personal favor or disfavor."[193]

Attention to the third pillar was necessary because it showed the physician those virtues that must remain with him until his death and support and complete the first two pillars. Underlying an allegiance to these three pillars is a question of the judicial principle "cui bono," that is, "who benefits?" The morally honest and humane physician was called to serve and benefit patients, first and foremost, and not intrude on their health nor interrupt the body's normal restorative power with ruinous interventions.

While criticizing the theory and practice of clinical medicine in the early ninetenth century, Jefferson was at the same time redefining the scope of healthcare in the United States, in effect expanding the remit of what medicine should accomplish at the individual and community level. His disdain for heroic unproven therapies stemmed not from an antipathy to treatment in general, but from the realization that most techniques applied by physicians were not up to rigorous scientific standards based on repeated testing.[194] Jefferson articulated his negative judgments seemingly without concern that they might cost him the connections he enjoyed with many prominent physicians, even a longtime and respected friend like Benjamin Rush. In terms of personal care, Jefferson was amenable, when necessary, to engaging a physician, but always ready to exercise his right of final refusal when dealing with doctors and their treatments.[195] In cases where techniques met Enlightenment standards of proof, such as vaccination, Jefferson not only endorsed treatments but promoted them with all the means at his disposal.

With remarkable acuity, Jefferson looked beyond the shortcomings of clinical medicine and emphasized aspects of medical care that would not become widespread until much later. At a personal and community level, he recognized the benefit of good health habits as a means of preventing disease, a position, at once medical and economic. Forestalling a disease presented a simpler challenge than curing it. In effect, he added a new charge to the province of healthcare: sustaining human well–being as opposed to treating illness. This shift was most pronounced in his political support of public–health initiatives, where Jefferson realized that psychological and mental equilibrium could be nurtured among citizens, thus promoting a sounder mind in many. For example, he understood that public building and space design could enhance the health of city dwellers. Even in the absence of a germ theory of disease, Jefferson saw that the health of a residential populace was safeguarded by regulating meat sales and installing infrastructure that, for instance, drained standing water and curbed the influx of contaminants into the environment. For persons unfortunate enough to be struck by disease, Jefferson used his political leverage to support facilities for merchant seamen, a policy that should be seen in light of his skeptical view of hospitalization.

Jefferson's attacks on intrusive and ineffective medical treatments were recorded largely in his correspondence and for the most part were carried on as a private conversation among an elite. By contrast, his numerous initiatives in promoting medical advances and public health were open and public. The founding of the University of Virginia, a project that occupied his final years, offered an opportunity to connect his privately expressed reservations about medicine with an institution that deliberately sought a profile in the public arena of science. In developing the University, Jefferson saw that his scientific ideals could be wielded not only as tools for criticizing physicians but as precepts for educating them, thereby altering the way medical education and medicine as a discipline were understood and, to some degree, practiced. This forms the subject of the next chapter.

Chapter 3

FOUNDING OF THE MEDICAL DEPARTMENT: IMPORTANCE OF PLACE, PURPOSE, AND PEOPLE

This institution will be based on the illimitable freedom of the human mind. for here we are not afraid to follow truth wherever it may lead, nor to tolerate any error so long as reason is left free to combat it.

Thomas Jefferson to William Roscoe, 27 December 1820[1]

THIS CHAPTER will explore how Jefferson the scientist became Jefferson the educator par excellence, as he spearheaded the founding of the University of Virginia, the beginning of which was intertwined intellectually and organizationally with the establishment of the University's medical department. The chapter will show how the University as a whole and the medical department in particular were not only realizations of Jefferson's scientific values and practices but also the result of organizational principles inspired by his lifelong observation of the approaches and offerings of universities in Europe and the United States.

The requirements of the curriculum, the selection of the faculty, and the setting of training standards not just for medicine but for all subject areas were supervised, and, in a sense, imposed by Jefferson and led to a far more rigorous concept of medical education than any found in America at the time. This chapter will also show that the advances in medical education at the University of Virginia stemmed less from deliberate interventions in the training of physicians and more from Jefferson's radically innovative changes to the nature and structure of a university. Officially chartered by the Virginia General Assembly on January 25, 1819, the University of Virginia, comprising eight distinct but highly integrated academic departments, opened its doors on March 7, 1825, after decades of planning by Jefferson.[2] A Literary Fund, which had been created by the state legislature in 1810, provided an annual sum of $15,000 for the establishment and support of the university.[3] Jefferson hoped for and obtained a small nonsectarian board of governors, a body of enlightened "gentlemen of distinguished worth and information" who would establish and enforce uniform standards for all eight schools. The first Board of Visitors, all appointed by then–governor James P. Preston, included three former or sitting presidents of the United States — Thomas Jefferson as rector, James Madison and James Monroe, as well as General John Hartwell Cocke and two state legislators, Joseph Carrington Cabell and David Watson.[4]

The Massachusetts-born historian Herbert Baxter Adams has termed the founding of the University of Virginia "the noblest work of Jefferson's life."[5] Others have said of the University, that it "quickly became the most admired institution of higher education in the southern states, and so remained throughout the nineteenth century," with innovations that included: implementation of university standards of instruction and scholarship; a constitutional government in academic form; a faculty composed mainly of professors brought over from Europe, complete rejection of any organized religion or theological dogma, a curriculum divided into separate schools, departmentally organized and uniquely specialized; and a novel elective system.[6] And of the Medical School, the historian William Norwood said, "That the Medical Department of the University of Virginia was a country school, characterized by deficient anatomical and clinical facilities, is unquestioned, but its plan of organization and curriculum lifted it to a level attained by few [if any] of its contemporaries."[7]

Preparation, Allies, and Founder's Influence

In correspondence spanning four decades, Jefferson identified deficiencies in the Colleges of Philadelphia, New Jersey (later Princeton University), and William and Mary; King's College (Columbia); Yale; and most big-city institutions, as well as American medical schools and several long–established European universities such as Oxford, Cambridge, and the Sorbonne. His reasons included outdated curricular content, insufficient time for reflective learning, limited choices of study, failure to comprehend the expanse of the arts and sciences and extend to the utmost boundaries of human knowledge, subject–specific teaching methods that were altogether inadequate, lack of academic freedom for professors and students due to domination by clergy who taught both political and religious "heresies," and ill–advised urban locations that were "sinks of voluntary misery" and "a Cloacina of all the depravities of human nature." Four institutions that Jefferson did hold in high esteem were the University of Edinburgh, the Institut de France, the College of Geneva, and the University of Göttingen. As early as 1779, Jefferson was exhibiting an interest in establishing an institute for liberal education in the vicinity of his own home.[8] Thereafter, he assiduously examined "the organization of the best seminaries" wherever they might be found, as well as a wide variety of educational proposals and theories of many "wise and learned men" in America and Europe.[9] From this "survey of the general field of science," and after many years of mature reflection, Jefferson refined his conception of the proper place and purpose of higher education, and "marked out the portion" that his university would occupy.[10] At the same time Jefferson was immersing himself in the intellectual life of the French Enlightenment and evolving his own concepts of science, he was empirically investigating institutions of higher education, so that it could be said his exploration of the proper way to teach science was itself the subject of his personal scientific inquiry.

Jefferson's educational philosophy was arguably more progressive and comprehensive than any conventional model in early–19th–century America.[11] It emphasized a unique organizational and operational construct in an exceptional architectural setting that tied learning and domesticity together; an unambiguous attention to rigorous academic instruction and scholarship and a philosophical pragmatism linking educational purpose to social action in a democracy; and the importance of academic autonomy and pedagogical process. In his long struggle to establish an institution of superior purpose, Jefferson repeatedly stated his aspiration that the University of Virginia would be far more impressive than just another petty academy, an institution that would become "the future bulwark of the human mind in this hemisphere," and a force that might resolve social ills, and thereby improve American prosperity.[12] To accomplish this, Jefferson gave little indulgence to precedent, especially if wrapped in themes of conformity and conservatism. In establishing the University of Virginia, the founding father considered venerable customs only when esteemed worthy of retention.[13] In conceiving the University, he borrowed from European models but was conscious of a need for novelty, in the context of a young nation that had not, in his opinion, achieved an intellectually satisfying solution to higher education.

Equally significant was Jefferson's "remarkable ability to command the services of faithful lieutenants and supporters, to fill them with the zeal of crusaders and the devotion of fanatics, and to hold them to their tasks through years of disappointment and defeat."[14] In his exhortations, he pleaded with them to stay the course in a cause for which he himself would willingly "die in the last ditch," and always to "be bold in the pursuit of knolege, never fearing to follow truth and reason to whatever results they led, & bearding every authority which stood in their way."[15]

Of all his allies, perhaps the most notable was Joseph Carrington Cabell (1778–1856) (see Figure 10). The scion of a prominent Virginia family, Cabell was educated at Hampden-Sydney, William and Mary, and several prestigious European universities.[16] He met Jefferson for the first time in 1806, quickly became attached to his educational philosophy, and soon thereafter embarked on an illustrious career in the Virginia legislature—where he became Jefferson's principal spokesman in Richmond and a critically important pillar of support in helping Jefferson overcome the criticism of his plan to establish the University of Virginia. The many factions who opposed Jefferson's efforts included: friends of the College of William and Mary, several religious denominations which railed that Jefferson was establishing a school for the purpose of promulgating infidelity, politicians who opposed almost anything connected with Jefferson, and others who believed the plan for the University was far too extravagant. Seeking to mute the hostility of political opponents, Jefferson was careful to disguise his labors and show his opponents as little of his logic and methodology as possible. Despite being the great exponent of democracy and majority rule, Jefferson was not above resorting to behind-the-scenes maneuvering to ensure that the University of Virginia would be located in Charlottesville.[17]

Jefferson had his hand in every essential part of the establishment of the University of Virginia. Unlike most philanthropists who bestowed their benefactions on other seats of higher learning in 19th–century America, Jefferson was not content to impart in a "general way only ... the trends and color of certain principles" to the aims of his university, and to its method of administration and instruction. As Philip A. Bruce points out, Jefferson did far more, and "He was not merely the father of it [the University] in the spiritual and intellectual sense: he was the father of it in a corporeal sense also."[18] He arranged the purchase of the 43.75–acre site for the university and surveyed its boundaries.[19] He meticulously planned the grounds and buildings and superintended the construction, drawing heavily on his experience abroad.[20] He contributed his own monies at a time when he was seriously burdened with debt, and he "wrung funds from a niggardly [stingy] legislature while he sought even the smallest economy in the cost of bricks."[21] Until its completion in 1825, Jefferson rode almost every day on horseback to watch the work of construction and when he could not ride he sat on his mountaintop terrace with a telescope to see the building grow.[22] The course of study, the plan of organization, rules for admission, graduation, and government were all products of his work, as was the nomination of faculty members, an important step, as we shall see, for the medical school. Moreover, Jefferson chose many of the textbooks, formed the library, and established a standard of participatory democracy for the faculty and of self–discipline built on integrity for the students. For these reasons, "no one thinks of Jefferson [merely] as the founder of the University of Virginia. He called himself its father. Scarcely an institution exists which can so aptly be described, in the words of Emerson as 'the lengthened shadow of one man.'"[23]

Jefferson envisioned the University of Virginia as a new model for American higher education, built "on a reformed plan,"[24] where "all the branches of science deemed useful at this day, shall be taught in their highest degree[25] and where future leaders would explore and expose "every subject susceptible of it's contemplation."[26] When he endowed the University with his uniquely purposeful ideology, in rural central Virginia, Jefferson declared it to be "the last of my mortal cares, and the last act of service I can render my country."[27]

Instruction in medicine was to reflect the same pedagogical priorities that governed the University as a whole. Jefferson, the ardent disciple of the Enlightenment ideals of secularism, useful knowledge and never–ending improvement, referred to medicine as "the most important of all" branches of science, being "that to which we commit the care of health & life."[28] In a letter to Dr. Thomas Cooper, Jefferson wrote that "no knolege can be more satisfactory to a man than that of his own frame, it's parts, their functions & actions."[29] To others, he said that "Health is the first requisite after morality" and wrote of "health, without which there is no happiness. An attention to health, then, should take the place of every other object."[30] By including medical education in the curriculum and general education of the University of Virginia, Jefferson demonstrated considerable foresight and wisdom. His goal in offering medical courses at the University of Virginia was not only to produce more professionally competent physicians but also to provide educated laymen with a basic understanding of contemporary medicine.[31] Unlike other medical schools of Jefferson's era, the School of Medicine in Charlottesville was an integral part of the University from its inception. It not only provided a secure home for the full–time pursuit of medical scholarship, but it fostered fluid intellectual and cultural exchange among other academic disciplines, and a sense of balance.[32]

In its structure and curriculum, the university Jefferson envisioned was more akin to modern graduate and professional schools than to the more limited "general" collegiate institutions of the day, and for this reason the University of Virginia did not offer baccalaureate degrees until long after his death.[33] The "honorary distinctions" established by the visitors in October 1824 consisted of three levels; (1) Books, to be awarded to those of the lowest grade deserving commendation; (2) Medals, to be given to the second tier of honored students; and (3) Diplomas for the highest achievers, divided in turn into "Graduate," signifying that a student had mastered an entire school's curriculum, and the highest honor, the coveted doctorate of medicine.[34] In 1831, a "Master of Arts" was added as a special award in recognition of students who had obtained graduate diplomas in five different schools—ancient languages, mathematics, natural philosophy (physics and astronomy), chemistry, and moral philosophy.[35]

Vision of Medical Education

Medical education was a special but not exceptional subject at the University of Virginia. As will be shown in the following sections, Jefferson's plan advocated the purest, most demanding academic model for medical education, a field with a particular socially responsible agenda, replete with students willing to meet the demands of a long and arduous curriculum that emphasized the preclinical sciences and proof of learning by rigorous examination, and a full-time salaried faculty, all scholars of the first order, who maintained an unequivocal and conscientious commitment to the discovery, aggregation and dissemination of medical knowledge for public benefit.[36]

Jefferson realized that medical teaching and scholarship was much better organized and conducted in European schools, especially in London, Edinburgh, Paris and Gottingen, than in America, but he surmised that the educational and professional problems peculiar to the special conditions of the new republic of America would not be satisfactorily solved by the simple transplantation of a foreign system to the United States.[37]

Jefferson's solution was to establish a university founded on principles that were the result of his analyses of teaching at other schools, as well as the fruits of philosophical and ethical thinking. These original concepts permeated all aspects of the new university, from the governance, curriculum, and graduation requirements to architecture and faculty compensation.

The Teaching of Science and Medicine Integrated into the University

First and foremost, Jefferson addressed the educational environment and chose to create a residential medical department that was an integral part of a genuine University from its inception. He regarded the environment for learning as critically important. Jefferson deplored the inadequacy of the apprenticeship and independent "proprietary medical school" models in America. He seemed to recognize that even "the best" medical schools in America (e.g., those loosely aligned with the University of Pennsylvania, Harvard, and Yale), had no credible relationship with their colleges except in using the authority granted to them to award medical and law degrees. Moreover, throughout the eighteenth and most of the nineteenth century in America, the public exercised virtually no control over the standards of medical training or practice. Medical schools were physically separate and virtually autonomous—fundamentally, "closed corporations" administered and controlled entirely by the physician owners, a situation akin to *"an imperium in imperio"* (an empire within an empire) with college and university functionaries assuming little or no jurisdiction over such matters as the medical–school curriculum, qualifications and instructional rigor of the teachers, proof of learning, or the establishment and collection of fees. Medical schools were "essentially private ventures, money–making in spirit and object."[38] And unlike the prevailing models of American medical education, Jefferson's university-based school would have a publicly advantageous agenda that was responsive to social needs.

Unlike other American medical schools, all branches of useful knowledge were united at the University of Virginia, where interdisciplinary curricular arrangements were encouraged, and to an extent required, giving student matriculates ample opportunity to become broadly educated in multiple fields of knowledge, and be better prepared for the community they would one day serve. The medical curriculum was one of several domains of knowledge in a setting where students were expected to explore and connect insights from different disciplines. According to Paul Barringer, Jefferson believed "the various branches [of knowledge], when opposed, all tend to emulate, illustrate and adorn each other … and when separated, a small part of the vital spirit [free–flowing inquiry leading to advance] goes with the dismembered part."[39] Far from being an inanimate thing, Jefferson saw learning as a living body whose different members belong together, as parts of a coordinated whole. The various academic branches and the elements of a finished education "cannot be quartered with the expectation that they will live" and flourish. Delving into subjects other than one's own was mandated. All students at the University were encouraged to attend courses in three or more schools and develop broad proficiency in different fields. To facilitate this, lectures in the different schools were purposely scheduled at different times, and tuition fees were discounted for students attending more than one school.[40]

Architecture as a conduit for intellectual exchange

The University's architecture reflected the interdisciplinary aspirations of the institution as a whole. When designing and arranging the buildings of his University, Jefferson proposed a series of pavilions (see Figure 11), one for each of the eight original academic departments that included Anatomy and Medicine, Natural History, Natural Philosophy, Mathematics, Law, Moral Philosophy, Ancient Languages, and Modern Languages. No fewer than fifty-eight subjects were to be taught.[41] All pavilions would have a spacious hall on the first floor for classroom activity, an office for the professor to be used for student counseling and personal scholarship, and chambers above for the faculty member and his family. Joining these pavilions would be a series of dormitory rooms for students, opening onto "a covered way to give a dry communication between all the schools." Room assignments were arranged so that students of a particular school would be located adjacent to their professor's pavilion, with "the whole of these arranged around an open square of grass & trees," which "would make it, what it should be in fact, an academical village" that "would afford that quiet retirement so friendly to study," be "more promotive" to "health, to study, to manners, morals & order." [42] As part of his idea of a university village, containing smaller communities of students, Jefferson's plan included six dining halls, which he called hotels. These were located behind the pavilions, along with additional dormitories."[42]

Jefferson recognized that much of the best medical training required exercises in both didactic and experiential learning that certain competencies could be taught in the classroom while others, such as integrity, compassion and empathy, and community consensus might best be learned in the culture outside the classroom. Faculty were expected to combine pedagogical, disciplinary, and paternal functions in their role as guardians of the students with whom they lived.[43] Jefferson intuited that the culture of a university encompasses what is today referred to as a hidden curriculum, present in all subject areas including medicine. At the University of Virginia, this hidden curriculum, which included the modeling of humanistic behavior, was also promoted by the layout of the academical village, where professors and students were channeled to social intercourse, from which a sense of common purpose might emerge. Where other contemporary medical schools provided little or no personal contact between student and teacher, Jefferson's unusual design linked learning and domesticity through the juxtaposition of pavilions for professors and adjacent dormitories for students that enabled near constant intermingling between teachers and pupils from all academic disciplines.[44] The architecture of the university transferred to academia a concept Jefferson had promoted for public health, namely that careful construction of the built environment could positively affect behavior and psychology.

Centrality of the Library

In its day the library of the University of Virginia was unique among institutions of higher education in its location, scope and cost, purpose, and organization. Unlike other colleges and universities, this was an integral part of the original organic plan for the institution from its inception, constituted to include a large and expensive collection that provided authoritative coverage in all specialized academic departments.[45] Jefferson realized that a great library, if properly organized and maintained to serve the needs of each academic department, was an indispensable element of university education. With holdings available to all, such a collection was not just one intellectual accoutrement among many at the University, but physically and symbolically its centerpiece. By locating it in the Rotunda, the tallest structure and central edifice in his academical village, Jefferson placed knowledge and reason at the center and heart of an institution he founded and grounded in "the illimitable freedom of the human mind."[46] To plumb the depth of every branch of science, students needed to do more than pay attention to lessons learned in the classroom; they must also be taught how to read and reflect on the best, most authoritative works of erudition, past and present, from every credible source. Unfortunately, this particular pedagogical practice of teaching students the tactics of lifelong education by doing library research was not embraced by many, if any, of the other American medical schools of the early 19th century, nor was much emphasis placed on establishing their own libraries.[47] The few medical libraries that existed were usually privately owned by hospitals, medical societies or individual physicians, and acquisitions were almost never by deliberate purchase of specific titles of merit. Rather, the collections were built by gift, by swapping duplicates, or by bulk purchase of used books. Cataloguing was minimal. Because little effort was expended to facilitate access and retrievability, books were in effect just "warehoused."[48] The University encouraged library use and the borrowing of books by students, albeit with some restrictions, including those in the medical school. In chapter 5, it will be shown just how extensively the library was used by students of medicine.

Medical Education Subject to University–Wide Jurisdiction

All academic departments at the university were subjected to the same polity and supervision. To ensure unity of purpose, fiscal integrity and educational quality, Jefferson insisted on university–wide oversight of all administrative affairs in each and every department. At the University of Virginia, the medical department was neither separate nor autonomous. Like all other academic departments, it was subordinate to the guidance and direction of a secular Board of Visitors whose members were duly appointed by the Governor and confirmed by the Virginia Senate and House of Delegates. The statutes of 1818–1819, of which Jefferson was the principle author, clearly show the supremacy of the Board in matters of organization, governance, property rights and preservation of all University assets, curricular content and rigor, the hiring and removal of professors, as well as all other agents of the University, the determination of salary ranges and other forms of compensation for all faculty ranks, the fixing of tuition charges, other fees and room rentals, establishing and regulating criteria for the public examination of students, the creation and awarding of degrees, and for the preparation and submission of annual reports and such budget request as might be required by the appropriate state agency.[49] Moreover, as rector of the University in its early years, Jefferson promoted a principle of informed stewardship that was unique for the time inasmuch as the same standard was applied across all departments, including the medical school. The 1819 statute creating the university required that Board members "once in every year at least visit the sd University, enquire into the proceedings and practices thereat, examine the progress of the students, and give to those who excel in any branch of science there taught such honorary marks and testimonies of approbation as may encorage & excite to industry and emulation."[50] This particular duty was designed to insure that the Visitors embraced their fiduciary responsibility to assess first–hand the fidelity of the professors and students, and truthfully disclose their findings in the annual report to the Virginia legislature.[51] The theory behind this enactment was that the members of the governing board were to confer with the teachers on pedagogical practices, attend classes and public examinations, give advice when necessary and show an intelligent interest in the day–to–day workings of the educational system.

Location of the University

The University was deliberately located in a nonurban area, which meant that physician training there occurred closer to the frontier of early nineteenth-century America than to its major cities. Jefferson claimed that situating the university in a decidedly non–cosmopolitan and putatively healthier area of Virginia would have many advantages.[52] In terms of the study of medicine, this was not a popular decision among other powerful Virginians who wanted the medical school in Richmond.[53] In establishing the University of Virginia in Charlottesville, Jefferson had to overcome multiple arguments which he viewed as driven by "ignorance, malice, egoism, fanaticism, religious, political & local perversities."[54] In logic expressed both by himself and his loyal friend and political ally, Joseph Cabell, Jefferson cogently laid out a belief that teaching, mentoring and the creation of publishable works of erudition were likely to flourish best in a small town environment, where the medical professors, removed from the commercialism of city life [meaning the financial lure of unfettered private practice] taught their subjects as did Latin professors and others.[55] In short, rural Charlottesville would allow professors to be scholars and devote themselves to the personal and professional growth of their students.[56]

In establishing the first university–based model for medical education in America, Jefferson promoted the concept that pedagogical methods and instructional rigor in the healing arts must be congruent with all other scientific disciplines, a position that did not become generally accepted for decades.[57] He was eager to create a unifying culture of professionalism and expertise across all academic disciplines. At the University of Virginia, the process of medical discovery and the dissemination of its useful products to students and the public at large would result not from chance, but from the expression of choices dictated by ideals of intellectual excellence. The starting point for research at this level was a faculty different from many others of the time.

Full-Time Professional Scholars

Throughout most of the nineteeth century, medical schools relied on part-time teachers. The vast majority of these practitioner-teachers felt little or no responsibility to conduct original research, advance the frontier of medical knowledge, and publicly disseminate their scientific findings for the good of the people. For his University, Jefferson insisted on a *full–time* faculty, which, when applied to medical education, was a new idea. Jefferson envisioned a professorate that encompassed persons who were publicly recognized for their intellectual accomplishments. This too was novel for American medical education as it automatically excluded physicians whose "credentials" consisted of a thriving practice and the capacity to lecture or administer apprenticeships on the side.[58]

No educator in America realized more fully than Jefferson that his oft–repeated ambition that his would be a university "in which all the branches of science useful to us, and at this day, should be taught in their highest degree," could be fulfilled only by the work of a superior faculty.[59] He emphasized that "we mean to accept for our institution no person of secondary grade in his science, if there be one of the first on either side of the Atlantic, who can be tempted to come to us," and that they would accept "either the ablest which America or Europe can furnish, or none at all." By April 1824, the Visitors had concluded "that to obtain Professors of the first order of science in their respective lines, they must resort principally to Europe." For every faculty appointment, Jefferson said, "The only question therefore we can ever ask ourselves, as to any candidate, will be, Is he the most highly qualified?" If "motives of favoritism and Nepotism" were allowed, they could not hope to "give our institution splendor and preeminence over all it's sister seminaries. " Jefferson thought that cronyism had led to the relative decline of the University of Pennsylvania and the University of Edinburgh.[60]

At the University of Virginia, the competency requirements for all professors, medical and nonmedical, were the same and went well beyond eminence in their respective fields of learning.[61] To Jefferson, the essential qualifications included: a broad education and culture combined with deep knowledge of one's specialty; an ability to teach the specialty effectively; industry and integrity in one's field of scholarship; and an unwavering commitment to innovation, collaboration, and service to others. Jefferson then imposed other considerations when he added that "we have determined to recieve no one who is not … of sober and correct habits and morals, harmonising tempers, talents for communication E^{t}c,"[62] and that "a man is not qualified for a Professor, knowing nothing but merely his own profession. he should be otherwise well educated as to the sciences generally; able to converse understandingly with the scientific men with whom he is associated, and to assist in the councils of the Faculty, on any subject of science on which they may have occasion to deliberate."[63] All of this should be done with "an accomodating and peaceable temper."[64] On the latter, Jefferson seemed to realize that petty squabbles and acrimonious feuds within and between departmental faculties, regrettably commonplace in 19th–century medicine, must be avoided if scientific advance and educational reform at his University were to be accomplished. The bar for being a University of Virginia professor was set perhaps higher than at any time thereafter, since it included exemplary personal moral ideals, knowledge in fields outside one's specialization, and a good measure of urbanity when dealing with colleagues and students.

Another aspiration Jefferson had for the University of Virginia was to create a "natural aristocracy of virtue and talent" – a professional class of socially aware men who, because its members had pursued learning to the highest level, might be entrusted with the highest offices and responsibilities in society.[65] These men, whom he considered "the most precious gift of nature,"[66] should promote public health, exert moral leadership locally and nationally, advance the importance of professional self–regulation, and help create reform coalitions and build practical consensus among otherwise competing groups. Jefferson hoped that those who chose careers in academic medicine would improve the health of Americans by fostering innovation in medical education that would better align the knowledge, skills and cultural ethos of practitioners with the needs and expectations of the public.

Jefferson promoted the concept of total devotion to academic life by establishing the first full-time salaried professorship of medicine in America.[67] He had no interest in part-time faculty or the so-called practitioner-teacher model common to all other medical schools at the time. In order to assure that faculty at the University of Virginia had adequate time to fulfill their academic responsibilities, Jefferson required that medical professors be restricted from the business of clinical practice, that they "follow no other calling." In his words, "The collegiate duties of a professor, if discharged conscientiously, with industry & zeal," were "sufficient to engross all his hours of business," and therefore, "he shall engage in no other pursuits of emolument unconnected with the service of the Univ[ty] without the consent of the visitors."[68] The overriding purpose of this innovation was to create a new breed of academically minded educators in America, who sought intellectual distinction rather than just monetary reward.[69] This required a policy that guaranteed a "living salary" and rent–free quarters for all professors.[70] Moreover, by limiting the portion of student fees that accrued to the professors, the School of Medicine could counteract the practice, common to other schools for many years to come, of admitting questionably qualified students to didactic lectures just to swell the teachers' income through ticketed attendance fees, or of graduating weak candidates to insure receipt of the graduating fees. A full-time salaried academic staff, first instituted at Virginia, is now widely regarded as a prerequisite for accreditation by national licensing agencies.[71]

Length and Pace of Academic Terms

Enrollment at Virginia entailed a commitment of considerable time. As with other Jeffersonian concepts, extended academic sessions represented a significant change for medical education, more than doubling the duration of instruction for aspiring physicians.[72] Jefferson boldly rejected tradition and made the length of each academic session the same as those of all other University departments. In the early years, terms of instruction were set at 10½ months with a mere six weeks off for vacation. Each session began on February 1 and concluded on December 14. At most other contemporary medical schools in America, including the University of Pennsylvania, the College of Physicians and Surgeons (later part of Columbia University), Harvard, Dartmouth, Yale and the University of Maryland, classroom instruction commenced in November and concluded in February or March of the following year, a total of only three or four months. These dates have customarily been attributed to a desire to avoid conflicts with seedtime and harvest and the comparative ease of preserving cadavers in the winter. Despite some lengthening by mid-century, the vast majority of American medical schools still had terms no longer than eighteen weeks. Virginia's ten months were still the longest, only approached by Michigan at seven months.[73]

Unlike most educators of the time, Jefferson believed that all students, regardless of their field of study, needed abundant time to review and assimilate material imparted by lecture, to engage in private reading and laboratory work, to buttress their understanding through dialogue and debate with peers and professors within and outside their academic school, and for physical exercise.[74] In relating the 10+ month semesters to medical education, Jefferson asserted that "time & experience as well as science are necessary to make a skilful physician," implying that if learners are pushed too hard, not giving them time for every step, they regress to a state of confused tumult.[75] In another passage that illustrates his appreciation of the irreducible element of time for the student to absorb knowledge and learn how best to apply it for the benefit of mankind, Jefferson wrote that "as far as I am acquainted with the colleges and academies of the U.S. … I have found their method of instruction very superficial & imperfect, carrying their pupils over the ground like racehorses, to please their parents and draw custom to their school." He contrasted this with William & Mary in his youth, where "whatever they learned, they learned thoroughly, and the principles in which it was founded.[76]

In the early years of the University of Virginia, the medical school offered only six lectures a week, two apiece on Tuesday, Thursday and Saturday, each about ninety minutes long. The plan was designed to give students ample time to absorb the information conveyed orally."[77] In the University catalogues of the 1830s, this lecture schedule was prominently featured and held to be a distinct advantage over the plan of large city schools, where attendance at six or seven lectures in rapid succession, every day, resulted in "confusion of thought and fatigue of mind."[78]

Foundational Learning in Basic Science

Jefferson was arguably one of the first Americans to understand the importance of what would today be called pre-clinical training in the basic medical sciences, meaning scientific courses in anatomy, human physiology in health and disease, chemistry, pathology and pharmacology (often called materia medica and pharmacy), should precede the more applied study of the practice of medicine and surgery. He believed that the primary function of a university-based medical department was to provide, through formal instruction, a broad and thorough foundation of medicine, which involved an intimate knowledge of the human body and an understanding of the effects of various climates, medicinal substances, and other interventions or extenuating factors on health and disease.[79] Jefferson freely conceded the value of practical experience but thought it an unprofitable use of time for first- and even some second-year students. Only when they were well versed in the principles of scientific inquiry and "basic" knowledge, a task that required a minimum of 1 to 2 years of intensive study, were students ready to benefit fully from clinical instruction. This policy of instructing students in the fundamental branches of medical science before directing them to its practical application was an innovation not followed in many other schools of the time.

Since there was neither a hospital in Charlottesville, nor a desire to build one, nor much opportunity for students to observe sickness at the domestic bedside, Jefferson anticipated that the young medical graduates of the University of Virginia would have to find their own ways of gaining advanced practical experience before they could reasonably expect to build a clientele of patients willing to pay for a doctor's services. He regarded this form of postgraduate professional development, even for physicians bound for rural practice, as a necessary step to ensure competent patient care.[80] He wrote in one of his last letters, "consider that we do not expect our schools [at the University of Virginia] to turn out their Alumni already enthroned on the pinnacles of their respective sciences; but only so far advanced in each as to be able to pursue them by themselves and to become Newtons and Laplaces by energies and perseverances to be continued thro' life."[81] This passage suggests that in Jefferson's mind, learning to heal was indeed a lifelong process that only begins with what one is taught in medical school. Jefferson did recognize the deficient opportunities for clinical training at his university and suggested a solution when he wrote,

> I have always had Norfork in view for this purpose. the climate, and Pontine country around Norfolk render it truly sickly in itself. it is moreover the rendezvous not only of the shipping of commence, but of the vessels of the public navy. The U.S. have there a hospital already established, and supplied with subjects from these local circumstances. I had thought, and have mentioned to yourself and our colleagues, that when our Medical school has got well under way, we should propose to the federal government the association with that establishment, and at our own expense, of the Clinical branch of our Medical school, so that our Students, after qualifying themselves with the other branches of the Science here, might complete their course of preparation by attending clinical lectures for 6. or 12. months at Norfolk.[82]

As previously described, Jefferson was familiar with the marine hospital system in his state and elsewhere, and he recognized its potential for postgraduate teaching.[83] Jefferson appointed Dr. Benjamin Waterhouse director of Boston's Marine Hospital, and during his tenure he "established a system of student internships and in effect turned the Boston Marine Hospital into one of the country's first teaching hospitals."[84]

At a time when physiology received little or no attention at American medical colleges, Jefferson believed it to be the linchpin of medical science, and he took steps to ensure that the discipline would be central to his school's medical curriculum.[85] A premium would be placed on the teaching of physiology as an ascendant science, worthy of concentrated study and advancement through research. The subject Chair would be expected to pay attention to the organ–specific branches of physiology, and his lectures would focus on the most current, scientifically sound physiological knowledge in health and disease. Moreover, the teacher of physiology would be expected to contribute new knowledge to the medical literature and see to it that pupils had access to good textbooks in the library. Where most medical schools possessed only a handful of English translations of European studies, by 1828 the University of Virginia Library contained more than thirty textbooks and fifty-six volumes in total on physiology.[86]

Unlike many contemporaries, Jefferson also had a high opinion of chemistry. He gave it a prominent place in the curriculum and took the visionary step of providing for a well-equipped laboratory in which students could take part in experiments.[87]

Required Course in the History of Medicine

A further curricular novelty was inclusion of a series of formal lectures on the history of medicine, with explanations of its successive theories and principles of practice from Hippocrates to the present.[88] This course was an integral part of the medical school curriculum from its inception.[89] Rather than focusing on fads in vogue, Jefferson insisted that to be effective in any academic sphere, one must be equipped with sound knowledge of the developmental background of the field. He believed that the curriculum, by blending the best ideas of the ancients with the more insightful of the perspectives set forth by the moderns, would not only enlighten but inspire youthful matriculates. It would also serve as a "moral exercise"[90] by revealing examples of aggressive and abusive behavior of men, institutions, and nations. Indeed, by informing students of past errors, including examples of outright fraud and quackery, the study of history would "qualify them as judges of the actions and designs of men," and thus "enable them to know ambition under every disguise it may assume; and knowing it, to defeat its views."[91] Throughout his adult life, Jefferson regarded history as both a guide to and model for a perfectible future. Also, through the study and sympathetic appreciation of the best things said and done in the history of mankind, students would experience a degree of inspired enculturation.[92] For these reasons, Jefferson considered the study of history essential for worldly success.

Ensuring a Broad Cultural Education

In nineteenth-century America, there were four ways to obtain medical education: medical school, apprenticeship, private courses, and teaching in hospitals and dispensaries. To avoid the insular perspective that most of these methods insured, Jefferson saw the university as a place where budding physicians could and should broaden their perspective to fields other than science.[93] In a letter to John Adams, he criticized the scholastic standards of "the petty academies, as they call themselves," which sent students out into society "with just taste enough of learning to be alienated from industrious pursuits, and not enough to do service in the ranks of science."[94] By most accounts, medical education in antebellum America was exceptionally casual and superficial. "No one worried about admission standards, for entrance requirements were lower than they were for a good high school."[95] Because even basic literacy was not required, the average medical tyro was often depicted as a dullard, barely able to express "vague and confused" ideas in "barbarous English" that was "at defiance with all rules of grammar."[96] Instruction in medical science was shallow and brief, focusing on rudimentary principles of practice. The terms lasted only three or four months per year, and after a second term (typically a repeat of the first), "the M.D. degree was automatically given, regardless of the student's academic performance."[97] Moreover, no medical school in America, or its student matriculates, paid attention to the humanities and social sciences. As a result, medical graduates "lacked the wide ranging cultural interests which are expected in educated men," and they "were consequently incompetent to fill their proper role as leaders in American society."[98] The idea of educating and cultivating medical students to become learned gentlemen was an unheard of scholastic principle for virtually all American medical schools in the eighteenth and most of the nineteenth century.

Seeking to ensure a thorough and broad cultural education and a fixed standard of scholarship, Jefferson imposed three unprecedented conditions on all candidates for graduation. The first has been mentioned. Students were to attend lectures in three departments. Second, all students had to pass an English examination to prove their ability to write in correct English, with proper regard for spelling, grammar and syntax. A high proportion of failures attested to the need for this test.[99] The third requirement was the most extraordinary. In 1824, Jefferson decreed, on behalf of the Board of Visitors, that

> no Diploma shall be given to any one who has not passed such an

> examination in the Latin language as shall have proven him able to read the highest classics in that language with ease, thorough understanding, and just quantity. and if he be also a proficient in the Greek, let that too be stated in his Diploma. the intention being that the reputation of the University shall not be committed but to those who, to an eminence in some one or more of the sciences taught in it, add a proficiency in these languages which constitute the basis of good education, and are indispensable to fill up the character of a "well educated man."[100]

These purposeful actions suggest that the University of Virginia wanted its medical-school graduates to display not just professional skill, but broad intellectual interests and reasonable fluency in their native tongue. But Jefferson's revolutionary plan for reforming medical education in America required much more.

Proof of Learning by Attendance Checks and Frequent Examination

Jefferson understood that days, months, and years spent at the university were by no means a sufficient condition for securing a degree, including the doctorate of medicine. To maintain high standards, a system that recorded performance was needed. Regarding time, detailed class–participation records were maintained for each student, and regularly reported to the chairman of the faculty. In the antebellum period, the University of Virginia regularly issued printed report cards throughout the academic term that graded students on "a scale of preparation" for "such subjects as anatomy, physiology, pathology, chemistry and materia medica, and medicine."[101] Any student who neglected his responsibility to attend each and every class, actively participate in all didactic and experiential exercises, and demonstrate a satisfactory "scale of preparation" throughout the ten–and one–half month academic term would be subject to censure, up to and including summary suspension from the school. This was another significant departure from most contemporary medical schools, where attendance was not enforced and there was "a very significant minority of students who did not attend a large majority of lectures."[102] The proper use of students' time inside and outside the classroom was reinforced by a network of formal examinations and informal review. Jefferson stressed that possessing knowledge and having the ability to communicate it were the primary criteria for education.

Instruction in the science of medicine would be conveyed, partly by courses of lectures and anatomical demonstrations, and partly by the study of approved textbooks, and in all cases the progress of the students would be tested by a system of oral, written and public examinations. For example, immediately before each lecture, students in all scientific departments were to be "subjected to a full and rigid examination on the subject of the preceding lecture and any assigned reading." This practice of daily examination, which was one of the many extraordinary features in the organization of the University of Virginia, was intended to spur hard study from serious students while stimulating competition among classmates to emulate the few who successfully achieved a measure of scholastic excellence and fame by being perpetually prepared for dialogue and debate whenever opportunity arose.[103] Of equal if not greater importance, daily examinations enabled the professors to revisit parts of the material that were imperfectly understood by the class, fill in gaps, and weed out those languorous students who failed to show a satisfactory scale of preparation throughout the nearly year-long term. The daily examination was largely a recapitulation of the previous day's lecture, intended to "fill in the vacant gaps" in the student's imperfect memoranda. The student would thus have a valuable opportunity to retain and reinforce correct information, while experiencing "an incidental advantage in familiarizing him with the mode of trial to which he is subjected in his final examination for graduation."[104]

From the start, the medical school administered two "general examinations": an "intermediate" (midterm) and a final exam. Both occurred in the one of the oval rooms of the Rotunda. The final exam was partly oral but mostly written and subjected students to "searching interrogations" upon the details in all aspects of the topics covered in each of the seven courses of lectures, textbook assignments and experiential demonstrations in anatomy, chemistry and pharmacy. These tests were patterned after the system used at Oxford University. They were administered and graded by an impartial "Committee of Professors" constituted to include both medical and nonmedical faculty, with the written English section taken into account as a specific condition for the degree of doctor of medicine. According to Robley Dunglison, the first medical professor recruited by Jefferson, the construction, implementation, and grading of the nine-element final exam was a thoroughly laudatory response to Jefferson's authoritative edit to protect the credibility of the Virginia M.D.[105]

Only those students who were ranked in the top scholastic quartile, based on their final examination score, were declared eligible for the coveted M.D., and then only if other criteria for graduation had been met.

They needed to have performed well in the classroom throughout their university careers, earned satisfactory grades on both the English and Latin examinations, and achieved recognition as honorable men of high moral achievement.[106] The academic demands of the University led one student to say, "I think it is the last place in the world for a lazy man to try to enjoy himself."[107] In the awarding of the M.D., no school in America required more than the University of Virginia.[108]

In 1825, the University of Virginia became the first institution of higher education in America to adopt a rigorous system of written examinations. It was also the first to introduce the "English system" of written examinations with a numerical grading scale. By contrast, other contemporary medical schools did not require proof of proficiency by written examination until much later in the century. Before then examinations that were given were oral, privately administered, and cursory, even farcical in form.[109] To graduate, students merely had to answer a brief set of perfunctory oral questions and pay all lecture and graduation fees to their practitioner-teachers. Some schools did also require that students write a thesis on a medical topic of their choice. Although these dissertations may have been a "necessary for the obtaining of a diploma," it has been said "that not one in fifty affords the slightest evidence of competence, proficiency, or ability, in the candidate for graduation."[110]

Not until the late nineteenth century did most medical schools adopt a rigorous graded curriculum.[111] One reason for this fundamental pedagogical deficiency was the perverse system of faculty compensation. It based a professor's income on the number of students matriculated, those enrolled in courses of lectures, and the number of candidates approved for the degree. In effect, the more students that graduated, the higher the instructors' incomes, thus almost ensuring a laxness in applying rigorous and public standards to pass students to higher levels. According to William Norwood, "this proved to be unsound and productive of educational policies that debased standards and made teachers mercenary minded."[112] With the American system of measuring medical-student achievement horribly flawed throughout most of the nineteenth century, the motivation among schools to reform did not come from institutional leaders, who lacked incentive to change. Rather, it stemmed largely from external social, political and economic forces, including the advent and growth of licensing legislation at the state level.

Virtually every school in Jefferson's time awarded honorary degrees, with Yale awarding the first honorary doctorate in medicine in 1720, almost a century before it established a medical school.[113] Jefferson strongly opposed the practice, even though he was awarded several such degrees himself, including doctorates of law from the College of William and Mary (1783), Yale (1786), Harvard (1787), the College of Rhode Island (later Brown University) (1787) and the College of New Jersey (later Princeton University) (1791).[114] In his mind, awarding a degree without proof of learning by rigorous examination would seriously compromise the reputation of his institution. At the University of Virginia, the granting of degrees would be based solely on merit that had been laboriously acquired and exhibited in the classroom. According to Bruce, Jefferson's "distrustful attitude towards honorary degrees was characteristic of a man who had struck fiercely at all artificial distinctions, and who was suspicious of men's disposition to create them where they did not already exist."[115] Jefferson's policy was an unprecedented academic virtue in his time, and to this day only a few institutions of higher education have adopted and sustained it since their inception.[116] By 1850, honorary M.D. degrees from American medical schools had become so common that the AMA recommended that the practice be severely restricted. In some cases, proprietary medical schools went so far as to grant honorary degrees to local practitioners in order to induce them to send their apprentices to their schools, simply to swell a professor's income through ticketed lecture and other fees.[117]

This section has shown that the requirements for an M.D. degree at Virginia were demanding. As was the case in Britain and all of Europe, medical professors at the University of Virginia were given a fiduciary responsibility to approve no one for graduation who was not broadly and well educated, and duly examined and certified by a legally chartered body, which in Charlottesville was the Board of Visitors appointed by the governor and approved by the Virginia legislature. One effect of such standards was a very low graduation rate. After awarding its first three medical diplomas in 1828, only 14 percent of medical–school matriculates at the University of Virginia received an M.D. degree between that year and 1861.

State Support and Oversight

Jefferson repeatedly expressed his conviction that "the field of knolege is the common property of all mankind" and that it was the duty of the state to provide every citizen with an education "proportioned to the condition and pursuits of his life." He consistently argued that the state, not public or private corporations, should sponsor schools. This separated Jefferson from Benjamin Franklin, even from John Locke, and most assuredly from all the physician–owners of proprietary medical schools.

Seeking to change the pattern of unregulated American medical education, Jefferson promoted the concept of state-supported scholarship—a mechanism whereby an annual appropriation, which he was instrumental in securing, enabled the professoriate in Charlottesville to engage in medical scholarship, especially physiological research and the scientific aspects of hygiene and public health.[118] He recognized that the medical scholar was more dependent than the doctor of letters on libraries and laboratories, endowments and salaries—expensive luxuries only remotely accessible in nineteenth-century America, and he encouraged government support of scientific research without interference therein.[119] In return for financial support from the state, Jefferson understood that the University and its medical faculty had a fiduciary responsibility to protect and promote the trust of the citizenry by supplying better physicians to serve the Commonwealth of Virginia,[120] and he pledged his support for an annual institutional assessment and accountability through full public disclosure. As University rector, Jefferson demonstrated this commitment by creating a culture whereby the "University should in all things, & at all times be subject to the controul of the [state] legislature."[121] Let others be the judge, Jefferson proclaimed, of whether "this institution of my native state" was fulfilling its public purpose in reaching upwards and outwards and providing those destined for the learned professions ample opportunity to pursue their education "with more minuteness and detail than was within the scope of the General schools," in a manner that would increase the health, power and prosperity of a growing nation.[122]

One effect of linking support of the University and medical education there to an elected body was to increase transparency. In nineteenth-century America, the concept of public disclosure was for the most part ignored by medical schools and the profession at large. Medical schools arguably have a greater fiduciary responsibility than any other schools within an institution of higher education. Yet the vast majority were autonomous silos, accountable to no one except the physician-owners who often had serious conflicts of interest and no publicly advantageous agenda for either increasing scientific knowledge or improving its application throughout their state or locality. Medical schools with few exceptions not only questioned but openly resisted the right of any other agency to collect and publish the facts concerning their operations.[123] This dynamic did not exist in Charlottesville.

Jefferson's proposals, including the pursuit of postgraduate medical education in a federally run marine hospital, may appear contrary to his long-held opinion that government should interfere as little as possible with the natural functioning of society, excepting "such acts only as are injurious to others."[124] Although he strongly favored small government,[125] clearly "spending on education constituted the grand and significant exception to Jefferson's minimal state, for this was precisely the kind of investment that would foster the welfare of the rising generation without wasting its future prospects."[126]

The University of Virginia was not the first state university in America, but it was the only one to offer rigorous instruction in medicine from its founding.[127] In terms of chronology, Virginia's charter in 1819 made it a later creation than the state universities of Georgia (1785), North Carolina (1789), Vermont (1791), Tennessee (1794), South Carolina (1801), Ohio (1804) and Michigan (1817).[128] Even so, the University's medical department was the first beneficiary of state sponsorship and financial support in a university-based medical school, and "the principles it championed almost alone at its inception have since been embraced by all leading state universities."[129]

Moral Values and Professional Ethics

Jefferson displayed an uncommon faith in the transformative powers of education to strengthen a person's capacity for virtuous behavior when he wrote, "Education generates habits of application, of order and the love of virtue; and controuls, by the force of habit, any innate obliquities in our moral organization." With proper instruction, one could engraft "a new man on the native stock" so as to improve "what in his nature was vicious & perverse, into qualities of virtue & social worth." Jefferson believed one goal of higher education was "To develope the reasoning faculties of our youth, enlarge their minds, cultivate their morals, & instil into them the precepts of virtue & order."[130] For him education was thus a moral action and an edifying activity, whether one was a teacher or student. He promulgated a view of science that, as we have seen, incorporated an ethics of knowledge, i.e., rules that one ought to follow to achieve both scientific truth and personal probity. To an extent, this mindset was a secular substitute for theological commands and religious ritual, which were not part of the University charter or daily life.

In organizing his university, Jefferson hoped to create an environment that would bring out the best conduct and habits of application on the part of the students.[131] As was mentioned above in conjunction with the University's architecture, his plan for an academical village in which professors and students would live and study in close proximity was a deliberate effort to promote discourse among the members of the university community. Such dialogue, carried out with cordiality and curiosity, was itself a moral phenomenon for Jefferson. Ever the optimist, he envisaged all graduates of his university being men of distinguished character, who would achieve success in society not by trickery or artful calculation, but by honest dealing.[132]

Jefferson consistently lauded honesty as the best course of action, for practical as well as moral reasons. As early as 1774 he wrote that "The whole art of government consists in the art of being honest," and late in life he affirmed that that "Honesty is the 1st chapter in the book of wisdom."[133] His conception of virtues that might perfect the American national character was arguably broader than that of many of his contemporaries. According to one scholar, Jefferson's vocabulary included: the "moral sense virtues" of justice, faithful duty to others, sympathy and enlightened benevolence; the "agrarian virtues" of industry, self–reliance, patience, moderation and independence; the "civic virtues" of vigilance and spirited participation against conduct and acts that are injurious or vicious; the "epicurean virtues" of wisdom, prudence, fortitude, temperance and friendship in political, philosophical and sentimental domains; and the "secular virtues" of charity, tolerance and hope.[134]

In regard to the training and maturation of physicians, Jefferson placed particular emphasis on honor, duty to others and responsibility as quintessential.[135] In his mind, this meant acting honestly and benevolently to all with the purist intentions, always showing regard for the welfare of others and a desire to serve others in a humanistic way.[136] These virtues were not abstract verbiage. At the University of Virginia, before a student could qualify for the M.D. degree, he had to demonstrate high moral character, determined by the faculty through observation inside and outside the classroom.[137] To Jefferson, intellectual achievement without moral correctness is nugatory.[138]

Jefferson believed that on its own, science was an inadequate basis for professional practice—that physicians must also possess a core of ethical values that included such attributes as allegiance to the do-no-harm principle, therapeutic restraint when evidence of benefit is lacking, and affectionate optimism.[139] He encouraged his nephew to pursue his studies with the "purest integrity, the most chaste honor," and he subsequently showed considerable confidence in the "pride of character, laudable ambition, & moral dispositions" of students at the University of Virginia when he instituted a system of self-government that encouraged students to assume personal responsibility for their conduct, on and off grounds.[140] Jefferson's plan promoted concepts of truth telling within and between the student bodies in all eight schools. In disciplinary matters students were not compelled to inform on other students. Faculty were instructed to remind students of the moral rule that "every one is bound to bear witness, where wrong has been done," after which students would not be compelled to testify under oath, but asked to speak up voluntarily, based on their "own sense of right." The original regulation of 1824 was revised the following year to remove the call on faculty to remind students of their moral obligations and simplified to read: "When testimony is required from a Student, it shall be voluntary, and not on oath, and the obligation to give it shall be left to his own sense of right."[141] Although labeled by some as a "fanciful idea" if not an altogether "erroneous impression,"[142] Jefferson's scheme of student self-regulation nonetheless had to be accepted by the faculty, which had no choice but to abide by the founder's wishes. This visionary plan would soon pose huge problems for the professoriate and Board of Visitors.

Jefferson was in the vanguard of a small cadre of enlightened thinkers who seemed to encourage the conceptual development and application of a higher form of professionalism among medical practitioners. His rhetoric reflected several modern-day precepts that give the profession legitimacy:[143] the demonstration by examination of up-to-date knowledge and exemplary communication skills; the importance of self-awareness and its associated mental power, self-control; the concept that all philanthropic healers must subordinate their interests to those of the patient; deference to technical competence and rational persuasion based on a commitment to evidence-based medical practice and lifelong learning; enough humility to admit one's limitations; a commitment to social reform through promotion of the public good; and professional self-regulation as opposed to government intrusion.

Academic Freedom Faculty Tenure, and Self-Government

Throughout his life, Jefferson devoted himself to the causes of freedom of thought and expression and the persuasive force of enlightened, evidence-based argumentation. Against both ignorance and undue enthusiasm, he argued, "education & free discussion are the antidotes."[144] At a time when conformity to the religious positions of sponsoring denominations was still expected from faculty in both English and American institutions of higher learning, Jefferson proclaimed that "I have sworn upon the altar of god eternal hostility against every form of tyranny over the mind of man."[145] He was steadfast in his belief that academic freedom was an essential ingredient for all colleges and universities committed to the discovery and dissemination of knowledge and truth. A striking example of Jefferson's vigorous defense of institutional academic freedom occurred in 1819 when he unsuccessfully attempted to hire Dr. Thomas Cooper (1759–1839) as the University of Virginia's first professor, persevering even in the face of widespread opposition from religious groups.[146] Jefferson feared that, without academic freedom, institutions of higher education would become instruments for indoctrination—for uncritical absorption and inculcation of particular dogmas. He realized that freedom of inquiry and expression was important not only to educational institutions but also to society as a whole, that "every difference of opinion was not a difference in principle." In his inaugural presidential address of 4 March 1801, he famously remarked that, "If there be any among us who would wish to dissolve this Union, or to change its republican form, let them stand undisturbed as monuments of the safety with which error of opinion may be tolerated, where reason is left free to combat it."[147] As a legal scholar, Jefferson had a keen appreciation for aspects of constitutional law that protected free-speech rights, and he hoped that his University would become a citadel for intellectual liberty—a place for robust debate (a back-and-forth conversational aspect) and a forum for the competition of ideas, where faculty and students would be expected to resolve conflict and policy through honorable challenge, critical appraisal of relevant facts and civil discourse.[148] In Jefferson's mind, the prohibition of the free exchange of ideas stops the full development of scientific knowledge and thus diminishes the quality of instruction.

Jefferson's profound antagonism to the debasing effects of tyranny led him to propose a number of changes that were designed to alter fundamentally the intellectual framing of personal freedom in an academic setting. He outlined his views on freedom of inquiry and expression, in reference to the research and educational enterprises of the University of Virginia, in a letter to William Roscoe, saying that "this institution will be based on the illimitable freedom of the human mind. for here we are not afraid to follow truth wherever it may lead, nor to tolerate any error so long as reason is left free to combat it." In a similar comment to Destutt de Tracy, Jefferson stated that the school's aim was to permit the mind "to explore and to expose every subject susceptible of it's contemplation."[149] In this inspired prose, Jefferson declared that his institution of higher education would not advance the old orthodoxies of any insular empire, nor would its governing board be a self-perpetuating, authoritarian aristocracy, brooding over its professors and students with overly restrictive doctrines, including the loyalty oaths required of the faculty at his alma mater, the College of William and Mary. Conformity to denominational modes of thought, always greater in the South, was also expected at other colonial colleges, including Harvard, Yale, and Princeton, and at some schools, trustees spent much time vigilantly scanning the writing and lectures of its faculties to ensure their orthodoxy. After the eighteenth century, enforced assent to religious doctrine gradually gave way to political ones.[150] Many of the steps that Jefferson took to replace repressive institutions with others free from sectarian control and enjoying democratic governance illustrate how prescient his vision was for one of the most cherished foundations of university life—the principle of academic freedom.

Firm in his belief that freedom is "the firstborn daughter of science," Jefferson promoted the concept that tenure, or election without term, is fundamental to achieving academic freedom in a university community, asserting that professors should not be easily dismissed for light or temporary reasons.[151] In a letter unsuccessfully urging Nathaniel Bowditch to accept the professorship of mathematics, Jefferson said that "the Professors of the University will of themselves comprise a scientific society. they will be removable only by a vote of two thirds of the visitors, and when you are told that the visitors are mr Madison, Presid[t] Monroe & myself, all known to you by character, Senator Cabell, Gen[l] Cocke, and mr Watson, gentlemen of distinguished worth and information, you will be sensible that the tenure is in fact for life."[152]

The medical faculty at Virginia enjoyed more than the assurance of lifelong tenure in their posts. Their authority in the conduct of scholarly work was unrestrained, and most professors received total freedom in the selection of textbooks to be used in their courses. Jefferson stated that while the trustees of most public institutions prescribed the textooks, at the University of Virginia this would be left to the professors, who were presumably better qualified, being "so much at the heights of science in the several branches as to undertake this."[153] The one exception was the School of Law. Fearing that Federalist works would contaminate the minds of impressionable students, the Board of Visitors mandated a required reading list in law, government, and history.[154] This decision was the one notable exception to Jefferson's otherwise absolute commitment to academic freedom.

Another safeguard of academic independence that Jefferson promoted was the democracy of the faculty within itself. All professors were to be on equal footing in rank, compensation and influence, and assignment to the various pavilions was by lot.[155] The University would have no president. At his last meeting of the Board, Jefferson objected strenuously to a proposal to lure a prospective law professor to the university by offering him the presidency. This hypothetical appointment failed when the candidate refused the offer, and the unusual administration of the affairs of the university by an annually rotating faculty chairmanship persisted until 1905.[156] Jefferson intended that each professor should hold this office, that of chairman of the faculty, in turn, and he attached much importance to the principle of rotation.[157] Believing that people were, on the whole, rational, moral, and benevolent social creatures, Jefferson argued that the day-to-day operations of the University should reflect the majority will of the faculty. He mandated, following his theme of self-government, that the University of Virginia would have no bureaucratic control other than a secular Board of Visitors—a small governing body appointed by the state legislature that would represent the public in its outlook and responsibilities. Jefferson wanted the professors and students to work together to run the schools themselves. At the University of Virginia, the duly certified members of the academic community, like the citizens of the United States, would each be called on to assume positions of leadership and do their parts to govern.

Jefferson gave students uncommon freedoms.[158] These included rejecting a prescribed course of learning, thus allowing students uncontrolled choice in what to read and which lectures to attend. Compulsory chapel attendance, a bedrock requirement elsewhere, was abandoned. At the University of Virginia, students were not subjected, at least initially, to police–like systems of surveillance of extracurricular activities. Finally, there was no fixed time schedule for completion of academic work. Exceptionally gifted students could accelerate through their course of study. However, Jefferson seriously doubted that many students, if any, could demonstrate sufficient proficiency to earn the coveted M.D. degree in less than two full academic terms. Indeed, between 1825 and 1870, only two medical students so distinguished themselves as to be awarded degrees in less than two years—John Staige Davis in 1841 and Walter Reed in 1869.

Jefferson's broad perspective on academic freedom and the actions he took to institutionalize his beliefs put him in the vanguard of his and future generations of reform-minded innovators of educational policy. Indeed, as Alan Barth so pointedly said in 1951, "it was not until the American Association of University Professors (AAUP) was established in 1915 that the right of the teaching profession to freedom in the classroom and tenure won general recognition, even in theory, and that the profession presented anything like a coordinated form in the defense of these principles." Even a tacit guarantee of tenure did not emerge until 1925. Before then faculty generally held one–year, at-will appointments.[159]

In endowing the University of Virginia with a uniquely purposeful philosophy and organizational structure, Jefferson sought to establish an institution that was far more impressive than any of his state's "petty academies & colleges"—one that could aspire to become "the most eminent in the United States," a destination for the best and brightest students and scholars, wherever they might be found. He described his plan in 1800 as "so broad & liberal & modern" that it would "be worth patronising with the public support, and be a temptation to the youth of other states to come, and drink of the cup of knolege & fraternize with us."[160] Such aspirations were not far-fetched. The foundational principles that governed Jefferson's vision of the University were a combination of ingenious organizational innovation and ethical belief, which in contrast to his earlier reforms at William and Mary, could be realized de novo, with the charter of the University starting from a blank slate.

Perhaps the overriding foundational principle was what can be called matrix-like planning, where the social, intellectual, and physical structures of the school were laid out in a way that individual structures, like cells in a matrix, could affect one another vertically and horizontally. Examples include the belief that porticos promote conversation, which could in turn engender collegiality among faculty and students, and making the library the visual focal point of the campus. In a more formal instantiation of cross–disciplinary dialogue, curricular rules established at Virginia encouraged attendance at lectures outside one's own field, with specific diplomas reflecting mastery across several disciplines. A third key innovation was the setting of high standards for faculty and students with homogeneous application to all intellectual departments, and quantitative feedback on whether the standards were met—via written tests, attendance checks, and public examinations. Standards could only be upheld and applied fairly when embedded in a routinely functioning monitoring system that produced written reports. Fourth, Jefferson espoused the need for a full-time paid faculty and endorsed a liberal, nonauthoritarian polity for professors. Such laissez–faire oversight gave them a fair amount of what one would today call a sense of ownership in the school, an attitude further secured by the fact the professors could not be dismissed for expression of their views. Both power and responsibility resided in those who taught, rather than in a bureaucratic administration. Moreover, the system was democratic in the sense that rules and changes could be proposed and voted on. The chapter also stressed Jefferson's fundamental insistence on a scientific epistemology, which was characterized as ethical to the extent that it required inquiry to be executed according to strict evidentiary methods. Debate was encouraged, but the final arbiter of defensible belief was not authority but rather empirical and logical proof. Finally, and more subtly, Jefferson expected social habits of moral uprightness and etiquette among all faculty and students. While such a demand could have been influenced by the gentlemanly code of the early 1800s, Jefferson also wanted those educated at the University to be or become good persons who would contribute to society.

The institution's foundational principles created a new form of education at Virginia's medical department, as it did at all the others. It was unique, revolutionary, and, at least theoretically, superior to what was on offer at American medical schools functioning in 1825. Notable among the groundbreaking innovations were a full-time faculty, which contrasted with part-time doctors providing medical instruction in addition to a private practice; professors residing on campus, which encouraged frequent contact with mentors and delving into subjects outside medicine; and a lengthy academic term, more than doubling the amount of classroom time required by the typical medical school. Finally, as will be seen in Chapter 5, medical students heard lectures in more subjects than preclinical and clinical science, thus availing themselves of an opportunity not to be found in almost any other medical school.

Jefferson did not set out to revolutionize medical education. Rather, what at the time might be seen as radical reforms were based on foundational principles constitutive of the university as a whole. The department teaching medical science was but one beneficiary of eight. However, the chapter also revealed Jefferson's interests in and recommendations for the study of medicine per se. These ranged from questions of where students might gain clinical experience to formal requirements such as the need for prerequisite science courses. Documents in this chapter showed that Jefferson was aware that medical education especially must inculcate ethical beliefs and social consciousness in students whose training, in contrast to that of most other students, was to result in technical skills with a direct bearing on human well-being. In Jefferson's view, a good physician or medical student must also be a good person. Since in medicine, one is bound to deal with life as a whole, a purely scientific education is inadequate. For the profession of medicine, medical education cannot ever lose touch with the humanities and the continuously changing social structure in America.

Finally, while Jefferson's concepts of university formation were astute and prescient, in 1825 they were also theoretical and hypothetical—that is, based on theories of higher education gleaned from years of observation but not yet subjected to proof or disproof by the experiment of actually opening and running a university, with its essential and arguably most critical investigators being present, namely the faculty and students. The revolutionary model he proposed was viewed by John Adams as potentially original and novel, who for this reason deemed it unlikely to succeed. He praised the "noble Tryumvirate" of Jefferson, Madison, and Monroe, whose eminence was such that, by their fostering the creation of the University of Virginia, "the World will expect Something very great and very new." To this, he added a grim prophecy that, "if it contains anything quite original, and very excellent, I fear the prejudices are too deeply rooted to Suffer it to last long, though it may be accepted at first. It will not always have three Such colossal reputations to Support it."[161] Adams made that observation eight years before the university officially opened its doors. Before that could happen in 1825, candidates for the faculty needed to be identified, vetted, and appointed. This process led to the inaugural members of the medical faculty, starting with the first professor, who wasted little time in translating Jefferson's ideas on medical education from paper to practice.

Part II

THE WORK OF JEFFERSON'S DISCIPLES: ROBLEY DUNGLISON AND JAMES L. CABELL

Chapter 4

RECRUITMENT, SELECTION, AND INSTALLATION OF THE FIRST CHAIR OF THE UNIVERSITY'S MEDICAL DEPARTMENT

Nothing is known in our profession by guess; and I do not believe, that from the first dawn of medical science to the present moment, a single correct idea has ever emanated from conjecture; it is right, therefore, that those who are studying their profession, should be aware that there is no short road to knowledge; and that observations on the diseased living, examinations of the dead, and experiments upon living animals, are the only sources of true knowledge; and that inductions from these are the sole basis of legitimate theory.

Sir Astley Paston Cooper, 1843[1]

JEFFERSON was meticulous in selecting the faculty of the University. His insistence that the professoriate should comprise only scholars at the apex of their field forced him and his agent to look for candidates in the English-speaking universities outside the United States. Although Joseph C. Cabell (see Figure 10) and John H. Cocke, fellow members of the Board of Visitors, wanted Americans to fill some of the positions, Jefferson, as its rector, wielded his considerable power and influence to ensure that only a "Professor of the highest order of merit" would be hired, recruiting in the United States if possible, but going overseas if necessary.[2] In the spring of 1824, when the Board of Visitors sent its envoy, Francis W. Gilmer, on a fateful recruitment mission to the United Kingdom, Jefferson wrote that "we have determined to recieve no one who is not of the 1st order of science in his line." If they could not be obtained in America, the University would "seek some of them at least in the countries ahead of us in science and preferably in Gr. Britain the land of our own language, habits and manners."[3] Besides, he reasoned, "To prohibit us from the benefit of foreign light, is to consign us to long darkness."[4]

When the University of Virginia opened its doors to students on March 7, 1825, the chair of the Medical Department was occupied by Dr. Robley Dunglison (1798–1869) (see Figures 12 and 13), who had been recruited from England. Jefferson felt fully justified in his decision to look overseas since his efforts and those of the various visitors had failed thus far to secure a single American scholar of distinguished character. In 1817 and 1818, with the consent of the Visitors of the University's forerunner, Central College, he had unsuccessfully attempted to recruit three scholars living in America, namely: Dr. Thomas Cooper (1759–1839), already mentioned above, Nathaniel Bowditch (1773–1838), a famed, self–taught mathematician and astronomer, and George Ticknor (1791–1871), a highly respected Harvard professor specializing in French and Spanish languages and literatures.[5] This quest to recruit reputable faculty members wherever they could be found set a new standard in the United States, following the practice of German institutions like the University of Göttingen (1734) and the University of Berlin (1810).[6]

This chapter recounts the background and appointment of, the first leader of the medical department. We contend here that Dunglison was selected not only because he met Jefferson's uncompromising standards but because the two shared key beliefs about the nature of medicine, derived in part from the fact that both were influenced by Cabanis and the French Idéologues, with Dunglison assimilating their effects on Parisian medicine. Dunglison went on to become the personal physician of Jefferson not only for his extraordinary competence but also because of an intellectual affinity with his sponsor that can be traced back to a common Parisian connection. More broadly, Dunglison's approach to medical science and his achievements in it mirrored Jefferson's epistemology and intellectual habits in scientific inquiry, as laid out above in Chapter 2. With few exceptions, Jefferson could perceive in Dunglison a facsimile of himself as an Enlightenment-inspired physician.

Dunglison's Background

Robley Dunglison was born in Keswick, Cumberland County, England on January 4, 1798. He initially trained to become a planter–merchant in the West Indies, where his uncle, John Robley, had extensive proprietary operations in Tobago and Saint Vincent. However, when this uncle died, Dunglison abandoned the idea of leading a commercial life and broadened his intellectual interests. He obtained part of his early education on

Solway Firth at the Green Row Academy in Holme Abbey, also known as Abbeytown, a celebrated classical institution where he "made himself a thorough master of the Greek and Latin languages and of the higher branches of English composition."[7] During this time, Dunglison gave serious consideration to law and medicine but ultimately chose the latter profession.

Dunglison began to study medicine in 1814 at the age of sixteen with an apprenticeship to John Edmondson, "a surgeon of repute" in Keswick.[8] As was then customary in England, he studied medicine with this village preceptor for one full year. Dunglison then moved on to London, where he completed much of his medical study as an assistant to Dr. Charles Thomas Haden (1786–1824), a respected surgeon-apothecary at the Chelsea and Brompton Dispensary. Trained in Edinburgh, Haden had studied in Paris and brought back a sound knowledge of French medicine and great enthusiasm for its innovations. Among his accomplishments, which surely had a profound influence on Dunglison, Haden is credited with: introducing the stethoscope to England; discovering in 1820 that gout and other inflammatory conditions could be treated with *Colchicum autumnale* (a treatment still in use); authoring important treatises on many other therapeutic remedies and the management of childhood diseases; and, editing several journals, including the *Medical Intelligencer* of London. Haden, like Jefferson, advocated preventive medicine, rather than potentially dangerous medical intervention, and supported improved female education in matters of health.[9]

While maintaining his connection with Haden, Dunglison subsequently attended courses of lectures at the University of Edinburgh during the winter and spring of 1815–1816. Topics included chemistry, by Thomas Charles Hope (1766–1844); structural and practical anatomy, by Alexander Monro III (1773–1859); and the principles of midwifery, by James Hamilton (1767–1839). He also came under the influence of Andrew Duncan (1744–1828), and learned clinical medicine from James Home (1760–1844), and Daniel Rutherford (1749–1819), the discoverer of nitrogen. Apparently sharing the view of some detractors that Monro was at best a mediocre anatomist, Dunglison elected to add a second course in the subject given privately by John Barclay (1758–1826), whose style was said to be extremely clear and illuminated by a thorough knowledge of the history of his subjects. The University of Edinburgh was prestigious and popular at this time, with class sizes often numbering in the hundreds. In 1815 Dunglison was among 423 students who attended Hamilton's lectures on midwifery.[10]

At the Royal Infirmary of Edinburgh, clinical appointments were available and many students, including Dunglison, availed themselves of this practical experience. A description by one student, Robert J. Graves (1796–1853), is especially revealing of the Infirmary's pedagogical style:

> Two clinical clerks, one for the male, another for the female wards, are selected by the [attending] physician from among the senior pupils; their business is to write an accurate history of the cases, to report the effects of medicines, and record the symptoms which might have occurred since the physician's last visit. At his daily visit the physician stops at the bed of each patient, and having received the necessary information from his clerk, he examines the patient, interrogating him in a loud voice, while the clerk repeats the patient's answers in a tone of voice equally loud. This is done to enable the whole audience to understand what is going on, but indeed, when the crowd of students is considerable, it is no easy task; it requires an exertion almost stentorian to render this conversation between the physician and his patient audible by the more distant members of the class; while the impossibility of seeing the patient obliges all who are not in his immediate vicinity to trust to their ears for information. This information is not indeed neglected, for every word so attentively listened to, and heard with so much difficulty, is forthwith registered most faithfully in each student's case-book; and afterwards all the observations the professors make in their clinical lectures, are taken down with equal care and fidelity.[11]

This form of integrated medical learning combined formal lectures with hospital and dispensary work. Particularly valuable for students, who were closely and properly supervised by professors from a medical school genuinely connected to a university, it did not exist in most European institutions of the time, or in any American school. Among other things, it stimulated students to pay attention in the classroom, knowing full well that their newly acquired scientific and practical knowledge would have immediate application at the bedside of the sick.

The Library of the College of Physicians of Philadelphia possesses the only extant documentary record of Dunglison's clinical experience at the University of Edinburgh and the Royal Infirmary. The most consequential evidence comes from a two-volume notebook compiled entirely by Dunglison that runs 923 pages. This amazingly detailed and orderly account of his two courses in clinical medicine reveals much about him, the pedagogical style of his teachers and their therapeutic strategies.[12]

The lecture notes amply illustrate Dunglison's all-embracing assiduousness in obtaining firsthand clinical knowledge from different but equally important sources. Formal instruction supplied in the lecture hall taught Dunglison that the ineffable components of the diagnostic art require a thorough history, including a comprehensive review of organ systems, and a good physical examination of the patient and their bodily fluids. Much emphasis seems to have been placed on acquiring an acceptable proficiency in interrogation, as well as an ability accurately to measure respirations and strength of pulse and rate, to percuss cavities (lungs and abdomen), and to assess their sounds by ear (students did not have the aid of the stethoscope). Outside the classroom, Dunglison benefitted from direct encounters with sick patients and the recording of their histories in minute detail, covering more than thirty of the most common Scottish afflictions; physical examinations of patients and their bodily fluids; lessons learned daily during bedside rounds with his preceptor-professor, to whom he was required to make a full report at least twice a week; autopsies on all but one of his fatal cases, which he did not perform himself but was permitted to attend; and readings from approved textbooks and essays written by some of the leading medical minds of his time, including works by William Cullen on nosology, and John Ferriar on diabetes, Joseph Adams on poisons, Thomas Bateman and Robert Willam on cutaneous diseases, Giovanni Morgagni on liver complaints, James Currie on typhus, and publications by John Abernethy on urethral diseases; John Pearson, John Hunter, and Richard Carmichael on syhilitic diseases.[13]

Dunglison's notebook entries suggest that, among his clinical preceptors, he had the greatest admiration for Professor Home. He appears to have been a dedicated teacher, vitally concerned with his patients and with transmitting the significant points of their illnesses to his students. Home "epitomized the Enlightenment–inspired physician of the early 19th century. He read widely in the current medical literature and applied his up–to–date knowledge to the care of his patients."[14] To students like Dunglison he passed on a scientifically informed and frequently skeptical attitude toward overly aggressive medical intervention. Home warned his pupils that the medicine of their day "was by no means static, that new remedies, new understandings of diseases, new terms and new instruments were constantly being introduced." Above all, he extolled the virtues of cautious conservatism when unsure of a diagnosis or the efficacy of some fashionable treatment; and he urged his students never to stop learning and to be active observers and participants in the ever-evolving debates concerning medical science. In terms of restraining judgment until justified by evidence and stressing learning as ongoing, Home's attitudes to medicine and to science in general mirrored Jefferson's.

Years after leaving the University of Edinburgh and the Royal Infirmary, Dunglison published *The Medical Student; or Aids to the Study of Medicine.* In this work, he presented his candid opinion on medical education, perhaps with his former mentor, Professor Home, in mind. Regarding training in clinical medicine he wrote:

> In respect to the best method of profiting by the *Clinical course*, a great deal will depend upon the method adopted by the professor,–as to the plan the student should pursue. Too often, perhaps, the clinical instructor selects the singular and the striking, rather than the common and more useful cases; and it has fallen to the lot of the author——as it must have done, more or less, to every one——to have had his attention directed chiefly to cases, during his period of hospital attendance, which he has rarely or never met with since. The object of the clinical professor should be to select mainly those cases, that must necessarily present themselves to all in their ordinary course of practice; to inquire aloud into the history of the case, and, at a fitting opportunity, to explain the etiology, semeiotics, diagnosis, prognosis and treatment adapted for the particular case, and for the class to which it belongs,—attracting the attention of the student to the more prominent points. With these views, acute cases should be first considered, as being most common and urgent; and, afterwards the more chronic. The young student is generally disposed to be over active in his treatment, and, if one remedy does not appear to be producing all the effect he anticipated, he is apt to fly at once to another; but if the professor be judicious, the student will soon learn that infinite mischief may be done in this manner, and that more reliance has to be placed upon the recuperative powers of the system, than he may have been disposed to imagine. It will be well for the clinical pupil to keep a journal of such cases as may merit the trouble; and never to permit an occasion to slip for verifying or disproving, by dissection, the views which he or his teacher may have been led to form of the precise nature of fatal maladies.[15]

Returning to London, Dunglison attended more medical lectures, presumably including those in anatomy by Astley Cooper, a friend of his mentor Dr. Charles Haden, who was then at Guy's Hospital.[16] Next he went to Paris, where he studied at the École de Medicine and took sundry private courses. Dunglison was certainly exposed in France to many of the great minds of the time, either through direct contact or their celebrated writings. Later, when Dunglison published his famous textbook on physiology, he referred to their important work frequently and was careful to cite them properly.[17]

Paris at that time was a highly advanced center of medical education and research, attracting students of means from England, other parts of Europe, and America.[18] It offered extensive opportunities to learn medicine by practice as well as professorial precept. By the time Dunglison arrived in Paris, medical hegemony had passed from Edinburgh to the French "Clinical School." The philosophical origins of the Paris clinical school owed much to the *Idéologues*, most notably Pierre Jean Georges Cabanis (1757–1808), who, as has been seen, corresponded with Thomas Jefferson. Under the influence of Cabanis, the hallmarks of Paris medicine were an aversion to theories in the absence of facts, adherence to empirical observation, therapeutic skepticism (the relative role of the physician and "nature" in the cure of disease), and the importance of principles of hygiene. The concept of scientific practice, based on the "intelligent empiricism" that Jefferson advocated, was emerging in the training of physicians. This development owned much to the groundbreaking clinical-pathological studies of French leaders, such as Marie François Xavier Bichat (1771–1802), which increasingly drew attention to specific body parts—first to entire organs and then to tissue within an organ. From this emerged the concept of "localized pathology," which enabled the construction and application of a nosology more attuned to surgical and medical practice.[19] French researchers had invented instruments and procedures that greatly facilitated bedside diagnosis. While Dunglison was in France, students were beginning to learn of Currie's practical thermometer, René Laënnec (1781–1826) was working with the stethoscope, which he invented, and actively engaged in teaching,[20] and Jean Nicolas Corvisart (1755–1821) was showing students how to percuss the chest. Pierre Charles Alexandre Louis (1787–1872) was starting his brilliant career, focusing on the value of statistics in therapeutic studies, and François Magendie (1783–1855), a pioneer of experimental physiology and a notorious vivisector, was shocking many of his contemporaries with his dissections of live animals during his public lectures. Dunglison apparently witnessed some of these experiments while in Paris, which "led to him being entirely opposed to vivisections; and his sensitive nature shrank so much from the infliction of pain, that he never could have practiced the surgical department of the healing art.[21] In common with his fellow medical students, Dunglison worked in Parisian hospital wards and special clinics in the mornings and listened to lectures and watched anatomical demonstrations in the afternoons, paying some heed to the battle cry of Antoine François Fourcroy (1755–1809), who helped devise the system of French higher education of France in the 1800's: "Peu lire, beaucoup voir et beaucoup faire" (read a little, observe and do much).[22]

The Idéologues had reinforced Jefferson's longstanding skepticism about medical theories and enhanced his desire to see a positivist epistemology applied to medical practice and pedagogy. This much can be inferred from his likely reading of Cabanis' 1791 book *On the Degree of Certainty in Medicine*. By the time Dunglison arrived in Paris, almost a generation later, what had been a revolution and reform of medicine, as Cabanis put it in a book title, *Sketch of the Revolutions*, in 1801, had begun to be institutionalized. The epistemology promoted by the Idéologues was being implemented in the training of physicians and the treatment of patients. Its novelty lay in its restrictions on theory, coupled with stringency of care and innovations such as the stethoscope and thermometer, improved hygiene, quantitative analysis of disease outbreaks, and a focus on observing disease in situ. As Jefferson had hoped, the ethos of science was finally being realized in medicine, and Dunglison was trained in accordance with these changes, with medicine now seen not as a physical handicraft but as a branch of science, derived from such underlying branches as chemistry and sprouting its own offshoots, such as physiology.

Certification and Doctorate of Medicine

Returning to London, Dunglison continued his medical studies under Haden and then passed two separate examinations in 1818 administered by the Royal College of Surgeons and the Society of Apothecaries in London. He began to practice his art the following year. At this time, three organizations largely controlled the practice of medicine in and around London: the Royal College of Physicians, the Royal College of Surgeons, and the Society of Apothecaries. They all required that physicians be licensed to practice.[23] In order to receive a license, practitioners had to pass an examination, and before they could take it, candidates were required to prove they had served at least five years as an apprentice to a reputable physician and attended courses of medical lectures. Dunglison's original certificate, in the archives of the Society of Apothecaries at the Guildhall Library in London, reads: "Qualified as L.S.A. (Country Practice), 1st January 1818. Apprentice to John Edmondson of Keswick and to Charles T. Haden of Sloan Street, London [more than 5 years total]. Presented testimonials from both as well as proof of lecture attendance: two courses in Anatomy; two courses on the Theory and Practice of Medicine; two courses in Chemistry; and one course of lectures on Materia Medica. Hospital attendance as probationer at the Royal Infirmary of Edinburgh – 12 months. Examined and approved by Mr. Johnson."[24] In 1823, after nine years of medical study, Dunglison received an M.D. degree from the University of Erlanger in Bavaria, Germany, "by written examination in the Latin language." At this time most British physicians obtained their degrees in Germany, since English universities were expensive and so backward that they graduated only a handful of medical students each year. His doctoral thesis was entitled "de Neuralgia" (see Figure 14).[25]

The breadth of Dunglison's education is noteworthy. Medical practitioners at the time in the United States were not required to pass any licensing examination. Indeed, most "doctors" in colonial America did not receive any formal university education or attend medical school. Only elite American physicians trained primarily in Europe or in a few Northeastern schools acquired M.D. degrees. Most others attended a few rudimentary lectures on anatomy and then served as apprentices to established physicians or surgeons. As early as 1765, Dr. John Morgan, founder of the first medical school in America, denounced this form of education as "lame and insufficient."[26] Jefferson was keenly aware of the deficiencies in the training of doctors, commenting that the state of medical education in America was "worse than that of total ignorance."[27] He was highly suspicious of most physicians trained in America—horrified by their superficial knowledge and their unwarranted assertions to medical authority. Clearly, Dunglison was of a different stripe. He was a remarkably well-prepared physician, having studied under "the most brilliant group of medical professors of his day"[28] while experiencing three different forms of medical education: formal instruction from university faculty in the fundamental branches of medical science and the basic skills necessary for taking histories and examining patients and their bodily fluids; practical experience in hospitals and clinics, enabling him to acquire proficiency in all aspects of patient care; and, experience in private laboratories of anatomy and surgery. Moreover, he was uniquely qualified and licensed to practice by formal examination.

Dunglison's Early Career as a Physician

When George Birkbeck (1776–1841), an enlightened physician, philosopher and philanthropist from Edinburgh, first brought Dunglison's name to the attention of Francis W. Gilmer (see Figure 15) and through him to Jefferson's scrutiny, he had proven himself to be an able medical practitioner, educator and scholar. Birkbeck noted that Dunglison had "habits strictly literary and a taste leading to actual investigation, with a decided tendency to prefer the contemplative species of occupation to the more bustling."[29] Within one year of graduation, Dunglison had won a prestigious appointment as *Physician Accoucheur* at the Eastern Dispensary, then one of the most extensive charities in London, located in one of the poorest areas in the city. There he devised his first medical course in 1824, on "The Principles and Practice of Midwifery," which included instruction in the diseases of women and children.[30]

Throughout his time in London, Dunglison tirelessly cultivated relationships with many of the leading medical men in England. He had a wide circle of friends and was admired, even celebrated, for his "conviviality as a host and jovial participant at social gatherings."[31] Dunglison gained the respect of his professional brethren before immigrating to the United States. He won election to several prestigious positions, notably, secretary for foreign correspondence and member of the governing council of the London Medical Society, a revered professional organization founded in 1773. He also belonged to the Royal College of Surgeons of England, the Society of Apothecaries, the Royal Humane Society of London, the Hunterian Society, and several French scientific organizations.[32] When Dunglison departed England, two different organizations—the London Medical Society and the Hunterian Society—passed resolutions wishing him good luck in America. The Hunterian Society even suspended one of its bylaws so that Dunglison might be "declared at once a corresponding member."[33]

Early Literary Contributions

The urge to write appeared early in Dunglison's life, and his prodigious literary labors "continued without interruption until within a few days of the close of his life, when bodily infirmity compelled him to lay aside his well–used pen."[34] In 1817 at the age of nineteen , he began to write for the periodical press.[35] One of his earliest medical works discussed the action of belladonna on the pupil of the eye.[36] In this inaugural investigation, Dunglison sought to clarify the observations made by Daries in 1776, by carefully describing the results of his own self-experimentation. He reported the timed onset of action, duration of effect and the mechanism of action of the mydriatic, thus providing a plausible explanation of the effect on both near and far vision. For a year or two thereafter, he was a regular correspondent of the *Monthly Magazine* of London, writing several articles that won him a reputation as a "practiced observer and writer." They included "The *Danger of Quack Medicines* "(1817)—an essay warning of the fatal effects of some of the more powerful quack remedies, especially when administered to children.[37] In 1822, Dunglison translated and edited Jean Dominique Larrey's *Essay on the Use of Moxa as a Therapeutic Agent.* He prefaced it with a long, erudite dissertation on the history and properties of various forms of moxibustion — an ancient Chinese medical treatment that presumably drew blood, pus or other impurities to the surface. This work, published at Dunglison's own expense, received highly favorable reviews. Later that same year, he translated and published his edited interpretation of François Magendie's *Formulary for the Preparation and Mode of Employing New Remedies*, and an edition of Robert Hopper's *The Surgeon's Vade-Mecum*. By 1823, in conjunction with his distinguished friend, Dr. James Copland (1791–1870), he was placed on the editorial board of the *London Medical Repository*, a prestigious medical journal published under various titles from 1815 to 1836.

One of Dunglison's more noteworthy contributions to the *London Quarterly Review* was a paper on malaria, in which he affirmed his belief that this intermittent fever was in no way associated with miasma from vegetable and animal decomposition.[38] "Certain strange statements" that Dr. John MacCulloch (1773–1835) made in an essay in the *Edinburgh Review* in 1823 prompted this controversial stance by Dunglison. MacCulloch based his "mischievous assertions" on a flawed interpretation of information obtained from an "animated miasmometer" during a devastating outbreak of malaria in 1809 among British troop at Walcheren, an island in Holland. After his own inspection of the data, Dunglison concluded that "effluvia from rotting organic material could not" by itself, "transmit malaria." In his refutation of the Edinburgh article, Dunglison discussed malaria in general and the comparative prevalence of this "fitful pest" in Rome and other locations at different periods of history. He took strong ground in maintaining, that if malaria was due to vegetable decomposition alone, "every farmyard ought to present evidence of it, as both vegetable and animal decomposition are perpetually going on" throughout the year—not limited as it was to specific periods of the year. Throughout his academic life, Dunglison maintained an interest in all endemic and epidemic fevers, and he was among the few early advocates in America of quinine instead of calomel in the treatment of malaria.[39]

Another early effort by Dunglison was a review of numerous articles published in the transactions of learned societies and in monthly and quarterly journals published in England and foreign countries, with critical remarks. This work helped create a concentrated record of the medical literature and contained a great deal of useful information.[40] In addition, before leaving England in 1825, Dunglison wrote literary pieces for the *Annals of Philosophy*, the *Quarterly Journal of Science,* the *Universal Review* and the *Eclectic Review* and published a work of 201 pages entitled *Commentaries on Diseases of the Stomach and Bowels of Children* (see Figure 16).

This work of erudition impressed Francis W. Gilmer and may have been an important factor in Dunglison's engagement to teach at the University of Virginia. The preface of this book included an excellent account of the "Physiognomical System," of Jean François Nicolas Jadelot (1771–1855), a theory that the scrutiny of an infant's face could lead to a diagnosis of internal disease.[41] Dunglison's book contains chapters on intestinal worms, constipation, acidity, flatulence and colic, diarrhea, procidentia ani, vomiting, cholera, aphthae, inflammation of the stomach and intestines, and one of the earliest chapters on intussusception. It exhibits an early propensity on the part of the author toward heroic intervention, views that Dunglison was soon to moderate under Jefferson's influence.[42]

Dunglison's early literary labors earned him much admiration and respect in England. In a notice in the *London Medical Repository* in October 1824, Dr. James Copland captured the sentiment of many of his learned countrymen:

> It is impossible for us to announce the departure of our Colleague, Dr. Dunglison, to occupy a highly honourable professional appointment in a foreign country, without expressing great regret at the loss we shall experience in the privation of that assistance we have been accustomed to receive in our Editorial labours. At the same time we gratify ourselves in stating our confidence that his industry and talents will be more advantageously and beneficially exercised for the promotion of Medical Science, and that we shall have, from time to time, opportunities of seeing the result. We part with him, on every account, reluctantly; and it would be a common–place, unworthy of the occasion, did we confine our public adieu to a mere expression of regret, or a simple record of good wishes. He is now Professor of the Institutes and Practice

> of Medicine in the University of Virginia–an University recently endowed by the American Congress, through the influence of Mr. Jefferson, the Ex–President of the United States: – and we are quite sure he will be well received among our Transatlantic Brethren.[43]

Later events show that this last prediction was not particularly accurate. Indeed, the reaction by some professional "Brethren" in America to Dunglison's appointment at the University of Virginia was openly hostile, likely driven by jealousy and self-interest.[44]

By the time Dunglison attracted Jefferson's attention, he had initiated a scientific career path similar to Jefferson himself, minus the politics. Before the age of twenty–five, Dunglison was a prominent member of multiple intellectual societies, had published a book and many articles, was an active and respected correspondent, and had in general both the intellect and convivial disposition to be recognized by the medical profession. But on a personal level as well Dunglison reflected Jefferson in his embrace of novel instruments and meticulous recordkeeping, disavowal of unverified theories, preference for hands-on observation, endorsement of lifelong education, and more. The two were brethren in curiosity and controlled inquiry, the older American in vertebrate paleontology, medicinal botanicals, insects, geography, climate and vaccine medicine, the younger Englishman in the locus and progression of disease. Small wonder that Jefferson found his candidacy appealing.

Recruitment, Journey Abroad, and Reception in the United States

One may wonder why such a talented and well-educated young physician at the outset of a promising career in London would leave that city to accept a teaching position at a fledgling university in the backwoods of rural Virginia, especially when one considers all of the obstacles that had to be overcome. Clearly, there were many unknowns and some serious barriers that might have dismayed all but the most zealous candidates.[45] Would the foreign professors find the strange and remote community in which they would be secluded congenial to their tastes? Would the Englishmen who were accustomed to stately colleges and universities with centuries-old buildings and traditions of scholarship running back to the mediaeval age be satisfied, at first, in a university of red brick too raw to be covered with ivy and boasting as yet no achievements to spur emulation and excite a sense of pride? How much latitude would professors have in controlling their own time? Would the foreign professors, being new to America, survive dangerous epidemic disorders? Would the expense of the overseas journey be covered? What was the cost of living and would all reasonable amenities be available in Charlottesville? Would the fixed salary of $1,500 be raised when the institution got fully underway? Finally, would professors be compelled to subscribe to any particular religious principle or aid in the propagation of any doctrine or speculative tenet about which sects differ? Additional, more general questions were being asked by both enlightened thinkers and enemies of the institution: Was the scheme of the University of Virginia permanent or simply an experimental proposition? Realistically, what would the size and intellectual aptitude of the first class of students be? How would the foreign-born instructors, most of whom were quite young, embrace Jefferson's mandate that each professor teach many different courses during a ten-and-one-half-month academic term while simultaneously pursuing productive scholarship? Was Jefferson's unconventional thinking about education and medical training, as well as his rejection of any religious grounding for the school, suited to nineteenth-century America?[46] Were his expectations of young professors too high, and the institution's resources insufficient?

A number of people, notably the Bostonian Oliver Wendell Holmes (1809–94), correctly surmised that the department head positions at the University of Virginia were not simply "Chairs," in any traditional sense, "they were full settees," requiring of the occupants an extraordinary depth and breadth of knowledge, as well as incredible industry.[47] Other concerns related to the short vacation (one six–week block) and the season at which it fell (from 15 December to the end of January). The requirement that faculty devote the majority of their time to their academic duties was especially troubling in the medical school, since "eminent" physician-educators, in the United States and abroad, had grown accustomed to retaining sizable incomes from lucrative private practice.[48]

None of these unknowns, potential barriers or restrictive employment conditions disheartened Dunglison. He readily consented to come to Charlottesville, and he provides the reason for his decision in his Autobiographical Ana, writing that when Gilmer offered him the position:

> it was a matter of serious deliberation on my part, and on that of some of my intelligent friends, ... whether I should avail myself of it. All agreed, that if I remained in England for a few years, my worldly affairs would be in a more prosperous condition than if I went to Virginia; one overwhelming reason, however, decided

> me. I was ardently attached to a daughter of Mr. Leadam, whom I could not expect to be able to marry if I remained in London, for years to come; whilst if I embraced the American offer I could do so immediately.[49]

As soon as Gilmer offered the professorship, specifying a salary and other benefits, Dunglison called at the residence of John Leadam, a prominent London apothecary, and asked his daughter Harriette if she would go with him to America.[50] She readily assented, whereupon Dunglison accepted the proposition of Mr. Gilmer and entered into a covenant with him on September 28, 1824. The original contract, a copy of which follows this paragraph, specified a "suitable" annual salary, use of one of the University pavilions free of rent and a portion of the tuition fees from students attending his classes. And it included an incentive clause allowing Dunglison to increase his annual compensation beyond the base salary of $1,500, by admitting more full-time and part-time students to the department of medicine. From the outset, however, it was clear that this incentive opportunity should not be abused; only properly credentialed students would be admitted. This was accomplished, in part, by negotiating a guarantee—"that, during the first five years, the remuneration of the incumbent was not to be allowed to fall below twenty–five hundred dollars."[51] Having already abandoned his earlier interest in a wholly commercial life, Dunglison thought $2,500 per year would yield a comfortable subsistence, at least at first, allowing him and his spouse to begin raising a family that eventually included seven children, four of whom were born in Virginia.[52] The contract also included language that suggests a certain reciprocity of responsibility, alluding to both a signing bonus and a default penalty.

The actual contract stated:

> This Covenant entered into on the 28th day of September in the year 1824, at London, between Francis W. Gilmer, attorney in fact for the University of Virginia of the one part, and Robley Dunglison of the other part, Witnesseth; that the said Gilmer attorney in fact for the Rector and visitors of the university of Virginia, doth hereby appoint the said Dunglison a professor in the said university, and covenants with the said Dunglison that he shall as professor aforesaid, occupy one of the pavilions of the University free of rent; and shall receive from the said university as a salary for his services, the sum of *fifteen hundred dollars* money of the united States, *per annum*, payable semiannually or quarterly, as the

> rector and visitors may prefer. and moreover, the said Dunglison shall be entitled to receive as a tuition fee, from each student who attends his class & no other, the sum of fifty dollars *per annum*; from each student attending his class, & only one other, thirty dollars *per annum*; and from all other students attending his class, twenty five dollars *per annum*; nor shall these fees be diminished for the space of five years during which this covenant shall last, without the consent of the said Dunglison, and the said Dunglison will proceed with as little delay as possible to the University of Virginia, & will there teach to the best of his ability & with due diligence, anatomy, surgery, the history of the progress and theories of medicine, physiology, materia medica, & pharmacy; that he will suffer no waste to be committed in his tenement, that he will maintain the internal of his pavilion, the doors, windows, & locks external, in as good repair & condition as he shall have received them; that he will conform to the rules & regulations of the visitors &c: and to secure the faithful performance of every of the above covenants, the said Dunglison binds himself to the said Rector and Visitors of the University of Virginia, in the sum of five thousand dollars money of the united States; and the said Gilmer binds the Rector and Visitors of the University aforesaid, to the said Dunglison, in the same penalty: In witness of all of which, the said parties have hereto set their hands & affixed their seals, on the day & year first above written.[53]

The financial arrangement worked out with Mr. Gilmer and Mr. Jefferson set a precedent, one very slow to take hold in American medical education. The concept of a guaranteed salary combined with rent–free quarters, sufficient to provide for a living in the United States, was unheard of in the early nineteenth-century, both in the United States and in Europe. In French medical schools, where hospitals were the historic focus, professors received little or no salary and had no financial stake in the size of their class, getting nothing from students. Their source of revenue derived largely from private practice or family wealth. In English and American schools, medical teachers received a stipend from students, each of whom paid a sum when they obtained a ticket to attend a specific course of lectures. Many of the students who were admitted on payment of their fees were at best marginally qualified, and in some cases wholly unprepared for a rigorous study of medicine. Although these fees belonged to the teacher, they were "hardly ever" sufficient for complete support. In virtually every medical school of the time, teachers supplemented their income by private practice, a situation that surely inhibited meaningful research and most scholarly writing.[54]

In line with Jefferson's belief that professors ought to focus on the educational business of the university and eschew outside career interests, Dunglison's employment agreement contained a provision restricting private medical practice. The original Board of Visitors resolution of April 1824 stated that each professor "shall engage in no other pursuits of emolument unconnected with the service of the Univ[ersi]ty without the consent of the visitors."[55] In limiting "this distracting privilege," Jefferson correctly surmised that Dunglison's maximum attention to his statutory duty, both as a teacher and medical writer, would be assured. Twice, the Board passed resolutions that partially eased the original restriction on clinical practice by its professor of medicine. A March 1825 revision permitted medical practice provided that it remained within the precinct of the University. The second resolution that autumn stated that "The Board, considering that it will be for the benefit of the school of Medecine that it's Professor should have opportunities of keeping in mind, to a certain degree, the practical part of his profession, and of acquiring moreover a knolege of the peculiarities of disease incident to our climate and country, are of opinion that, besides the habitual practice within the precincts of the University, allowed by a former resolution, he be permitted also to act as a consulting physician elsewhere, so timing these avocations, however, as not to interrupt the regular business of his school."[56] Coincidentally or not, this final change freed Dunglison to make house calls as Jefferson's personal, trusted physician at the same time that it enabled him to obtain a broader view of local disease. Although the original, restrictive employment covenants at Virginia proved to be an "insurmountable obstacle" for virtually every other potential candidate from Great Britain,[57] Dunglison readily accepted them. Moreover, when engaged in limited clinical practice, Dunglison typically rejected any form of remuneration. This latter point is illustrated below.

Voyage to Virginia

After agreeing to Gilmer's terms, Dunglison immediately began making preparations for the voyage to America. Haste was necessary because Jefferson had clearly indicated that he expected all of the foreign professors to arrive in Charlottesville well before the start of classroom activity on February 1, 1825. First, Dunglison had to marry Harriette Leadam, which he did on October 5, 1824. The couple then departed from London on October 27 to board the ship *Competitor,* an ordinary merchant ship docked at Gravesend downstream from London and bound direct to Norfolk, Virginia. Two other newly appointed professors, Charles Bonnycastle (professor of natural philosophy)[58] and Thomas Hewitt Key (professor of mathematics),[59] along with his wife, were also passengers on this ship.

The decision to sail to America on the *Competitor* proved unfortunate. The voyage, which required fourteen weeks instead of the usual thirty-seven days, was "most uncomfortable," at times mortifying and "much delayed." Dunglison observed that passengers on the merchant ship were but "incidents" to "administer to the cupidity of the Captain," a Mr. Godby, who was "unpolished, selfish and had no great liking for philosophers." Foul weather hampered the voyage from the outset, so much so that the passengers were first detained at the Downs for several days. After leaving the mouth of the Thames, they were forced to disembark at Motherbank between the Isle of Wight and Portsmouth harbor, and remain there for weeks, exposed to the "worst storm ever experienced on the southern coast of England." The hurricane nearly capsized the "old log of a ship with rotten sails." More than six weeks passed before the repaired vessel was able to clear the English Channel on December 16. Poor food, incompetent navigation, estrangement between the captain and his passengers, contrary winds and a violent storm off Cape Hatteras, characterized the remainder of the voyage, which finally ended in Norfolk on February 10, 1825. The three-and-one-half-month long journey on treacherous high seas must have prompted Dunglison and his bride to wonder at the wisdom of their decision to venture to a new land. It certainly "excited the greatest apprehensions for our safety in the mind of Mr. Jefferson; and in all those who felt concerned in the success of the new University."[60]

But the ordeal was not over even then. The winter trip to Charlottesville by stagecoach was not inviting, taking the party along the "vilest roads," worse than any of them had encountered "in all our previous experience in England or on the Continent of Europe." The stage overturned in a deep muddy rut, forcing the party to walk the last two miles to Charlottesville. Dunglison, who apparently possessed a spirited sense of humor, recalled this last mishap: "The accident occurred at a short distance from Moore's Creek, over which there was no bridge, and we were, consequently, compelled to ford it, bearing the ladies over; and such was our unpropitious introduction to the neighbourhood of the University. A Roman would have regarded it as a bad omen, and been disheartened. We were not Romans, however, and the affair only excited amusement."[61] After a brief stay in a

University hotel (its term for student cafeterias), the Dunglisons moved into their own pavilion on the grounds of the campus. Although he was quite impressed with the exterior design of his pavilion, he recalled later that the living quarters seemed to have escaped Jefferson's attention to detail, for the space "would have been far more commodious, had Mr. Jefferson consulted his excellent and competent daughter—Mrs. Randolph—in regard to the internal arrangements."[62] There they slept on the floor until their bedsteads arrived. None of these travel adventures diminished the resolve of the new medical professor. Nevertheless, the late arrival of the medical, mathematics and natural philosophy professors obliged the Board of Visitors to delay the opening of the University until March 7, 1825, which occasioned "enemies of the institution" to "whisper in public places that this dilatoriness would be certain to damage its hopes of permanent success."[63]

Seven of the eight original professors at the University of Virginia were foreign-born,[64] and of these seven, four were Englishmen: Dunglison, the aforementioned Charles Bonnycastle and Thomas Key, and George Long (1800–79), who was a Craven Scholar at Cambridge University and a fellow at Trinity College at the time of his appointment to the chair of ancient languages.[65] The other European-born professors included Dr. George Blaettermann, (1782–1850), a German educated at the universities in Leipzig, Heidelberg, and Göttingen;[66] John Patten Emmet (1796–1842), who, although born in Dublin, Ireland, was educated in America, first at the United States Military Academy at West Point and later at the College of Physicians and Surgeons of New York City, where he received an M.D. degree in 1822;[67] and George Tucker (1775–1861), the oldest appointee at the age of fifty, who was born in Bermuda and there obtained his initial training in the profession of law in the office of the island's principal barrister before immigrating to America at age twenty to study at the College of William and Mary.[68] Tucker was the one most familiar with the habits of Americans, and was chosen Chairman of the Faculty for the first session.

Nativist Criticism of the Selection of Dunglison

In choosing Dunglison, Jefferson was severely criticized for this supposed "slight of American Medicine."[69] Medical and political writers alike described Jefferson's action as: "invidious," an unmitigated "violation of propriety," and as "most injudicious and subversive of the general good of our citizens, and especially of the dignity and interest of our professional brethren" of the United States. Several northern newspapers, including the *Boston Courier*, the *Connecticut Journal*, The *New York Monthly Chronicle of*

Medicine and Surgery, and the *Philadelphia Gazette*, published scathing criticisms of Jefferson's recruitment decision and suggested that "Mr. Gilmer could have fully discharged his mission, with half the trouble and expense by a short trip to New England, or by a still shorter trip to Philadelphia." Others asserted that "The sending of a commission to Europe to engage professors for a new university is, we think, one of the greatest insults the American people have received," and "there can be no stronger proof of the occasional thoughtlessness; of a great man; than his attempt to place importrd mediocracy in a situation which could be filled by native talent "[70]

Despite such calls for censure, Jefferson's determination to obtain, at any cost, men of unquestioned capacity and demonstrated scholarship never wavered. Unperturbed by journalists imbued with an intense nationalist fervor and several Northern politicians, Jefferson's defense was simple—that Dunglison and the other foreign-born men represented the best talent available; only inferior men could be recruited to a new university unless capable ones were enticed by "considerable temptations" from some other institution. Jefferson believed that it was "not honorable or moral to endeavor to seduce" the best men from American universities, and he strongly opposed the alternative course of attracting men "unemployed and secondary characters." The latter would have been unfaithful both to his ideals and promises and to public expectations. Jefferson also noted that he had "been much squibbed for this" by disappointed applicants in America.[71] Nonetheless, not only did he refrain from compromising his standards for the faculty, he also respected the professorates of other universities.

Rather than poach the best and brightest scholars from American institutions of repute such as Yale and Harvard, Jefferson pursued a "minor brain drain" of Europe. In a letter to J. Evelyn Denison, penned in 1825, Jefferson said,

> I have no reason to regret the measure taken of procuring Professors from abroad where science is so much ahead of us. you witnessed some of the puny squibs of which I was the butt on that account. they were probably from disappointed candidates whose unworthiness had occasioned their applications to be passed over. … the Professors brought from abroad were as happy a selection as could have been hoped, as well for their qualifications in science as correctness and amiableness of character. I think the example will be followed and that it cannot fail to be one of the efficacious means of promoting that cordial good will which it is so much the interest of both nations to cherish … for these two nations

> holding cordially together, have nothing to fear from the United world. they will be the models for regenerating the condition of man, the sources from which representative government is to flow over the whole earth.[72]

Unlike Jefferson, Dunglison was depressed by the hostile response to his appointment to a professional chair in America. This may have been due, in part, to the fact that the most scathing criticism had appeared in the *Philadelphia Journal of the Medical and Physical Sciences*, which at the time was perhaps the most prominent medical periodical published in America. (See Figure 17). The article was written by its editor-in-chief, Dr. Nathaniel Chapman (1780–1853), who was also professor of the theory and practice of medicine at his alma mater, the University of Pennsylvania. In 1820, he founded the Philadelphia journal to counter an attack on American culture and science made by Sydney Smith in the *Edinburgh Review No. LXV*. Smith had disparaged American culture in general, but Chapman was particularly incensed by Smith's provocative question "What does the world yet owe to American Physicians and Surgeons?" He kept this quotation on the title page of his journal for many years to impress on patriotic Americans their duty to support home–grown science."[73] Due in no small measure to Chapman's plea that others join him in protesting "against this act of injustice," Dr. Charles Caldwell as late as 1842 complained of the supposed gall of Dunglison, who, having scarcely as yet "felt an American pulse, or made a single visit to an American sick room," dared to think, shortly after arriving in the United States, that he had "a complete knowledge of American diseases, and was perfectly competent to their treatment and care, and also to become an instructor in them to others." Dunglison retorted in his memoirs that excellence rather than nationality should be the criteria for the selection of scholars, extolling this as the practice at the University of Virginia.[74]

After stewing privately for a few months, Dunglison received a decided boast when he was "agreeably surprised" to learn, on September 23, 1825, that Yale University had conferred on him the degree of doctor of medicine, honoris causa.[75] The man who orchestrated this honor was himself an eminent scholar, Dr. Nathan Smith (1762–1829), who had founded three of the first eleven medical schools in the United States: the medical schools of Dartmouth (1798), Yale (1810) and Bowdoin (1820). Smith and Dunglison had much in common. Both men had received their medical education abroad, and both were considered "more modern" in their thinking than the Dr. Benjamin Rush of Philadelphia. They were also among a small group of American educators who had won election as "corresponding members" of the prestigious London Medical Society. This acclaim, it seems, came largely because of their "literary celebrity."

Jefferson's decision to recruit the most able persons possible, wherever they might be found, was a valuable one. It kept the University from mediocrity in its early years. As he wrote to Joseph Cabell, "you know that we have all, from the beginning, considered the high qualifications of our professors as the only means by which we could give our institution splendor and preeminence over all it's sister seminaries."[76]

In conclusion, in Dunglison, Jefferson found a medical leader who resembled him in intellectual heritage and interests, the ethics of scientific belief, professional recognition, and prolixity of scholarly output. In agreeing to appoint Dunglison to head the medical department, Jefferson chose a candidate who reflected and practiced the medical ideas he himself had espoused for decades, with the exception of heroic intervention, which, as will be seen, Jefferson probably taught Dunglison to eschew. The following chapter will recount how Jefferson and Dunglison worked together in launching medical education at the University of Virginia's very beginning and how, after Jefferson's death, Dunglison continued to apply the scientific creed both men shared.

Chapter 5

ESTABLISHING ACADEMIC MEDICINE IN VIRGINIA—1825–1833

The object of a public teacher is no longer to inculcate a particular system of dogmas, but to prepare his pupils for exercising their own judgments, to exhibit to them an outline of the different sciences, and to suggest subjects for their future examination.

Dugald Stewart[1]

WHEN DUNGLISON arrived in Charlottesville, conditions were discouraging at first. There was no instructional equipment, no amphitheater for large-group lecturing, no facilities or cadavers for anatomical dissection or any other type of demonstration exercise, and no medical library. The Medical Department was "as yet unprovided with it's proper subjects and apparatus, not possessing even a skeleton to begin with."[2] Dunglison later described "the duties assigned to this chair" as "more multifarious than are attached, so far as I know, to any professorship of medicine in this, or in any other, country."[3] Nevertheless, Dunglison was quick to channel his energies and mobilize support from Jefferson and other members of the Board of Visitors in correcting these early deficiencies.

This chapter will show how Dunglison cooperated with Jefferson during his life and continued his legacy after the first University rector's death in July 1826 by growing the University's teaching apparatus as a whole and creating a science-based medical curriculum with the requisite infrastructure. Specifically, Dunglison's energy and vision led to an enhanced and well-curated library collection, a new anatomical theater, rigorous but supportive classroom instruction, including a multitude of practice-based learning exercises, and a campus dispensary. Throughout his career at Virginia, Dunglison continued to publish nationally and internationally in the medical field, further enhancing his and the University's reputation for advanced study and a rigorous academic culture.

Initial Priorities

In the years leading up to the opening of the University, Jefferson set in motion a plan for building a first-in-kind collegiate library and having it strategically placed in "the noblest of all buildings," in the most handsome and spacious dome room of the centrally located Rotunda at the northern end of his educational institution, "where, in alcove after alcove, galley upon galley, the large collection of volumes was to be arranged."[4] Indeed, the library of the University of Virginia was unique among institutions of higher education in its location, scope and cost, authoritative quality, purpose, and organization.[5] While Jefferson clearly looked to the special knowledge of the professors in selecting the books and periodicals for their respective schools, he "manifested as much solicitude about the acquisition of a carefully chosen library as he did about the employment of competent professors; and he foresaw, from the start, that the books, like the men, would have to be imported from foreign countries."[6] This latter point should not be surprising. Books of great erudition in early nineteenth-century America were scarce, and the country's scientific literature was generally judged to be meager and inconsequential, especially by European observers.[7]

Most antebellum colleges and virtually all medical schools in America placed little or no emphasis on establishing an excellent library. Like Jefferson, however, Dunglison understood the differences between compulsory and higher learning, agreed that the success of higher education required proper facilities, and regarded a well stocked and serviceable library, similar to those in the English universities, as essential for higher learning and meaningful scholarship. A great library, if properly organized and maintained so as to serve the needs of each academic department, and *used by learners*, was seen as an indispensable educational tool.[8] Throughout his eight years at the University of Virginia (1825–1833), Dunglison took an unusually active interest in the affairs of the library, more so than any other of the original professors. His efforts included: (1) promoting the passage of many policies concerning library operations; 2) monitoring the performance of the book-buying agents in New York and Europe, and apprising the Board of Visitors of any dilatoriness in carrying out Jefferson's plan; (3) superintending the complete inventory of the library collection and its printing in an 1828 catalogue; (4) pushing Jefferson, the Board of

Visitors, and even the governor of Virginia, for an annual appropriation of funds for additional new works of erudition in order to keep pace with advancing science in other countries; (5) purchasing medical journals from his own purse and encouraging other professors to do the same for the benefit of their respective schools; (6) serving as the first "inspector" of the library, "whose duty was to report any cause of complaint to the general faculty;" and, (7) taking steps to resolve problems with moisture from a perpetually leaking Rotunda roof so that serious injury to library material would be avoided.[9]

Because the task of organizing the library was not completed in Jefferson's lifetime, much of the work fell to Dunglison and the university librarian, William Wertenbaker. Under Dunglison's guidance, the task of acquiring and making accessible the works on Jefferson's original list was completed, albeit with several significant alterations.[10] The 1828 Catalogue, the preparation and printing of which he supervised, contained many modifications of Jefferson's original library plan. Most of the changes were made to ease the path of discovery for the diligent learner. New titles made the collection more up-to-date, and some books from Jefferson's original list were deleted; all foreign-language titles were translated in the catalogue, which included bibliographical data on author, title, place and date of publication, language, number of volumes, and size; and the number of subject categories was reduced from 42 to 29, although in the case of the medical book collection the number was actually expanded from 2 to 11, as will be discussed below.

By 1828, the collection had reached massive proportions, totaling slightly more than 8,000 well-chosen volumes, prompting one observer from New York City to describe the library as "larger and more beautiful than the library in the capital."[11] A later historian remarked that "no University or other library in this country was planned [and assembled] with so wise an understanding of its purpose," and that "no other institution in the United States had expended on its library in the year of its founding so large a sum."[12] The cost was substantial and surely exceeded Jefferson's original estimate of $24,076.50, probably by at least one-third.[13]

Curating the Collection of Medical Books and Journals

In constructing the medical library, Dunglison displayed considerable insight, taking great care to include the best, most current editions,[14] a collection of "facts and reflections, which may be looked upon as constituting the existing state of the science, without wandering into idle speculation."[15] Of the 710 volumes acquired, comprising 435 different medical titles, the vast majority (81 percent) were published between 1806 and 1827. The medical collection was larger than Jefferson had proposed[16] and organized in narrower categories that aligned the collection better with the needs of the student learner. Instead of Jefferson's two very broad groupings (Anatomy & Surgery, and Medicine), the revised plan contained eleven. They consisted of the History of Medicine: its theories and principles of practice from Hippocrates to the present; Hygiene, or the art of preserving health; Materia Medica & Pharmacy; Medical Jurisprudence & Toxicology; Anatomy – Sound and Morbid; Physiology in health and disease; Pathology and Therapeutics; Operative Surgery; Obstetrics; Veterinary Medicine; and General Medicine, comprising dictionaries, transactions of medical societies and periodicals. Of critical importance, these library subject areas corresponded to required courses in the medical department. Students could thus match library holdings with topics being explored in the lecture hall.

In keeping with Jefferson's plan, 93 percent of the medical works were imported from Europe. Of the foreign titles, 51 percent came from France (Paris, Montpellier and Lyon), reinforcing the hypothesis that Jefferson and Dunglison both perceived medical advances in Paris as cutting edge. Thirty–two percent of the books were from Great Britain (London, Dublin and Edinburgh), with the remainder from the Netherlands (Leiden, Amsterdam, Utrecht), Germany (Berlin, Leipzig, Nürnberg, Frankfurt and Göttingen), Italy (Venice, Florence and Milan), Switzerland (Geneva) and Austria (Vienna). American titles comprised fewer than 7 percent of the total collection. The 1828 catalogue included seven authors from Philadelphia: William Paul Crillon Barton, Nathanial Chapman, John Redman Coxe, William Potts Dewees, John Syng Dorsey, John Eberle and Benjamin Rush; two from New York: Theodric Romeyn Beck and David Hosack; and five from Boston: Jacob Bigelow, William Cheseldon, James Jackson, Benjamin Waterhouse and John C. Warren.

The library was widely patronized from its inception, due in no small measure to the pedagogical practices of the original professoriate, who all demanded much more of their students than classroom work. According to Philip A. Bruce in his *History of the University of Virginia*, "The first year the completed library was open to readers, thirteen hundred and forty–five volumes were taken out," and "the numbers of volumes withdrawn in the following year were thirteen hundred and twenty-four."[17] Another scholar observes that "during the first session, all but 10 of the

123 enrolled students had borrowed books."[18] A more detailed analysis of the book—borrowing records for the better part of the first two years, March 1825 through December 1826, reveals that a total of 2,238 library titles were individually checked out by students.[19] Of these titles, 724 were circulated solely to students enrolled in the medical department. Book loans to the latter accounted for roughly 32 percent of the total number of books checked out for this almost two-year period. This total is impressive, given that the medical students during this time made up only 14 percent of the total enrollment. The average medical student checked out fifteen titles representing a wide range of materials, from classics to chemical tables to ancient histories. For example, Edwin Drummond borrowed versions of Dryden's Plutarch, the works of the Earl of Chesterfield, Cicero, and Shakespeare, Edward Gibbon's *History of the Decline and Fall of the Roman Empire*, and Mercy Otis Warren's *History of the Rise, Progress, and Termination of the American Revolution*. He also read widely in the sciences, covering atomic theory, William Cheselden's *Anatomy of the Human body*, Thomas Thompson's Chemistry and John Murray's *Elements of Materia Medica and Pharmacy* along with many other titles. Drummond's book-borrowing habits indicate that at least one medical student was reading in subject areas outside his specialty, and thus realizing Jefferson's hope that matriculates at the University of Virginia would be well versed in a range of subjects.

Equipping a "Museum" for Teaching Anatomy and Pathology

Dunglison's second task, begun within months of his arrival in Charlottesville, was to create an outstanding teaching museum of anatomical preparations, not from a single source but from all over the new and old world.[20] The collection of samples of both normal and morbid conditions was used to illustrate lectures on anatomy and surgery. It was eventually housed in the Anatomical Theatre, an edifice that at Dunglison's arrival was more a set of sketches by Jefferson than an actual building.[21] This effort was consummated through the purchase of materials, most but not all of which were imported from Italy, France, England and Scotland.[22] The collection included dried body parts from dissected cadavers, wax and plaster models, castings and carvings, various anatomical plates, and elaborately detailed paintings—"imitations of every part of the human body under various circumstances"[23] — and an exhibition of the "diversified instruments and apparatuses of modern surgery." The expanse of Dunglison's vision is partially revealed in an undated list he sent to Jefferson, received May 21, 1825.[24] The anatomical items that he most coveted included (1) male and female skeletons; (2) John Lizars's extensive collection of anatomical plates of the human body, from Edinburgh, accompanied with descriptions of physiological, pathological and surgical observations; (3) models of a head, likely a series of plaster craniums, laid out according to the system of Franz Joseph Gall and Johann Gaspar Spurzheim; (4) a head injected so as to exhibit the course of the carotids, as well as the vertebral arteries; 5) sections of the head to exhibit the falx cerebri carried down through the face; (6) an injected preparation of the heart and the adjacent vessels and the thoracic duct as well as a dried preparation of the heart to show its valves, cavities and chordae tendineae; (7) a dried preparation of the larynx and trachea; (8) a preparation of the lungs "in Spirit" to illustrate their vascularity; (9) a preparation of the stomach, wet or dry; (10) injected preparations of the intestines, liver, spleen, pancreas and kidneys; (11) any preparation to shew the mesenteric vessels and lymphatics; (12) a prepared penis, and testes with the artery, vein and vas deferens injected; (13) a dried urinary bladder; (14) urinary and biliary calculi; (15) a dried preparation of the uterus, bladder, rectum, etc., in situ; (16) male and female pelvises (two or three female); 17) a preparation of ligaments, especially of those of the pelvis; (18) bones injected and rendered transparent to show their vascularity; (19) a preparation to show the cancelli of bone; (20) a wet preparation to show the thoracic and abdominal viscera in situ in a child (anterior view); (21) fetal pelvis and skeleton; (22) an injected fetus to exhibit the fetal circulation; and (23) any morbid preparations with the histories attached. Regarding this last item, the intended use may have been for clinical-pathological correlations.[25] Jefferson demonstrated his responsiveness to Dunglison's desire to build an excellent teaching museum in his correspondence with purchasing agents in the United States, England, and Italy. In October 1825 Jefferson reported on behalf of the visitors that $3,157.50 had been deposited in London for the acquisition of materials necessary for anatomical education.[26]

The assemblage of teaching tools was so extensive that it included a "decomposable brain" — a model that could be separated into many parts to demonstrate its most striking features, as well as models, on an enlarged scale, of the intricate auditory apparatus and the organs of vision, speech and deglutition.[27] Dunglison later specified in his *Valedictory Lecture* that the unique stages of existence are infancy up to the seventh year, adolescence, the period after puberty, manhood, and incipient old age. He evidently intended to use these specimens and models to teach his students about fetal development and show them the structural changes that separate children from adults.[28] The collection was comprehensive in scope and consisted of anatomical preparations and other materials from the best sources in Europe. For this reason, it differed from collections at other medical schools in America, which were largely obtained from a single source, typically a personal collection donated by a retiring physician or surgeon.[29] Southern medical museums generally did not obtain specimens, models, and illustrations from European sources until the 1850s.[30]

The Anatomical Theatre

Another essential priority for Dunglison was construction of an Anatomical Theatre on the grounds of the University. Jefferson stated in 1818 that "the practical aspects of human anatomy" were to be "fully covered" at the University of Virginia, an indirect but clear reference to dissection.[31] Dunglison agreed.[32] Although considerable knowledge of the human body, in health and disease, could be gained by cohesively combining lectures, readings from carefully selected textbooks[33] and study of the anatomical and pathological specimens in a well-stocked museum, students needed more. In keeping with other medical schools, Dunglison realized that those learning to be physicians would benefit most by dissecting freshly procured cadavers, or at least observing "expository dissections" prepared by a professor or a prosecting demonstrator. In any case, hands-on dissection of human cadavers was from the start considered to be a standard element in the Medical Department's curriculum and was thus integrated into the rules and oversight of the University.

Another consideration, albeit one of secondary importance, was Dunglison's belief that he should not be expected to carry out all of his teaching activities in his residence. Under Jefferson's original plan for his university, all professors were expected to teach all of their subjects in the pavilion where they lived, in lecture rooms designed for roughly 150 students. The professors of disciplines with a laboratory component soon pointed out the shortcomings of this approach[34] Mrs. Dunglison found it particularly irksome, since it entailed the possible dissection of cadavers in her home during her first pregnancy, which culminated in the birth of a daughter, Harriette Elizabeth, on October 29, 1825. Fortunately, Jefferson quickly took steps to correct the problem. Even before Dunglison arrived in America, Jefferson advised Cabell, a member of both the University of Virginia's Board of Visitors and the Virginia General Assembly, that an anatomical theatre would be "indispensable to the school of anatomy" and added that "there cannot be a single dissection until a proper theatre is prepared giving an advantageous view of the operation to those within, and effectively excluding observation from without."[35] In this same letter, Jefferson also predicted that the cost would be "about as much as one of our [dining] Hotels," which he reckoned at approximately $5,000. As with most other buildings at the university, the actual cost wound up being much higher.[36] Shortly thereafter, the building of an Anatomical Theater was approved by the Visitors and Jefferson's design for it was accepted.[37] The inspiration for Jefferson's architectural plan came from several sources. It drew on existing European anatomical theatres and was quite similar to the early seventeenth-century design of Vidus Vidius (Latinized name for Guido Guidi), whose posthumously published plan also featured an octagonal surgical theatre on the top floor and emphasized strong lighting provided by rooftop skylights.[38] Dunglison played a role, later recalling that Jefferson agreed on the need for a building dedicated to anatomical purposes and offered to "choose the position and the architectural arrangement externally, whilst all the interior arrangements should be left to me."[39] Benjamin Henry Latrobe may also have been an influence, having designed the first anatomical theatre in America in 1805 for the medical school associated with the University of Pennsylvania.[40] Construction began in May 1825, but the theatre was not ready for occupancy until July 1827.[41] When completion extended to a second year, Dunglison was greatly frustrated, inasmuch as he favored a cycle during which "a course of lectures on [descriptive] anatomy should be followed, before practical anatomy [dissection] is prosecuted, – upon the principle, that it is well for a traveller to possess some knowledge of the geography, names, &c. of a district, before he undertakes a journey through it."[42]

The University of Virginia's Anatomical Theatre was a perfectly square, three–story building situated on a steep slope that descended from east to west, in close proximity to the Rotunda (see Figure 18). Its internal floor plan included 1,735 square feet of usable space on each level. The top level housed the octagonal–shaped theatre and featured tiered seating arranged in concentric circles to enhance sight lines and acoustics for everyone attending lectures and anatomical demonstrations. (Figure 19). The middle story contained the "teaching museum" mentioned earlier, and the lowest level was the "charnel," where cadavers would be stored and later disposed of. In 1833, after students in the vicinity of the Anatomical Theatre complained of an "extremely offensive odor," the Board of Visitors directed the professor of anatomy to use a distantly located small brick building "across a ravine" for "a boiling house and receptacle for subjects immediately after dissection." In 1837, all dissection work was moved to this facility, and it became known as the "stiff house."[43]

According to Richard Guy Wilson, professor of architectural history at the University, the Anatomical Theatre departed significantly from the classical order and symmetry of Jefferson's academical village. "It was an appendage – stuck on at the last minute," but a structure that nevertheless showed Jefferson to be "open to change and suggestion."[44] More importantly, it represented a belief, shared by both Jefferson and Dunglison, in the value of experiential learning. Furthermore, the University's Anatomical Theatre with its attached dispensary was evidently unique in early nineteenth–century America since it was owned and operated by the university; fully funded through a state appropriation; housed in a permanent building suitably constructed for consolidation of all medical teaching from its inception; and strategically placed on the main grounds, not separated from the residential university precinct.

Dunglison realized that cadavers would be difficult to obtain, especially in a small town like Charlottesville, and when dissection was done, it would *have* to be a fast-paced affair, because of the lack of facilities for chemical preservation and cold storage. Procurement records are lacking for the early years, and the exact number of anatomical dissections performed is unknown. It appears that only in the 1850s did cadavers (predominately Black) become plentiful at the university, and that access to such bodies may have been much greater in the Deep South than in Charlottesville.[45] Throughout most of the nineteenth century, human dissection in America was severely "frowned upon as immoral, irreligious, and a posthumous disgrace, and was seriously impeded by state laws prohibiting the legal acquisition of cadavers."[46] Because of this, most cadavers were obtained by the "heinous practice of grave robbing to secure bodies," or by requesting in advance the bodies of criminals condemned to execution.[47] Northern schools, typically located in large urban areas, used agents who pilfered corpses from potters' fields. In the South, grave robbers concentrated on procuring bodies of enslaved and free people of color, as well as corpses of destitute and friendless whites. The acquisition of black bodies for medical research and education in the South probably did not result from a conscious, organized plan on the part of white southerners to learn more about differences between the races in order to subjugate and support the existing social hierarchy, as some have suggested.[48] The simpler and more plausible explanation is that the bodies of deceased Blacks were more readily available and accessible, in part because their survivors had no effective recourse to judicial authorities to enforce protection of their graveyards.

Accordingly, every medical school in the South and West, as well as some in the North, relied heavily on cadavers of Blacks, often obtained in the large cities of the Deep South by mercenary-minded body snatchers and sold and shipped elsewhere.[49] The rampant practice of robbing the graves of these legally invisible and socially voiceless individuals resulted from blind indifference to the dignity of the dead of a different race, consensus about the educational merits of dissection, and the existence of a cottage industry focused on the grim trading of corpses for money.

Novel Approaches to Teaching Medicine

Dunglison perceived it as a duty to establish a pedagogical practice that would enable his students to acquire the knowledge and skills, including the intellectual and moral discipline, necessary for a lifelong career of scientific inquiry leading to merited distinction and honor.[50] In the most basic language, Dunglison articulated his duty as one that was intimately intertwined with his pupils:

> It is, moreover, the business of the medical professor to lighten the labors of the student. It is for him to collect and condense the existing knowledge of the subject he teaches, to explain away difficulties, and to suggest materials for reflection – trains of thought – that may tend to expand the minds of his hearers; but this reflection and these trains of thought ought to accompany the well devised lecture, and the chief labor of the [student's] evening should be, to embody the information, that has been acquired through the day, and to investigate the facts and arguments on which it reposes.[51]

Dunglison embraced his role in stimulating discovery and critical thinking among his students and assumed that his job as a teacher of a professional discipline was skillfully to analyze, synthesize, and present in the clearest possible way information gathered from, or generated by, past and present observation, experience, logic and reasoning, by himself and others. But, by the same token, he expected students to labor to construct their own understanding through inquiry-based study and reflective analysis. In other words, the professor was to facilitate and guide, challenge, and motivate, but the students needed to assume personal responsibility for the quality, depth and scope of their learning experiences. Thus, Dunglison's teaching philosophy employed strikingly modern pedagogical principles, such as constructivism, inquiry–based learning that was collaborative, and the importance of reflective analysis by students.

Since lectures were the primary mode of organized medical education, Dunglison took them seriously. Much like Jefferson, Dunglison understood the purpose of lectures as two-fold—to impart vital knowledge on what was known and unknown (content), and to teach students how to learn for themselves (process). Lectures alone were not to take the place of private individual study, but to inform the pupil how that study might be pursued to advantage. Both men believed that learning is not something that one can do for another, and that much of the weight leading to thorough comprehension must fall upon the learner. A pedagogical approach demanding frequent independent study was supported by the presence of a reasonably accessible and well-provisioned lending library, which as noted above was guided by Dunglison, who was thus in a position to ensure that the reading materials available for students coincided with the subjects of his lectures.

From the outset, colleagues at other medical schools considered Dunglison's teaching load to be unusually heavy,[52] and it was. He was expected, according to the original enactments of the Board of Visitors, to undertake with due diligence "the whole domain of medicine."[53] Every week, throughout the ten and one–half months of the academic term, he covered all of the subjects assigned to him in two lectures, each about ninety minutes long, on Tuesday, Thursday, and Saturday. In the beginning, Dunglison was the only professor in the Medical Department, although from the commencement of operations on 7 March 1825, Dr. John Patten Emmett (see Figure 20), the professor of natural philosophy, taught chemistry—a subject also considered essential for medical students seeking an M.D. Even so, Dunglison's heavy course load comprised physiology, descriptive and practical anatomy, pathology, materia medica and pharmacy, the history of the progress and theories of medicine, and surgery. By modern standards, this expectation was truly prodigious, and Dunglison carried it out with uncommon distinction and to the great advantage of his students. Moreover, he recognized the advantage of having one professor in charge of all medical students, arguing that, "These various subjects, embracing the departments of the healing arts… are usually assigned, in medical colleges, to at least four professors, but there is this convenience in having them taught from the same chair, that they are more likely to form one harmonious and consistent whole, and, consequently, to be better understood by the student than when his mind is distracted, as is too often the case in literary institutions, by the discordant sentiments of different teachers."[54]

The University Dispensary and Clinical Instruction with Patients

In addition to lectures and various exercises, Dunglison's teaching included a prescribed amount of clinical instruction on ambulatory patients. During the first session of medical instruction at the University of Virginia, he proposed the construction of an outpatint clinic with pharmacy to Jefferson, who quickly offered his full support and drafted a statute for Dunglison's review before obtaining approval by the Board of Visitors in April 1826. The following year, this "University Dispensary" was established as an adjunct to the Anatomical Theatre. There, in accordance with action taken by the Board of Visitors in April 1826, Dunglison was to remain after his lectures on alternate days, in order to render medical and surgical care to the people of Charlottesville and surrounding counties. This enactment also required that a monthly notice to this effect be inserted in the Charlottesville *Central Gazette* "for the purpose of keeping under constant notice, all those who may wish to avail themselves of the benefits of the Institution." "All poor, free persons" were seen "gratis," whereas all others, "bond or free," were charged 50 cents. The money so collected by the institution was used to purchase surgical instruments for ordinary operations, medicines and salves, and to cover the cost of the cowpox vaccine, with vaccinations administered free of charge to "all persons," with university students particularly encouraged to participate.[55] Medical students were required to attend these clinics and assist in their ministrations. Under Dunglison's supervision, they were enjoined "to examine the patients by the pulse, and other indications of disease, to ask them such questions as the Professor shall think pertinent and shall permit, and to acquire a practical knowledge of the process of pharmacy by taking part in the preparation of medicine."[56] The latter requirement is noteworthy. In contrast to many other American schools, the chair of the Medical Department of the University of Virginia emphasized the importance of a comprehensive "pharmaceutical education," which included hands-on instruction in "the art of compounding," of bringing together ingredients to make pills and potions. Dunglison sought to avoid the all-too-common circumstance of a young practitioner who found himself in a rural setting where there was no apothecary and no one properly educated in "the sensible properties of the various articles of the Materia Medica, and with the mode of preparing the different formulæ – officinal and extemporaneous."[57] He did not want his graduating pupils to be deficient in pharmaceutical preparation. They should be able, if needed, to assemble on their own the medicines they prescribed. In stark contrast with this, when the Philadelphia College of Apothecaries was founded in 1821, the medical school associated with the University of Pennsylvania stopped teaching pharmacy, "except in a limited way as part of the medical course."[58]

As a supplement to this hands-on experience, Dunglison probably also encouraged his students to read in American and European pharmacopoeias, easily accessible in the university's library, which contained 76 volumes and 47 different titles in its materia medica and pharmacy section, including numerous textbooks and treatises by prominent Americans and Europeans. They were not, however, to accept all formulations contained therein as useful, safe, or effective. Dunglison informed his students that the "London Pharmacopoeia contains about 230 articles; *the* pharmacopoeia of the United States about 280, and the Parisian upwards of 900—yet there are few practitioners who employ a fifth part of those that are comprised in the London Pharmacopoeias which is only one-fourth as copious as the French codex." Seeking to safeguard public health, both Jefferson and Dunglison wrote about the need to purge the materia medica of ineffective and dangerous drugs. Dunglison, in his lectures and published works, said that far too many formulations "that crowded the shop of the apothecary" had been "admitted into the catalogues of the materia medica," only to be quickly "discharged from them as injurious or inert." He spoke out against the "faulty reasoning which occasioned the admission of numerous articles into the lists of materia medica," arguing that "there must be a still further diminution to get rid of those articles that possess no advantage … relics of ancient ignorance." The lists should "embrace those agents only whose virtues and applications are understood."[59]

Philip A. Bruce, in his History of the University of Virginia, provides further insight into Dunglison's pedagogy: "The thoroughness of his system of teaching was illustrated in his course on materia medica . . . he first discoursed at length on the virtues and uses of the different articles, and then recapitulated the whole lecture; or else he recapitulated, equally as fully, at the end of the description of each article. In addition, he examined his pupils once a week on the subject of that week's lectures,—not, as he said, to catechise them, but to bring back again whatever might have been forgotten."[60] Dunglison himself said, "In this manner, the facts and theories of a science are impressed three times, upon the memory of the pupil; and if, after this, he is unable to retain them" and demonstrate sufficient learning throughout the academic term, then "he must be pronounced incorrigible," or at least, an academic laggard.[61]

In all of his courses, Dunglison's creative approach to teaching epitomized

Jefferson's objectives for university education, with due emphasis on the scope and rigors of academic study. Dunglison nurtured his students to become steady, disciplined and intelligent, in applying "the three great methods of acquiring medical knowledge." These were listening to lectures that were judiciously prepared and clearly presented; reading that was efficient and profitable to the learner; and cultivating individual powers of observation, reflective thought, and inductive reasoning.[62] His pedagogy emphasized discovery and explorations of the unfamiliar rather than drill and recitation of age-old knowledge.[63] Like Jefferson, Dunglison did not want his students chained to the present state of medical knowledge, to any inappropriate veneration for the supposed superlative wisdom of past generations, nor to the preposterous idea that it is always good to look backward for better principles rather than looking forward.

Dunglison often spoke of "obstacles and stumbling blocks in the path of the young student," and he sought to "to remove everything of mystery from the science" that it was his lot to teach; "to separate fact from hypothesis, and to attempt to exhibit it, as far as it is capable of being exhibited, as a demonstrative science."[64] Much of his academic writing, especially at the University of Virginia, was completed so that he would be able to offer his students an up-to-date, highly organized and analytical review of the existing state of the medical sciences, free from mystical and subjective contaminations.[65] He never distorted the science of medicine with heterogeneous and confusing nomenclatures, which he called "unintelligible" and "jargon."[66] Instead, Dunglison's style was one that always sought to put before the student terms and phrases that conveyed precise and authentic principles, which everyone could understand. To young medical aspirants, he was a purifier, a simplifier and a unifying organizer—a man whose whole aim was "to strip away all technical mystery, to illuminate every dark recess," so that his students could gain free access to all sources of useful knowledge, "with a view to improve them on rational principles."

Samuel X. Radbill, who edited and published Dunglison's memoirs, recognized his abilities as a teacher of medical students, saying that "He was a teacher in all he did, a friend to the young, devoted to his students and their interests, being always associated as a pedagogue with the young medical students."[67] Dr. Samuel D. Gross (1805–84), a distinguished surgeon at Jefferson Medical College in Philadelphia, added "Dunglison was remarkable for his fluency, the choice of his language, his melliferous voice, and the ease and grace of his manner," and he emphasized how conscientious he was in preparing his lectures and how few disciplinary problems he had. Available records suggest that Dunglison's students were diligent learners and well behaved outside the classroom, in marked contrast to those in other schools within the university who became notorious for violent attacks on enslaved laborers, hotel keepers, faculty, and local residents.[68] As a lecturer, Dunglison was lucid, entertaining and instructive. He held the attention of his class and brooked no whispering, lounging or disorderly conduct on the part of his students."[69]

Tests and Examinations, a Gauntlet to Graduation

Dunglison recognized that one of the most important drivers of student learning is how that learning is assessed. Student attitudes toward their studies are strongly influenced by the nature and timing of fair, yet challenging, examinations. His personal experience of the rigorous requirements for obtaining a medical degree in European universities made Dunglison critical of the American testing system. He quipped that the oral examinations in effect were so farcical that the term "Doctor" meant not "a learned man, but a man who will have to be learned." Fueled by Jefferson's authoritative edict to protect the credibility of the University of Virginia degree, Dunglison implemented a rigorous system of oral, written, and public examinations, so as to impress on his students the necessity of disciplined study from the very beginning of the academic term. He did not believe oral examinations alone were adequate, as the method made it difficult to determine the standing of a student relative to his peers and, if the class size was large, impossible to put a sufficient number of questions to each individual.[70] All who sought the title of M.D. in Charlottesville would have to run a gauntlet of examinations that tested the severity of their devotion to medical study, in each and every department of the science. Daily questioning was intended to reinforce ideas. As mentioned in Chapter 3, immediately before each day's lecture, students were quizzed on the preceding lecture and any assigned textbook reading. Their preparation, thus tested, was recorded numerically, and the mean of these numbers, indicating a student's average standing in each class, was communicated to his parents or guardian in a circular notice that was sent home at the close of each month. The assigned numbers, which in effect measured a student's day-to-day learning, were defined as follows:

5. Signifies very well prepared

4. Signifies well prepared

3. Signifies tolerably prepared

2. Signifies badly prepared

1. Signifies very badly prepared

0. Signifies entirely unprepared

Daily examination enabled Dunglison to revisit material as needed and gave students an ongoing metric for identifying and retaining correct information throughout the term, thereby avoiding the hazards of cramming, before a midterm or final examination, which Dunglison regarded as unhealthy, ineffective, and unlikely to result in long-term retention of course material.[71] This system of regularly assessing the assiduity of each student and weeding out the "incorrigibles" set the Medical Department apart from all other similar institutions in early nineteenth- century America.[72] "One happy result" of the graded curriculum of the University of Virginia, was "the enviable success" of its graduates in securing positions "for medical service in the army and navy and for hospital and other appointments."[73]

From the start, the medical school administered two "general examinations" – an "intermediate" (midterm) and a final. The final examination was a written test that complied with Jefferson's authoritative expectations outlined in chapter 3. It was patterned on the rigorous Oxford system of written examinations with a numerical grading scale. In an 1831 publication, Dunglison described each element of the final examination, including anonymous grading of the results to avoid favoritism, and his system of assigning a point value to each question that was in line with its difficulty, as well as the length of time they were likely to take and the importance of the skills they assessed. In formulating the final examination: "1. The chairman of the faculty shall appoint for the examination of each school, a committee consisting of the professor of that school, and of two other professors. 2. The professor shall prepare, in writing, a series of questions to be proposed to his class, at their examination, and to these questions he shall affix numerical values, according to the estimate he shall form of their relative difficulty, the highest number being 100. The list, thus prepared, shall be submitted to the committee for their approbation. . . . 3. The times of examination for the several schools shall be chosen by the chairman [of the faculty]. 4. At the hour appointed, the students of the class to be examined shall take their places in the lecture room [elliptical room of the Rotunda], provided with pens, ink and paper. The written questions shall then, for the first time, be presented to them, and they shall be required to give the answers in writing with their names subscribed. 5. A majority of the committee shall always be present during the examination; and they shall see that the students keep perfect silence, do not leave their seats, and have no communication with one another or with other persons. When, in the judgment of the committee, sufficient time has been allowed for preparing the answers, the examination shall be closed, and all the papers handed in. 6. The professor shall then carefully examine and compare the answers, and shall prepare a report, in which he shall mark, numerically, the value which he attaches to each; the highest number for any answer being that which had before been fixed upon as the value of the corresponding question. 7. This report shall be submitted to the committee, and if approved by them, shall be laid before the [entire University] faculty, together with all the papers connected with it, which are to be preserved in the archives of the university. 8. The students shall be arranged into three separate divisions, according to the merit of their examinations as determined by the following method. The numerical values attached to all questions are to be added together [i.e., maximal possible score], and also the values of all the answers given by each student. If this last number exceeds three–fourths of the first, the student shall be ranked in the first division; if it be less than three–fourths, and more than one–fourth, in the second; and if less than one–fourth, in the third." Only those who scored in the top quartile were deemed eligible for graduation, and only if they met other conditions.[74]

To receive an M.D. degree, each student ranked in the top quartile had to be declared "eminent" by the committee of professors, an honorific based on their performance in the classroom throughout their careers at the University, a satisfactory grade on both the Latin and English exams, and recognition that they were honorable men of high moral achievement. If all these conditions were met, the name of the student was presented to the Board of Visitors for a final decision. In the awarding of the M.D., degree, no school in America required more than the University of Virginia. Indeed, the system of examinations and requisites for graduation at the University of Virginia as a whole were far broader and more rigorously enforced than in any other American school of higher education.[75] It had the highest standards of scientific and literary scholarship – standards that were not surrendered even in the darkest days of the school's need.[76]

Dunglison's views on medical education were widely disseminated through his writings. Like Jefferson, he believed that the study of medicine required untiring industry in the acquisition of principle-based medical knowledge, including standards of ethical behavior and professional etiquette for which he drew heavily on the writings of Dr. John Gregory and Thomas Percival.[77] Only those "whose minds have been properly tutored for its investigation" should enter upon the study. Not surprisingly, both men favored a strong preliminary education of the student in mathematics, the literary classics and languages, especially English, and in the natural sciences. They lamented the "prevalent belief . . . that a less degree of talent is required for a physician than for a lawyer," commenting, "strange enough! we sometimes hear a parent speak of placing a son – of the strength of whose intellectual powers he has some doubt – to the study of medicine, because he [the guardian] is apprehensive that his talents might not enable him to succeed in the profession of law. Occasionally, too, we hear the remark, that a certain individual 'has a natural turn for physic;' is 'born, as it were, a physician.'" The exercise of the healing arts is not a "gift," and it was and is misguided to think that physicians "were born, not made." In this regard, Dunglison's pattern of thought was clear; "it may be laid down as incontrovertible, that he whose intellectual manifestations are generally feeble, cannot carry with him the necessary qualifications to the bed of sickness." The ability to minister to the sick requires a truly immersive University education, not merely an apprenticeship supplemented with a few rudimentary courses. Indeed, "no department of science or of art demands greater judgment, a higher reach of intellectual qualifications, or a deeper preparation, by physical and moral culture, than medicine."[78] Unfortunately, preparation for a career in medicine throughout most of the 19th century was mainly guided by the old saw – "a boy too dumb to study classics, too immoral for the pulpit, or too dishonest for the bar should study medicine."[79]

Physiological Science in the Curriculum

Jefferson advocated the teaching of physiological science as an essential element in medical education, and he found a willing partner in Dunglison, who was keenly aware that this subject received much more attention at European colleges and universities than it did in America, and that the works published overseas dwarfed the meager literature of American medical authors. Most medical schools in the United States throughout the eighteenth and early nineteenth centuries paid little more than fleeting lip service to the study of physiology. Rather than teach it separately, it was woven into other, supposedly more important courses.[80] The subject was, however, said to be Dunglison's "special delight," and he considered himself a pioneer in the systematic and detailed teaching of the subject in America. He always took pride in the belief that the University of Virginia was the first institution of higher education in America to deliver a full course of lectures and practical demonstrations on the general principles of physiology in health and disease from its inception. Moreover, in 1830, he influenced the Virginia Board of Visitors to offer physiology as an elective for students in the other schools of the university.[81] Through his familiarity with the work of von Haller, Magendie and other enlightened thinkers well represented in the University library,[82] Dunglison recognized the exigent importance of inculcating principles of physiology and functional pathology—of moving beyond "dead anatomy," which many eminent professors in the early decades of the nineteenth century still deemed to be the sole foundation of medical study. Even in Philadelphia—considered to be the mecca of medical education in America—only anatomy stood out, in the opinion of practical-minded faculty, as really important in the preclinical training of medical students.[83] In all of his teaching activities, Dunglison emphasized the importance of coherence and integration of subject material, as well as a strong foundation in the basic biological sciences. In one of his published works, he wrote that,

> it is not only essential, that proper books should be placed in the hands of the students; there should be an appropriate selection of subjects, to be investigated by him in due sequence. It often happens, that the very first book, put into his hands, is on the 'practice of physic' …which cannot be comprehended without an adequate knowledge of its elements. . . . In other words, when an important organ is diseased, we must know the structure of the organ; the function which it executes in health; the characters of that function, when in a state of aberration; the indications to be laid down for transmuting the diseased into the healthy condition; the agent capable of carrying into effect such indication; and – if we put more than one article into the prescription – we must know, that the articles are not incompatible, unless we desire the chemical results of such incompatibility.[84]

Dunglison's stress on physiology represented a shift from viewing the human body as a series of parts to understanding organs as functioning components of a system. This was essentially a move from a taxonomic and specimen view of organs to one that stressed the relation of anatomical form to systemic function. Disease itself became not just tissue deterioration but rather the interruption of processes, within a single organ and among other organs.

History of Physic as a Medical School Course

In addition to his pedagogical philosophy regarding the preclinical medical sciences, which was unique in early nineteenth–century America, Dunglison was also among the first to advocate study of the history of medicine.[85] He believed that it should be given as a course after the student had completed a series of introductory lectures on the various branches of physical sciences, preferably in the second half of the first year, or between the first and second year. This was not to be, for the original enactments required that the teaching of this subject commence on the first day of classroom work. As was the case with his other five courses, Dunglison gave one lecture per week on the history of physic, for a total of up to forty-five lectures during the ten-and-a-half month academic term.[86] The decision to teach medical history fits in well with Jefferson's broad cultural concepts of education, according to which the student was not merely to be taught the novelty of the day but also "something of the earlier progress of the science and the art."[87] In conformity with Jefferson's desire, Dunglison became the first academician to include formally and clearly a comprehensive course of lectures on the history of physic within a medical–school curriculum in the United States.[88] Dunglison's own series of lectures on medical history, as delivered at the University of Virginia, was published posthumously in 1872 by his son Richard, who recalled that his father had "deplored the fact" that the historiography of medicine had been "wholly neglected" in virtually every medical school in America. Even later, only three of fourteen leading medical schools offered a substantial course of lectures (from 8 to 16 lectures) on the history of medicine at the turn of the twentieth century. Although the University of Virginia was listed among the leaders, by then it had discontinued its seventy-five-year tradition of teaching medical history.[89]

Dunglison derived the content of his conspicuously detailed course on the "History of Medicine from the Earliest Ages to the Commencement of the Nineteenth Century" from two main sources: *The History of Physic* by John F. Friend (1675–1728), which had been published in 1725 and earned the author fame as the first English medical historian, and the widely celebrated *Versuch einer Pragmatischen Geschichnte der Arzneykund* (Attempt at a Pragmatic History of Pharmacology) by Kurt Sprengel (1776–1833) of the University of Halle. Dunglison went as far as to translate and condense Sprengel's works for the benefit of his students at the University of Virginia and the other schools at which he taught.[90] Sprengel, a keen classical scholar regarded as the finest, most learned and erudite professor in Germany, was an outspoken critic of speculative medical theories. His four–volume "pragmatic" history of medical therapeutics, published in 1800, undertook to portray the past with all of its errors and pitfalls, so that these aberrations might provide valuable lessons and reveal basic truths on which a more rational medicine could be developed. Sprengel's work deemphasized the strictly biographical aspects of medical history, stressing instead the connections between medicine, contemporary cultural, and philosophical forces, the moral sciences, and with great gravity, its communion with the world of mysticism, superstition, outright fraud and obfuscation by practitioners throughout ancient and more modern times.[91]

Like Jefferson and Sprengel, Dunglison believed students would profit from historical study, learning both from the successes and the failures of what others did or neglected to do in their time. He wrote in 1831 that "The mind of youth cannot be better engaged, during the early period of their university career, than in becoming acquainted with the classic models of antiquity, and practised in the habits of discrimination which the study engenders."[92] With innumerable examples, Dunglison demonstrated in his lectures that scientific advance was far from being a straight-line event, that the chart of human progress had been a stumbling affair, up and down, uncertain and sometimes devious—first a sudden leap forward, then a pause followed by a purposeless wandering, leading at times to actual retrogression. A favorite example was Hippocrates. Among the first to recommend therapeutic restraint, Hippocrates believed in diligent study of the natural history of disease and in placing trust in the sanative power of nature, "the first of physicians." He taught that excesses of all kinds are dangerous, that those in perfect health should abstain from all forms of medicine, and that for the sick, physicians ought to pay attention to the age of the patient, the nature and severity of their affliction, and the climate and season in order to judge whether depletive treatment would be salutary or harmful. Unfortunately, as Dunglison pointed out, these teachings were not heeded. "If the route traced and pursued by Hippocrates with so much success had continued to be followed up, Grecian medicine would have attained in a short time a degree of perfection of which we can scarcely form an idea."[93]

Although Dunglison encouraged his student to learn from the staggering history of bad choices so as to avoid repeating past mistakes, he also instructed them to contemplate, celebrate, and be inspired by the high ideals, elevated talents and achievements of the great men of the past, in his words by their "accurate and faithful observations . . ., and by the sober and diffident reasonings of men of true medical and philosophical genius."[94] History could help students gain an awareness of the importance of medical and social ethics, as well as an understanding that the embryo of much of the most advanced contemporary medical practice could be found in the past. Moreover, Dunglison asserted that the study of history should not be regarded simply as decorative, expressing umbrage against the dismissive attitude of several prominent professors in Europe and America, notably John Gregory of Edinburgh.[95] As with any course in the medical department, the one on history featured rigorous written examination.

Medical Learning as a Lifelong Discipline

Dr. Samuel D. Gross (1805–84), a surgeon and colleague of Dunglison at Jefferson Medical College, observed that "Dunglison did not intend that the instruction he gave his students should be conclusive, but felt that they should continue their medical education with actual clinical experience."[96] Dunglison realized that the study of medicine extended beyond graduation and encompassed a commitment to professional education at all stages of life.[97] Quoting from an esteemed colleague, Dunglison wrote that, "the moment a practitioner ceases to be a student, he is no longer worthy of the confidence of the public, and that the life of a physician can only be truly useful and honorable, when it is unremittingly employed in study, in determining the truth of theoretical opinions by observation, and improving the value of practical suggestions by the test of experience. Collegiate honors, as has been justly observed by Montaigne, may form the pedestal: it is the man who forms the statue."[98] Dunglison went on to say that, "Academic instruction and University degrees may place the candidate for professional eminence in the best road for the attainment of distinction, but, unless he continues to toil, he can never reach what ought to be the height of his ambition."[99] In other passages, Dunglison stated:

> When the student has attained the *summi honores* of his profession, he ought not — it need hardly be said — to imagine, that he has arrived at proficiency, — that he has attained all knowledge respecting the intricate movements of the human economy, in health and in disease. The diploma, in reality, only shows to a discerning public, that the mind of the young practitioner has been imbued with the principles of medical science; and that he is prepared, at the outset, to profit by every opportunity for observation; to trace the nature of disease from indications that

> may be afforded him, and to apply his remedies to such disease, guided by all the lights, that illumine the profession in its present improved condition.[100]

Dunglison believed passionately that scientifically prepared physicians must at every stage of their careers do everything in their power to avoid becoming merely an "unsophisticated observer":

> Instead of vague and disconnected observations, unsuggested by rational hypothesis, the philosopher now — as he ought always to have done — sets out with a preconceived idea, the result of profound thought, and careful examination of every fact or phenomena, that can have any — the most remote — bearing on the subject of his inquiry. He observes, and compares the recorded observations of others with his own, and if, after a sedulous examination into every possible source of fallacy, he finds, that observation confirms and establishes his hypothesis, he correctly infers, that he is justified in regarding that which was, at first, put forth hypothetically to be a law of phenomena, and a solid addition to science. If, on the other hand, the results of reiterated observation of phenomena do not support — and, *a fortiori*, if they negative — his preconceived hypothesis, he unhesitatingly rejects it, and substitutes another, which has to be subjected to the same scrutiny; and thus he proceeds, until, at length, he succeeds in framing and establishing one, that receives unquestionable support from observation.[101]

Like Jefferson, Dunglison thought that learning was a never-ending process that requires "untiring zeal and industry" in the pursuit of the skill and habits of a genuine investigator. Indeed, a requirement for successfully transitioning from a competent novice on graduation to a masterly practitioner is the scientific method—the exercise of which must involve deep and comprehensive thinking, especially analytical reasoning, and of "every faculty that exalts the mind, and of every feeling, that adorns the heart."[102]

Recommendation of Residency

In order to attain the necessary and correct experience before entering independent practice, Dunglison recommended as "very desirable — where it can be effected," a residency "for a time in some hospital, infirmary or almshouse," especially one where "the attending physician and surgeon" are learned gentlemen, "well acquainted with their profession; faithful observers, good therapeutists, and able and willing to communicate to the student all that they themselves know, the grounds for their judgment, and the mode in which they propose to carry into effect the suggestions of such judgment." For clinical training to be profitable, whether in medical school or a postgraduate environment, instruction should be structured around useful cases that are commonly encountered in ordinary practice, rather than those that are singular and striking, and pupils should be taught to employ all "valuable auxiliaries in the discrimination of disease," including but not limited to "the gifts of modern times," such as auscultation. And if the goal is "*medicina efficax*," a phrase Dunglison used to emphasize therapeutic efficacy, the judicious and moral professor will readily eschew heroic agency of unproven benefit, and instead promote therapeutic restraint while constantly reminding his students of the sanative power of nature, good hygiene and healthy living.[103]

Expansion of the Medical Curriculum

In 1827, with the completion of the anatomical theater, three new courses were added to the curriculum of the medical department. Additional faculty were recruited or transferred and the department organized as follows: Robley Dunglison, M.D., chair and professor of physiology, history of the theory and practice of medicine, obstetrics, and medical jurisprudence; John Patten Emmet, M.D., professor of practical chemistry, botany, materia medica and pharmacy; and Thomas Johnson, M.D., demonstrator of anatomy, pathology and operative surgery.[104] The course on operative surgery was largely designed by Dunglison, possibly because the newly hired demonstrator of anatomy was inexperienced in pedagogy and needed direction.[105] As a result of this expansion, classroom teaching became more vigorous. With two new faculty members, the corps of professors was able to specialize, with each instructor now having "no more under his care than he can attend to with advantage to his pupils and ease to himself."[106] As a result of this redistribution of teaching, Dunglison was able to devote more of his time to literary and administrative endeavors. Not only did he become a prolific medical writer, but he also continued to shape and grow the teaching apparatus and reputation of the school.

This change of emphasis enabled Dunglison to begin teaching on medical jurisprudence or forensic medicine, the application of medical knowledge to legislative and judicial inquiries. Although not the first, this was an innovation that few schools offered in early nineteenth-century America.[107] Unsurprisingly, the course attracted many students from the School of Law that opened in July 1826.[108] Dunglison started this lecture series with a brief history of European legal medicine dating to the early sixteenth century. He covered (1) extinction of life, including procedures to be followed when investigating death in a healthy individual, sudden death without question of criminal agency, and death when there is a question of personal agency, such as suicide, murder from poisoning (a subject in which he displayed deep knowledge of chemistry, materia medica and, pharmacy, and therapeutics), strangulation, suffocation, drowning, foeticide, and infanticide; (2) injuries not leading to extinction of life, including maiming, mutilation, unnecessary surgical operations, corporal punishment—for example, child and spousal abuse, judicial flogging, and chastisements of slaves—rape and accidental injuries; (3) moral and physical conditions that were disqualifying for performing social or civil functions, including service in the military, matrimony, and government-sanctioned work; and (4) miscellaneous questions, such as those relating to feigned illness for personal gain (for example, pretended lunacy to escape punishment), the jurisprudence of insanity, deafness, and mental retardation, the legal and forensic aspects of deviant sexual behavior (that is, sodomy), sexual ambiguity and gender identity, and such reproductive issues as pregnancy, assessment of fetal viability, accidental and criminal abortion (medicinal and mechanical), virginity, impotence, and sterility. The course material also addressed divorce, survivorship issues, insurance contracts, physician warranties of health, medical evidence, and morally reprehensible situations such as practitioners who displayed false certificates of competency or performed unnecessary surgery.[109] In constructing his course on the principles and case law of medical jurisprudence, Dunglison borrowed much material from British, Spanish, French, and American authors, relying most heavily on notably the writings of John Gordon Smith (1782–1833).

In 1827, provisions were made for teaching obstetric science. Dunglison's inaugural course on obstetrics included didactic lectures and experience with the practice of the art. The content of his lectures focused on "the physiology of the pregnant and parturient states; embryology; as well as the different diseases to which the sex are subject, with the physiology and pathology of infancy." Dunglison introduced a form of simulated instruction in his section on demonstrative midwifery, writing that "the student should embrace every opportunity for noting the different presentations on the 'mannekin;' and for rendering himself familiar with the various obstetrical instruments, and their application. The young practitioner is apt to become confused, if, in applying his forceps, the locking parts of the blades do not correspond. Familiarity with the instrument, which can be acquired by very slight attention, will prevent this; and if he practise frequently on the mannekin, he will not have much difficulty in the adaptation of his knowledge to the living female."[110] Reliance on such methods was necessary because his students had no access to a lying–in hospital or even private deliveries in a home. Typical of most contemporary American medical schools, few graduating students had ever examined a pregnant patient or witnessed a birth. As in his other courses, Dunglison therefore expected students to supplement their comprehension of obstetrics with library research, and he took steps to make available the most highly regarded textbooks on the subject, including William Potts Dewees' pioneering American *Compendious System of Midwifery* by (Philadelphia, 1824), and the writings of the most esteemed French and English practitioner-teachers.[111]

In 1832, Dunglison secured the first regularly recurring appropriations from the Board of Visitors for the annual purchase of cadavers. In the same year, he helped produce the first University catalogue, which described the work in his department. It emphasized an extensive teaching museum, mentoring and quizzing as features, the ten–month course of study, and his belief that the theoretical instruction in basic medical science at the University was unexcelled.[112]

The Faculty Colleagues of Dunglison

John Patten Emmet (1796–1842 (see Figure 20) was born in Dublin, Ireland, the second son of a well-known Irish physician, nationalist lawyer and orator, Thomas Addis Emmet, and nephew of the famous Irish patriot Robert Emmet.[113] He was brought to the United States by his father at an early age and received all of his schooling in this country. Initially, this included a classical education in New York under the tutelage of Richard W. Thompson, a graduate of Trinity College in Dublin, until a "severe pneumonia" forced him to suspend his studies when he was sixteen. This and previous attacks of smallpox, measles, and whooping cough permanently undermined his health. After recuperating he spent three years at the United States Military Academy at West Point, serving as an "acting assistant professor" of mathematics in addition to being a cadet. When ill health again plagued him and prevented his graduation with a military commission, he went to Italy for a year, studying music, sculpture, painting and the Italian language. Afterwards, he returned to New York and began to study medicine at the College of Physicians and Surgeons under the direction of Dr. William James MacNeven, professor of chemistry, who there orchestrated the construction of a magnificent chemical teaching complex with laboratories and lecture rooms that would later attract Jefferson's attention.[114] Throughout his medical studies, Emmet's health remained so impaired that during the winter months he was frequently confined to his father's house. But this time was not lost, as he fitted up his own laboratory there in the house and applied himself assiduously to the study of chemistry, carrying out experimental research while absent from class.[115]

In 1822, Emmet received an M.D. degree from the College of Physicians and Surgeons after defending a 125–page dissertation entitled "An Essay on the Chemistry of Animated Matter," in which he argued for the application of chemical concepts to physiology and explicitly denied any function to a "vital force."[116] Although Emmet was careful to speak in terms of "proximate cause"—implicitly leaving room for an "absolute cause" or "first cause" underlying scientific phenomena—several religious leaders were outraged at its attribution of the formation of organic matter to chemical factors, a concept not widely accepted until 1844.[117] Dr. Henry W. Ducachet, writing in July 1822 in the *American Medical Recorder*, denounced Emmet's work as "materialism and infidelity." Although Ducachet admitted that inaugural dissertations were traditionally immune from public criticism, he felt that an exception had to be made in this case. He branded the essay as destructive to the "high and holy sanctions of morality" and went so far as to petition the medical school to renounce its acceptance of the dissertation. Much of this controversy derived from the theological position that ecclesiastical revelation must have primacy in all aspects of mind and body. Emmet's work was accepted, nonetheless, he graduated with distinction, and the entire faculty attested to his character and his prowess as a chemist.[118] The Ducachet article was widely circulated, however, and made it very difficult for Emmet to secure an academic position for several years.

Following his graduation, Dr. Emmet moved to the warm climate of Charleston, South Carolina, to protect his fragile health and establish a practice in general medicine. His clientele was slow to grow, however, leaving him ample time to compose and deliver a series of public lectures on practical chemistry to the townspeople. The highly favorable reaction to these lectures, as well as strong recommendations from John Torrey at West Point and Francis W. Gilmer, led to his hiring by the University of Virginia as professor of chemistry and natural history in 1825. During his first two years there, Emmet's annual teaching load consisted of a dozen lectures each in botany, zoology, mineralogy, and geology, and *eight dozen* in chemistry. His course on chemistry was unique in early nineteenth-century America in its length, its inclusion of both inorganic and organic chemistry, and its requirement that students perform experiments themselves, rather than simply observing the professor's demonstrations. Both Jefferson and Emmet believed that verbal instruction alone "is altogether inadequate." In order "to give to our Students the advantage of all the auxiliary appendages of a literary institution," a chemical-teaching complex constructed in the basement of the Rotunda included lecture rooms and a separate laboratory equipped with all essential accoutrements for research and instructional purposes.[119] The facility was modeled in part on MacNeven's chemistry laboratory at the College of Physicians and Surgeons. In planning this laboratory, Jefferson also consulted the work of other eminent chemists in America and Europe, including Thomas Cooper, then at Carlisle (later Dickinson) College, Robert Hare of the University of Pennsylvania, John Griscom of Queens College (later Rutgers University), John Torrey of West Point, and William T. Brande of the Royal Institution of London.[120]

Sometimes enrolling nearly a third of the student body, chemistry was one of the most popular courses at the University of Virginia, quite possibly because students were allowed to "practise all the operations of Chemistry relating (among others) to the analysis of Minerals, the reduction of ores and the Preparations employed in Medicine."[121] Between 1820 and 1870, students elsewhere rarely engaged in "actual laboratory instruction." Instead, they merely "witnessed the experiments performed in the lecture room, but were not permitted themselves to handle the apparatus." Exceptions were the previously mentioned William James MacNeven, and Amos Eaton at what would become Rensselaer Polytechnic Institute, in Troy, New York.[122]

Dr. Emmet remained at the University throughout his academic career, enjoying great success as a teacher, researcher and skillful administrator during his eighteen-year tenure. He contributed frequently to *Silliman's Journal* and the *Journal of the Philadelphia College of Pharmacy*, and, like Dunglison was elected to the American Philosophical Society. His published works demonstrated that iodide of potash affords a ready test for the presence of arsenic (1830), suggested that certain solutions of potash would give gypsum the solidity for which heat had previously been thought necessary (1833), discussed a new method of exhibiting the magnetic power of the horseshoe magnet (1833), inquired into the cause of voltaic current produced by the magnet (1834), wrote on caloric as a cause of galvanic currents (1834), and showed that formic acid could return metals in solution to their original state (1837).[123]

Dunglison held Emmet in very high regard, in part because of his many extracurricular attainments, such as fluency in multiple languages, skill as a musician, mechanical aptitude, and a becoming modesty.[124] Together, Dunglison and Emmet collaborated in many articles published in the *Virginia Literary Museum*, and performed original research, discussed below, on the physiology of gastric digestion, using the well–equipped chemistry laboratory in the basement of the Rotunda.[125] Emmet died in 1842, at age forty-seven with some of his failing health attributed to various accidents and mishaps suffered while he was conducting chemical experiments.[126]

Thomas Johnson joined Emmet and Dunglison on the full–time faculty of the Medical Department. Unlike Emmet, he did not receive high marks from Dunglison. Johnson was the first incumbent demonstrator of anatomy, pathology, and surgery. He lectured on anatomy and surgery, conducted dissections and demonstrations, and acquired cadavers for dissection, duties previously part of Dunglison's responsibilities, which he seemed pleased to surrender because "he could not bear the sight of blood."[127] Johnson may have owed his appointment in part to being a nephew of Chapman Johnson, who was one of the University's visitors. Johnson's career in Charlottesville was undistinguished. According to Dunglison, "he did not give entire satisfaction," and he resigned his position in 1834 when the Board of Visitors refused to raise his salary. Johnson then became associated with a short-lived Richmond Medical School before joining the newly organized Hampden-Sydney College Medical Department in 1838, the forerunner of the Medical College of Virginia established in 1854.[128] According to Blanton, Johnson's tenure at Hampden-Sydney was cut short as a result of "charges preferred against him, and he resigned in 1844."[129] Little is known of Johnson after this. He died at an almshouse in Richmond.[130]

The Number and Nature of the First M.D.s

In 1828, the University graduated its first class in medicine. Only three students were deemed qualified at that time to receive the M.D. degree.[131] Joining two Virginians, George W. McCulloch of Albemarle and Gessner Harrison (1809–62) of Rockingham, was Thomas Jefferson White of Florida. Harrison was the most distinguished student of the inaugural graduating class, having received diplomas from three separate schools—Medicine, Ancient Languages, and Modern Languages. He soon began a long and distinguished academic career in classical philology as professor of ancient languages at the University of Virginia, 1828–59, during which he used his medical knowledge "to elucidate, with special interest and success, the anatomical and physiological elements of language—to explain its relations to the human organs of speech, as well as the faculties of the human mind..[132]

By the fifth session, tweny-two students were enrolled in the medical school, and eight graduated (see Table 1). In this year, 1830 the first external recognition appeared, when the University of Pennsylvania acknowledged the high estimation in which it held medical graduates from the Charlottesville school.[133] Table 1 shows the number of students and graduates in the earliest years of the Medical Department.

Table 1. Matriculates and Graduates: 1825–1833

Session	Enrolled Students	M.D. Graduates
1825–26	20	0
1826–27	16	0
1827–28	16	3
1828–29	23	4
1829–30	22	8
1830–31	29	2
1831–32	25	5
1832–33	41	8
Totals	212	30

The small number of medical graduates from the University of Virginia in its early years inspired some critics to attack the worthiness of Jefferson's scheme of education. Many schools located in large Northeastern cities claimed that the best measure of success was the number of matriculates and graduates. The two largest medical schools in the 1830s were both in Philadelphia, with the University of Pennsylvania and Jefferson Medical College each boasting enrollments in the hundreds, later growing to more than a thousand between the two schools. One of the major factors attracting large quantities of students was the short length of study demanded of them.[134] The relatively modest Virginia totals showed, critics argued, that the "experiment in Charlottesville" was not working; few came to "drink of the cup of knowledge" and even fewer stayed the course. But it was precisely the high scholastic standards that kept the numbers in Charlottesville low. The unusually lengthy and arduous curriculum, coupled with the requirement of demonstrated competency by "rigid" examination, were unheard-of prerequisites for graduation in nineteenth-century America, and it should thus not be surprising that fewer than 25 percent of Medical Department matriculates at the University of Virginia, between 1825 and 1858, received an M.D. degree.[135] Indeed, the University of Virginia stood alone in its intentional exertions to provide a medical education of exceptional quality. Not until 1859 did a second school follow Virginia's lead, when the Chicago Medical School, later the Northwestern University School of Medicine, adopted reforms that elevated academic standards and included a graded curriculum, even though this put it at a competitive disadvantage with other nearby schools with lower standards. In 1870, Harvard joined the improvement crusade when its president, Charles Eliot, decided to lengthen the term of study, institute a graded curriculum, and subsidize faculty compensation with university funds.[136]

Although only 30 of 212 medical matriculates (14 percent) received the M.D. degree between 1825 and 1833, these graduates had unique characteristics when compared either to graduates of the other academic branches in the University or to virtually every other medical school in America. On entry to the school, they were older, with an average age of twenty-one years, suggesting that they had already devoted more time to study as a preliminary to their formal medical education. They spent more time at the University, averaging 3.2 academic terms, meaning that successful matriculates had devoted more than thirty months to classroom work as compared with the usual four to eight months in most other medical schools. The typical graduate of the University of Virginia Medical Department in its early years was a native Virginian (28 out of 30), 24 years old, and proficient in at least two other academic disciplines. The majority pursued postgraduate studies outside of Virginia, most often in Philadelphia, with others completing their medical education in New England or Europe. Many (24 of 30) then returned to Virginia to practice their art, usually in the four counties surrounding Charlottesville. The six graduates who settled elsewhere chose Missouri (3), Mississippi (1), Arkansas (1), and California (1). The group included one of Jefferson's grandsons, Benjamin Franklin Randolph, who graduated in 1831 from the University of Virginia with a doctorate in medicine.

Dunglison's Use of Enslaved Laborers

The construction of Jefferson's university, beginning in 1817, and its operations during its first half-century depended on the labor of enslaved people, both skilled and unskilled. At any given time between 1825 and 1833, 100 or more such persons worked on Grounds. The University owned very few of these individuals. Instead, the vast majority (that is, 97 to 99 percent) were purchased or leased from local residents by hotel keepers, administrative staff, or faculty. Each of the original eight professors used local slave labor to meet the domestic needs of their households,[137] Dunglison was no exception. His domestic needs were substantial and growing, owing to the birth of four children, the tenuous health of his wife, and his numerous professional responsibilities. On three occasions—in 1827, 1828, and 1832—he successfully petitioned the Board of Visitors to secure additional space for his servants. At first he rented enslaved laborers, beginning with a renewable contract with John Hartwell Cocke, a member of the Board of Visitors, to hire his slave, Nelson, for labor in Pavilion X's garden and stables.[138] Subsequently, Dunglison became a slave owner at the January 1827 Monticello sale of Jefferson's estate when he purchased Fanny Gillette Hern and her youngest daughter Bonneycastle, and two years later he added her husband, "Waggoner David" Hern, thereby keeping that enslaved family together.[139] By the time of the 1830 Census, Dunglison owned 11 of the 146 enslaved people on Grounds.[140] The fate of these enslaved laboring families following Dunglison's move to Baltimore in 1833 remains unknown. On leaving the University at least one faculty member, George Tucker, hired his enslaved servants out to other professors or local residents and later freed all of them.[141] Perhaps something similar happened in Dunglison's case.

Dunglison's Medical Practice in Charlottesville

Dunglison recalled that "During the whole period of my residence at the University of Virginia I practised my profession within the walls; but was not permitted to exercise it out of the University except in consultation—a restriction, which I greatly preferred."[142] This arrangement for professors was continued throughout much of the antebellum period. Some of the physicians on the faculty may have had a much larger practice than Dunglison, but surely none had more distinguished men as patients; his practice included four presidents or former presidents of the United States. While at the University, he was personal physician to Thomas Jefferson, James Madison, and James Monroe, and he was called into consultation in the treatment of Andrew Jackson.[143] Dunglison provided episodic care to Governor Randolph's family, to his faculty colleagues and their families, including obstetrical service, and to the student body. Beginning in

1827, when the campus dispensary was opened, Dunglison also offered a limited service to the community at large, doing so in part to help himself understand local diseases.[144] His on-campus practice included students, professors and their families, enslaved laborers, free people of color, and indigent whites. Unfortunately, no clinic records survive, making it impossible to know the exact proportion of free black, enslaved, and white patients treated. Dunglison typically rendered his professional services with no expectation of compensation. Certainly, this was true for indigent whites and free people of color. Enslaved individuals were usually treated at company expense, meaning that owners were expected to pay a modest dispensary fee of 50 cents for each episode of care.[145]

On medical matters, Dunglison came to admire Jefferson's progressive health views, and he could not help but be influenced by Jefferson's visionary thinking and forceful personality. Dunglison's publications reveal a sharp turning point after he came under the spell of Jefferson, who repeatedly emphasized medical enlightenment and education of the public as the best means of combating superstition, medical delusion, and outright quackery. His encounters with Jefferson evidently convinced Dunglison to moderate his use of drugs, giving up the fearsome and heroic therapy recommended in his book, *Commentaries on the Diseases of the Stomach and Bowels of Children*, published the year before he left London in 1824. Incidentally, this book may have been a reason, among others, for his invitation to come and teach at Mr. Jefferson's academical village.[146] And in contrast to most physicians practicing in Virginia at the time, Dunglison sought to classify and treat disease based on the affected system of organs rather than simply the symptoms that were produced. By attending the sick, and carefully observing the various occurrences in diseases, Dunglison believed information could be acquired that was critical to resolving the differential diagnosis of symptoms and to applying sensible and specific remedies aimed at combating the root cause of the affliction. Much like Jefferson, Dunglison came to realize the mettlesome futility of plying the patient with "shotgun" prescriptions. The therapeutic restraint adopted by Dunglison while in Charlottesville did admittedly lead local physicians to regard him as an "inert" practitioner. because he eschewed the "energetic and heroic treatments" that were universally deployed throughout Virginia. This criticism did not bother Dunglison, since he believed his parsimonious attitude toward "remedial agencies" would in time belong to an enlightened philosophy of "masterly inactivity." He was among a very small cadre of enlightened medical teachers who took the laudable position that "Every organized being is as a general principle, capable of repairing its own injuries when not excessive, and of exerting a sanative power in the cause of disease."[147]

Dunglison as Personal Physician to Jefferson and Other U.S. Presidents

Shortly after his arrival at the University, Dunglison was called to evaluate Jefferson, who was then eighty-two years old and suffering from a "great irritability of the bladder," meaning unusual frequency of urination.[148] After examination, the diagnosis was clear—an enlarged prostate accompanied by a urethral stricture. Dunglison prescribed the use of the bougie, a device that he described in his Medical Lexicon as "a flexible cylinder, variable in size, to be introduced into the urethra, œsophagus, rectum, &c., for the purpose of dilating these canals, when contracted. A simple bougie is composed of solid and insoluble substances; as plaster, elastic gum, catgut, &c. It acts of course only mechanically."[149] Jefferson soon learned to pass the device himself, and over time as the urethra became gradually enlarged, his "inconvenience" greatly diminished. Jefferson expressed his pleasure with the outcome, in part because of his personal participation in its solution and his enchantment with the mechanic arts. In his memoirs, Dunglison recalled, "whatever may have been Mr. Jefferson's notion of physic and physicians, it is but justice to say, that he was one of the most attentive and respectful of patients. He bore suffering inflicted upon him for remedial purposes with fortitude; and in my visits, shewed me by memoranda the regularity with which he had taken the prescribed remedies at the appointed times."[150]

Jefferson frequently sought Dunglison's medical attention and he fully expected to remunerate him. In the span of five months, between May, just three months after his arrival in Charlottesville, and September 1825, Dunglison traveled to Monticello on at least thirty-one occasions to render professional service, sometimes two or three times a week.[151] From the outset, he showed no interest in any form of payment. This prompted Jefferson to write a series of letters to Dunglison, asking that he be informed of "what compensation I shall make you," adding that "in this I pray you to do justice to yourself."[152] Dunglison replied:

> I know not how to express the gratification which I feel, at the subsidence of your troublesome affection [illness], nor the fervor with which I hope the favorable prognostication in which you have indulged may be verified. With respect to the subject of

> compensation for any trifling attentions which I may have been able to pay you – I beg that I may be allowed to fix my own terms, and to declare most firmly but respectfully, that the only compensation which I shall accept of, is — that which has already afforded me the greatest satisfaction – the being able in any respect to add to the comforts of one whose existence is so valuable to all but perhaps as much so to the Alumni of this Institution as to any.[153]

In nineteenth-century America, almost all practitioners expected payment for all "duly acquired" service, either in the form of a yearly contract or a set fee for each individual visit, with add-on charges for prescriptions as well as any device or instrument used in the care of a patient, and surgical procedures. Physicians in one region sometimes banded together and published a list of charges to which they would adhere.[154] That Dunglison refused a fee from Jefferson, except possibly on one occasion,[155] was not an abnegation of professional ethos but rather a sign of his respect, gratitude, and to a limited extent, friendship. It shows that Dunglison saw Jefferson as a scientific colleague, and from this alone it might be expected that he waive his fee, not as a professional courtesy among physicians, but from their shared roles as scientists and professional educators.

Dunglison continued to attend Jefferson until the latter's death on July 4, 1826. From the outset of their relationship, Jefferson gave Dunglison his entire confidence and at no time requested a second opinion. On one occasion, Mr. William Short, a longtime friend and former American diplomat, wrote Jefferson urging him to consult Dr. Philip Syng Physick, a renowned physician in Philadelphia. The former president promptly replied that his trust in Physick was "equal to yours, were he on the spot to judge for himself. I am however in very able hands, Dr Dunglison Medical Professor in our University"[156] And on another occasion, Jefferson's daughter showed her own confidence in Dunglison when she expressed her displeasure that Henry Lee, the son of General Henry "Lighthorse Harry" Lee, a bitter critic and political foe of Jefferson, had said that the family "ought not to trust the life of such a distinguished individual wholly to the hands of a foreigner!"[157]

In the spring of 1826, Jefferson was attacked by dysentery and suffered from its attendant weakness and malnutrition.[158] Dunglison traveled frequently to Monticello to comfort and minister to Jefferson at the close of his life, noting that his intellect remained vigorous even though his diarrhea was having a decidedly ominous effect on bodily power, reducing the former president to skin and bones. Most of those who visited the elderly statesman expressed apprehension that the illness would prove fatal, and Jefferson agreed.[159] During the final week of Jefferson's life, Dunglison spent all of his time at his patient's home, creating comfort when he could, and observing Jefferson's every behavior—how he carefully arranged his private affairs without regret, laying his well-used pen down only a few days before his death.

Even as he lay dying, Jefferson was consumed by the potential failure of his university. To bolster its chances of future prosperity, he stated that he wished James Madison to succeed him as rector, and he did so with cheerful confidence. This came as no surprise to Dunglison, who, as chairman of the faculty, had frequent occasion to consult both men, one-on-one, and recalled that "it was a common interrogatory—what did the other say of the matter?"[160] In a letter Jefferson wrote to Madison a few months before his death, he expressed his deep feelings for his friend of many years:

> the friendship which has subsisted between us, now half a century, and the harmony of our political principles and pursuits, have been sources of constant happiness to me thro' that long period. and, if I remove beyond the reach of attentions to the University, or beyond the bourne of life itself, as I soon must, it will be a comfort to leave that institution under your care, and an assurance that they will neither be spared, nor ineffectual. it has also been a great solace to me to believe that you are engaged in vindicating to posterity the course we have pursued for preserving to them, in all their purity, the blessings of self-government, which we had assisted too in acquiring for them. if ever the earth has beheld a system of administration conducted with a single and steadfast eye to the general interest and happiness of those committed to it, one which, protected by truth, can never know reproach, it is that to which our lives have been devoted. to myself you have been a pillar of support thro' life. take care of me when dead, and be assured I shall leave with you my last affections.[161]

That Jefferson desired to extend his life until the anniversary of his country's birth, is evident from this description in Dunglison's memoirs:[162] "In the course of the day and night of the 2nd of July, he was affected with stupor; with intervals of wakefulness and consciousness; but on the 3rd, the stupor became almost permanent.[163] About seven o'clock of the evening of that day, he awoke, and seeing me standing at his bedside, exclaimed, 'Ah! Doctor are you still there?' in a voice, however, that was husky and indistinct. He then asked 'Is it the fourth?' to which I replied 'it soon will be.'"[164] Two hours later, Dunglison woke him up to relieve him with another dose of laudanum to which the patient allegedly responded, "no, doctor, nothing more." Thereafter, Jefferson fell back asleep, "wholly unconscious to everything that was passing around him." According to Dunglison, Jefferson's circulation gradually became "more languid; and for some hours prior to dissolution, the pulse at the wrist was imperceptible." He died, in his own bed, at 1:50 P.M. on July 4, 1826. Jefferson's death is doubly memorable because his ninety-year-old compatriot in political hostilities, John Adams "chose" the same day to die, outliving the Virginian by several hours. By a remarkable coincidence these two past presidents, Jefferson and Adams, died on the same day, exactly fifty years after signing the Declaration of Independence. Only one man who signed this document, Charles Carroll of Carrollton (1737–1832), lived longer.

Since no postmortem exam was performed on Jefferson, one can only speculate on the cause of his death. Jefferson's diarrhea reportedly appeared first in 1801 after he bathed in and drank the sulfur waters of the Virginia springs "for a psoric," thus raising the possibility of chronic amebic dysentery, which can be mild in character and of very long standing.[165] Other considerations, given his diarrhea, constipation, and intermittent pain, include: spastic colon exacerbated by stress and possibly self-medication with calomel to which Jefferson was occasionally prone, noninfectious inflammatory enteritis, or prolapse of the rectum produced by repeated bouts of diarrhea. Perhaps the most likely diagnosis is cancer, either gastrointestinal or prostate. The actual cause of death was undoubtedly a combination of ailments: exhaustion from intense diarrhea, toxemia from a kidney infection, uremia from acute-on-chronic kidney damage, and finally orthostatic old-age pneumonia.[166]

Outbreak of "Typhoid Fever" at the University

In January 1829, Dunglison faced his most serious medical crisis, when an epidemic of what he called "a malignant typhoid fever" struck the University. At that time, typhoid was a descriptive term, not the name of a specific disease as it is to us now. Twenty of 117 students were infected and four died. Seven "others," likely free or enslaved servants, experienced the illness, but none died.[167] As the professor of medicine and then chairman of the faculty, Dunglison was expected to deal with the outbreak, both medically and administratively. He advised that academic exercises be suspended. The visitors agreed and the students were dismissed for several months until the University reopened on the 1st of April.

Dunglison's anxiety and his feeling the full weight of a dreadful responsibility can be understood when one realizes that he was compelled to act in almost total ignorance. Not until 1880 did Karl Eberth, a German pathologist, identify the causative organism *Salmonella enterica*. Human transmission is by the oral-fecal route, either through contaminated food or water. Typhoid fever is even now a major, worldwide, public-health concern. Before the development of antibiotics, mortality rates often exceeded 15 percent.[168] As Dunglison commented at the time and in several later publications, "we were totally unacquainted with the cause of every endemic and epidemic disease of every kind, and consequently, the fever could not be directly combatted."[169]

Some "righteous" citizens in the community, including the Reverend William Meade, an Episcopal minister who later became bishop of Virginia, were not at such a loss to explain the epidemic.[170] They understood the malady as an affliction visited on the University because it had no religious affiliation or instruction within its walls. Many regarded the epidemic as a sign of divine displeasure brought on the institution's supposed hostility to religion.[171] From the outset, however, Dunglison correctly assumed a "physical cause" and warned that the disease might be contagious, perhaps even "highly infectious," with unclean dormitories and hotels where meals were served, poor ventilation in the residence rooms, and problems with the water supply and privies possibly to blame.[172] Although many of the initial cases were mild, he was careful to have all of the dormitory rooms belonging to infected students fumigated with chlorine. In addition, these rooms as well as all uninfected dormitories and other buildings, including a vacant hotel that had been transformed into an infirmary for sick students, were scoured with a lime whitewash, an agent commonly used to clean unsanitary buildings, and a nurse was hired to care for the sick, at the University's expense.[173] Eventually, Dunglison summoned the students to resume academic exercises, but only when he was confident that all proper precautions had been taken and all the signs of the disease had disappeared from the precinct. No fresh cases were reported, and the Board of Visitors commended Dunglison for his efforts.[174] Several faculty members and their families left Charlottesville at the onset of the outbreak. Such was not the case with Dunglison. He never considered deserting his post and, along with his entire family, remained at the institution throughout this distressing period. Herein lies another similarity with Jefferson. In 1793, during the terrible outbreak of yellow fever in Philadelphia when it was the seat of the federal government, Jefferson went into town every day for weeks to fulfill his obligations as secretary of state, only giving up and retreating to Virginia for the duration after the desertion of the city made it impossible to conduct business.

The reputation of the University was a major concern for Dunglison, and he acted quickly and with dignity to squash an onslaught of unfounded speculation "full of sly malevolence" by enemies of the University who seized on the occurrence of the epidemic to "spread an alarm through the Country," via newspaper articles, which were intended "to make permanent impressions injurious to the University."[175] In order to "relieve public anxiety," Dunglison first communicated with parents and guardians, and the University's rector (James Madison), about containment efforts in order to build and maintain trust.[176] He then drafted a narration of "the beginning, progress, and present state of the disease, as well as the proceedings which the Faculty have from time to time taken concerning it," which was published "from time to time" in the *Richmond Enquirer* and the Washington *National Intelligencer*, so that the University could set the record straight.[177] The third step in Dunglison's crusade to protect the University's reputation was taken to assuage still further public and parental fear. On March 12, 1829, the chairman, with unanimous faculty consent, boldly proposed to the Visitors that a committee be appointed to inspect the grounds and report back on the salubrity of University facilities. The resolution stated:

> Resolved, that as the best means of relieving the public anxiety and of ascertaining what may be the cause of the disease, and especially of ascertaining whether there exists any permanent cause thereof, that it be suggested to the Rector that in the opinion of the faculty it is expedient that there should be a minute survey & inspection of the University, its buildings, and its environs – which inspection & survey should be entrusted to some three or more persons selected from the neighboring counties, whose disinterestedness, respectability, and intelligence would entitle any report they may make to the full confidence of the public – and that the same persons be also requested to take into consideration the dieting, lodging & the exercises & habits of the students, and to ascertain whether these are likely to cause or promote disease in the University.[178]

Dunglison's Medical and Nonmedical Writing at Virginia

In addition to being a superb lecturer in medicine and a compassionate practitioner of the art, Dunglison was widely regarded as one of the most prolific and authoritative medical writers of the nineteenth century. After moving to America, he continued to publish pieces that reflected broad views, a wide general education, wonderful energy, and versatility. Hugh Blair Grigsby, a notable historical scholar, said of Dunglison in 1858 that "more copies of his works have been issued from the press and diffused through this country and Europe than those of almost all the medical writers of the Union put together," and, "In the number and popularity of the volumes of his works no single European writer in ancient or in modern times can vie with him."[179] Dunglison's most significant works appeared while he was at the University of Virginia between 1825 and 1833. Many of his scholarly pieces were written to address the literary and scientific needs of his students. In 1827, Dunglison wrote a text titled *Syllabus of Lectures on Medical Jurisprudence*, including in it the treatment of accidental poisonings and suspended animation. This text was designed to accompany his pioneering course on medicine and the law described above. In 1832, he published the first American textbook of *Human Physiology*, (see Figure 21), which he dedicated to his venerable friend and patron, James Madison, in recognition of his "talents and philanthropy," and his being "a zealous promoter of science and literature, and the friend of mankind."[180]

Moving beyond the treatises of François Magendie (1783–1859), Anthelme Richerand (1779–1840) and John Bostock (1773–1846), which had been reprinted in America between 1817 and 1825, Dunglison's 1,058 page textbook on physiology was far more comprehensive in scope and illustrated by numerous engravings, so that it "might prove attractive . . . to the student more especially."[181] The last of its eight editions, published in 1856, contained 1,484 pages and 532 illustrations. The work earned the author the title of "Father" of American Physiology."[182] Samuel Gross, in describing the importance of Dunglison's textbook, says that "What Albert von Haller's great work accomplished for physiology in Europe in the 18th century Dunglison's accomplished for it in America in the 19th century. Each textbook [edition] affords a complete summary of the literature of the science at the time at which it was written; each is analytical and rich in learning, accurate and logical in its statements, exhaustive in matter, philosophical in its deductions. Each marks an era in the history of physiology."[183] And in a review from *Silliman's Journal*, the text was declared to be "a work so abounding in important facts, so correct in its principles, and so free from prejudice to favorite opinions."[184] To this can be added that Dunglison was generally quite "careful to give exact references both for facts and opinions," especially those that are not usually consulted by the student. Like Jefferson, Dunglison believed "that a treatise on the existing condition of any branch of science, which is not founded on the accumulated observation and reflection of an author's predecessors and contemporaries would be an absurdity, and therefore of but little or no value."[185]

In 1833 Dunglison published his second major book, *A New Dictionary of Medical Science and Literature* (see Figure 22).[186] The first indigenous medical lexicon in the United States, it was recognized widely as a work of immense intellectual effort and erudition. The two-volume first edition totaled 1,239 pages and contained more than 30,000 medical terms— all with explanations. More than 70,000 copies of the various editions were sold, and the sixteenth edition, published in 1860 was deemed so important during the Civil War that the United States surgeon general issued it to the Medical Corps. Dunglison earned a worldwide reputation and the nickname "The Walking Dictionary" among his friends and students in Virginia. One of the important features of the work was "its extensive synonymy, not only in the Greek and Latin, but also in the French and German languages." In Dunglison's words, "I endeavored, indeed, to make it a complete Dictionary of French medical terms, so that the medical students engaged in the perusal of a French medical author need not seek in a French Dictionary for the explanation of any medical term he might meet with." In 1903, the tweny-third edition of this dictionary appeared. As seen in the comment below by Osler, the dictionary was so widely consulted, it was referred to simply as "Dunglison," similarly to Webster's. Every new edition incorporated medical advances that had appeared since the previous one. As an example of the work that went into each new version, the volume he edited before his death in 1869 contained 6,000 new words or terms.[187] On the utility of this textbook, Sir William Osler commented, "there is no such literature as a dictionary, and the twenty-three editions through which Dunglison passed is a splendid testimony to its usefulness."[188]

Dunglison wrote rapidly, but in a well-organized manner. Dr. Gross observed that, "as a scholar, using the term in its most exalted sense, he was without a rival in the medical profession of the United States, he was well-versed in Latin and Greek as well as French, Italian and German." His works had their effect on nineteenth-century medicine, for, as Dr. Gross also noted "There was hardly a respectable medical man in the country, during the 19th century, that was not indebted to him, in a greater or lesser degree, for some of his professional information, derived either from his works or from his oral instruction. No physician on this continent has surpassed him in the extent of his erudition, in the variety of his information, or in the magnitude of his labors."[189]

At the University of Virginia, Dunglison's writing was not confined to medicine. He also contributed unsigned essays on numerous occasions to the *American Quarterly Review*, which was started in Philadelphia in 1827.[190] A remarkable breadth of interest is revealed by his contributions, which included: "Introduction to the Study of Grecian and Roman Geography," published in 1829 in association with George Long (1800–1879), a faculty colleague and the chair of ancient languages at the University of Virginia; "Gastronomy of the Romans," a piece that required vast research on the diets and culinary preparations of the Romans, Greeks and early inhabitants of Britain; "Longevity," a paper that examined the arguments for and against total abstinence from alcohol; "Infirmities of Men of Genius," in which Dunglison maintained that intellectual work is not harmful if due attention is paid to good diet, exercise, sleep and a regular schedule; and "College–Instruction and Discipline," an effort by Dunglison to "canvass the great questions of instruction and discipline in our higher schools, and to bring the [educational] plan adopted in the University of Virginia more prominently into notice."[191] Working with Professor George Tucker (1775–1861), chair of moral philosophy and political economy, he also edited several periodicals and journals, including the *Virginia Literary Museum and the Journal of Belles–Lettres, Arts and Sciences,* which Dunglison established in 1829 as a medium for publishing science and history, especially the history of Virginia, as well as literature of a diverse nature for general readers. It excluded discussion of party politics and theology. Sadly, this journal lasted only one year because Dunglison could not get enough of his colleagues at the University and throughout the state to contribute articles.

Dunglison's Bench Research at the University

When the University of Virginia was founded, biomedical research of any meaningful sort was rare in America. Dr. Dunglison undertook one of his experimental projects at the request of James Lovell (1788–1836), surgeon general of the United States Army, and William Beaumont (1785–1853), an army surgeon who was studying the physiology of gastric digestion in a Canadian, Alexis St. Martin, who had a fistulous opening into the stomach (see Figure 23).

Dunglison was an experimental scientist only in this one instance, which occurred in 1832–33 while he was at the University of Virginia. Beaumont had no formal medical education beyond a two-year apprenticeship with a local practitioner in St. Albans, Vermont. He evidently sought out Dunglison because he knew that "Professor Dunglison's work on human physiology, taken as a whole, is perhaps the most comprehensive," and that "his excellent treatise" on the "subject of gastric functions and fluids" was replete with "principles, reasonings and suggestions, and irrefragably established physiological facts."[192] Dunglison and his fellow professor John Patten Emmet performed microscopic examinations and many chemical analyses and provided Beaumont with valuable direction and critical interpretation, in contrast to three other scientists who were sent gastric samples but whose help was of little value. Dunglison and Emmet have sometimes been credited with the discovery of free hydrochloric acid and a second digestive substance subsequently identified as pepsin. This finding was one of the most important medical advances in antebellum America. It proved that gastric digestion was truly a chemical process, and, along with the brilliant subsequent investigations of Claude Bernard (1813–78), helped usher in a new biochemical point of view with regard to physiology, namely, that all life processes result from chemical reactions.[193] Despite this important work, Dunglison received what he regarded as inadequate recognition in Beaumont's *Experiments and Observations of Gastric Juices and the Physiology of Digestion* (Plattsburg: Printed by F.A. Allen, 1833). When Dunglison expressed his dismay, Beaumont responded "that I did not think you would care to be associated with so humble an individual as I."[194] One recent historian has concluded that "Beaumont was wise to rush to press, leaving his colleagues [at Virginia] in dire distress. Beaumont gets credit for collecting the juice, but Dunglison discovered the 'acid' truth." This interpretation is not entirely correct. Certainly Beaumont's "peculiar" oversight did not keep Dunglison from supporting a petition to Congress to grant $10,000 for Beaumont's research. The bill, however, failed, because at the time Congress objected to appropriation of money for any scientific or philanthropic purpose.[195]

After this experience with Beaumont, Dunglison never again engaged in bench research. In contrast, Emmet did much to advance scientific research at the University of Virginia. At the request of the Board of Visitors in 1827, Emmett began plans to build a chemical laboratory for his own research and pedagogical purposes. He apparently purchased most of the apparatus and equipment himself, for in July 1829, the Board advised that he be reimbursed. Emmet published the results of many of his original experiments while at the University, with most of these articles appearing in *Silliman's Journal* and the *Virginia Literary Museum*. In addition to those mentioned above, Dr. Emmet performed numerous scientific studies on magnets and on electricity, as well as producing a vacuum apparatus to generate propulsive power long before the "atmospheric railroad" was invented. He also exercised his ingenuity in the field of scientific horticulture, experimenting with flowers, fruits, and various manures. Emmet's interests extended to the cultivation of grapes, the manufacture of wines, the use of pyroligneous acid as a shorter and better way of curing hams, the raising of silkworms and the use of chemical agents for coloring of silk threads, and the development of a particular kind of kaolin which he discovered on his city property and adapted to the manufacture of pottery and porcelain vessels. And in 1840, Emmet began a study of the "phenomena" of optical physics that might have extended the Newtonian theory of refraction had he not died prematurely in 1842. In his relatively brief career, cut short by weak lungs, he was "a cultivator of Physical Science" whose "talents for original investigation won him a high place among the scientific [men] of our land." As pointed out in several memoirs, written by his son and a faculty colleague, "The life of Dr. Emmet presents an instructive example of what may be accomplished by an ardent and energetic spirit in overcoming difficulty. When but a child of seven years, before immigrating to America he was afflicted by a severe attack of small–pox which was nearly fatal, and before he had convalesced he had the measles and whooping cough." Throughout the remainder of his life, his constitution was "delicate and susceptible" to pulmonary disease. "Against the approaches of the dread malady [probably tuberculosis] he was made to struggle through life; yet, under this disadvantage, he was always a zealous and a diligent votary of science." And "he lived [long enough] to be the esteemed and successful instructor of more than 1200 young men in the principles of the useful science he taught."[196]

Dunglison as "Chief Executive Officer of the University" in its Early Years

At the first organizational meeting of the faculty in April 1825, Dunglison was asked by his colleagues to play a significant role in University governance. During its inaugural academic session, he served as secretary of the faculty. Later he was elected chairman of the faculty, a post defined as "the chief executive officer of the University; and as such charged with superintending the execution of all laws made for its government."[197]

Dunglison's election as faculty secretary had received Jefferson's unqualified approval. However, as this section will illustrate, he endorsed several initiatives that ran counter to Jefferson's ideals.

In addition to being an exceptional teacher and scholar, Dunglison was an administrator whose actions helped guide the fledgling University through a number of early crises. During his eight years at the University of Virginia, he participated in no fewer than 342 administrative meetings of the faculty, far more than any of his associates.[198] Dunglison's input on matters of importance was highly valued and always given. Faculty colleagues were quick to recognize his integrity, vast erudition, and natural inclination towards consensus building. He never quashed dissent, but he did demand decorous and gentlemanly behavior during debate. During faculty meetings, he displayed an inordinate ability to sift through information and testimony, to know what was practical and useful, and to see where the common ground lay. A natural conversationalist who was informative and convincing, he was decisive, leaving no doubt of his position in the minds of his faculty colleagues or other university officials.

Dunglison served as chairman of the faculty for three one-year terms between 1826 and 1830. Unlike him, George Tucker, and, to a lesser extent, Charles Bonnycastle and John Emmet, three of the original faculty members (Thomas Key, George Long, and George Blaettermann) "showed little disposition to cultivate the society of the other professors" and were not valued in the practical affairs of the institution beyond the thresholds of their classrooms. Key's irritable behavior bordered on fierce hostility, whereas Blaettermann's radical personal defects created so much tension that he eventually became an embarrassment to everyone.[199] Although the duties of the chairman garnered an additional stipend of $500 per annum, Dunglison found the work to be sometimes "disagreeable." This undoubtedly was because one of his main duties was to oversee the discipline of the institution. This meant monitoring, and "calculating," the performance of every professor in each of the eight schools and ensuring that reports were prepared on: how often an instructor had failed to lecture on the scheduled day appointed for his lectures; how frequently teachers had neglected to question their students in the classroom after each lecture; how much time the professors had spent delivering lectures and giving examinations; and, how often a professor had omitted sending in his weekly class reports showing the number of student absences and the degree of their attention and progress. He was also expected to submit annual reports to the Board of Visitors summarizing these findings, and "to communicate with each parent & guardian the standing of his son & ward, without informing him of the standing of any other student."[200] In current public–education jargon, Dunglison was called upon to be an "instructional leader," even though his duties were largely confined to recording the delinquencies of his fellow professors. He did not view these administrative functions as encroachments on the academic freedom of the faculty. Dunglison did not regard tenure merely as an academic sinecure with no standards of conduct. It should not, he wrote "be altogether independent" of a professor's behavior toward colleagues and students, his energetic attention to self–improvement, and the gentlemanly honor he displayed in complying with the rules and regulations set forth in the enactments of the University. All professors should "be held rigidly responsible" for their work and behavior. And if a professor should fail consistently in these responsibilities, then "he is unfit for his situation, and the trustees should have moral courage enough to remove him."[201] On this matter, Dunglison's views were both broader and more specific than those of Jefferson.

The chairman's most important functions included acting as the voice of the faculty during the deliberations of the Board of Visitors, so that the legislative authority of the University "would have the advantage of the voice of experience." To Dunglison, the faculty were "unquestionably the best judges," and "no non–resident" member of the Board of Visitors could "possibly have the necessary experience" of the day-to-day operations within the University precinct. Without faculty input, rules were "apt be enacted" by the "superior board" that were "either wholly inoperative, unfeasible, or impolitic."[202]

One example of the need for faculty input concerned the issue of student self-government and discipline. Jefferson and the visitors had "fancifully believed" that "the students themselves might be induced to form a part of the government" of the University, for instance, "to constitute a court for the trial of minor offenses, and to inflict punishment on a delinquent colleague," or to testify willingly against a fellow-student who had engaged in behavior that threatened the "reputation and prosperity" of the institution, or "injures the cause and saps the very foundation of education." This utopian code of discipline, ratified by the Board without faculty or student input in 1824, that is, prior to the actual opening of the school, reflected Jefferson's belief that his University would be populated, not by raw boys shirking their studies and running after irregular pleasures—indulging in adolescent pranks and wild profligacy—but by sedate young men with erect characters who would engage themselves in "a fierce schedule of scholarly labor." Since he evidently assumed "that the youthful matriculates would, as a body, belong to the oldest, wealthiest, and most cultured families of the South, he took it for granted that their instincts would be gentle; that they would disdain to violate those precepts of upright conduct which they had learned at home; and that if there were to found among them, as in the whitest flock, a small number of black sheep, these degenerates would be shamed into decent behavior by the compelling example of the great majority." In essence, Jefferson's liberal, albeit impractical, views on student discipline not only demonstrated his noble faith in abstract rights but also his belief in the ultimate perfectibility of humanity, including the late–adolescent male. Dunglison more realistically viewed this scheme of student self–regulation as formed under "an erroneous impression that more might be done with the students by an appeal to their patriotism and honor, than by positive punishment." But one could scarcely expect cooperation from the students themselves so long as "the *esprit du corps* or Burschenschaft, prevails amongst students, which inculcates that it is a stigma of the deepest hue to give testimony against a fellow student."[203]

Almost as soon as the University admitted its first class, Jefferson's idealistic scheme of student self-government proved unworkable, a fact that both Dunglison and Emmet quickly realized and eventually acted to correct. Almost as soon as the first academic session began, it became apparent that many of the students in Charlottesville were not prepared by temperament or prior education to accept the scholastic rigors, laws of conduct, and associated freedoms of the University. The majority of the students were not only quite young (two-thirds were 19 years old or less) but the sons of affluent parents. Expecting to be wealthy in turn by inheritance, they had never acquired habits of self–denial and self–repression. The students' exaggerated sense of self–importance, imbedded in their class upbringing, led some to act out in the classroom and beyond. They verbally and physically assaulted professors, walked out in the middle of lectures, swore, chewed tobacco, gambled, drank ardent spirits, partied with abandon, discharged firearms on campus, and brutalized the slaves who made the university run. Neither Dunglison himself nor his family ever experienced a student assault, but John Patten Emmet was the first of several professors to be punched by a student.

Even in the face of such outrages, moreover, the body of students declined, sometimes in an openly hostile manner, to "act the part of Informers" or sit on a Board of Censors. In their view, taking up this role—a responsibility imposed on them without their consent—would have put them in an unpopular and dishonorable position, acting not only as judges of, but also spies on the conduct of their fellows. Because they refused to sit in judgment on their peers, and as some faculty were reluctant to assume the neglected duty, possibly out of respect for Jefferson's plan, student demeanor in the earliest days of the University fell into a state of insubordination and lawlessness. Eventually, a few "vicious irregularities" climaxed with a series of major disturbances in the autumn of 1825, which included riots in which the students expressed their "objection to the European professors." In the worst to date, a nighttime riot on October 1 fueled by alcohol included yelling profanities and launching missiles (sticks, bricks, and bottles filled with urine) at professors and their pavilion windows. Many of the student participants wore masks to hide their identity. Faculty members were attacked, and property was damaged. Jefferson accordingly assembled the students, faculty, and visitors in the Rotunda and began to admonish the students for their disgraceful conduct.[204] As by the historian Jennings Wagoner, "Choked with emotion and unable to go on, the eighty-two-year-old Jefferson yielded the floor to Visitor Chapman Johnson, who rebuked the students and asked for the leaders of the disturbance to confess their guilt. Fourteen stepped forward in admission of the part they had played in the riotous behavior, one of whom was one of Jefferson's grandnephews. Upon seeing a member of his own family admit guilt, Jefferson could not disguise his grief."[205] He was clearly upset that one of his most cherished convictions, student self-government, was not working. Jefferson's disillusionment did not keep him from agreeing promptly to the faculty's plea for "a vigilant & efficient police,"[206] and he presumably encouraged the Board of Visitors to appeal to the General Assembly in Richmond for authority to tighten regulations within the University. In the years that followed Jefferson's death, the faculty and visitors multiplied the rules, as the students multiplied their offenses. In a way, the tightening of the codes of student conduct reflected Jefferson's belief that laws and institutions needed to change over time as background political circumstances changed.[207] As pointed out by Wagoner, "the tide began to turn back towards Jefferson's idealistic vision of student self–government when in 1842, two years after the murder of a popular Law professor [John Andrew Gardner Davis] by a drunken student, Virginia students adopted an 'Honor Code' which contained the essence of Jefferson's belief in individual integrity and self-discipline. It remains as one of the most distinctive and significant features of the university—and a point of continuing tension."[208]

In contrast to student discipline, where events forced Dunglison and Jefferson to revise policy, Dunglison directly challenged one of Jefferson's treasured beliefs, that "no Diploma shall be given to any one who has not passed such an examination in the Latin language as shall have proved him able to read the highest classics in that language with ease, thorough understanding, and just quantity." This resolution was passed by the Board of Visitors on October 24, 1824, with the stated intention "that the reputation of the University shall not be committed but to those who, to an eminence in some one or more of the sciences taught in it, add a proficiency in these languages which constitute the basis of good education, and are indispensable to fill up the character of a 'well-educated man.'" In a letter to the rector and visitors dated April 3, 1826, Dunglison petitioned for a modification. He argued that the enactment was too strict and should not apply to the medical school as a condition for graduation. Indeed, as he later commented, "To be able 'to read the highest classics in the Latin language, with ease, thorough understanding, and just quantity,' would, of itself, require as much time as the majority of our youths are capable of devoting to their collegiate instruction."[209] Dunglison pointed out that no medical school in America required any knowledge of the Latin language, and that even in the best schools of Europe, "a much slighter share of classical learning is required." As in the universities of Edinburgh and Glasgow, and the Royal College of Physicians of London, etc., all decisions on the attainments of medical students, "classical as well as medical, should be left to the medical professors themselves," who could be relied on to "act with becoming strictness" concerning the classical knowledge of their students. Requiring advanced skills in Latin was already retarding the progress of the medical school in Charlottesville by inhibiting enrollment, and thus also diminishing "the amount of emolument" for the professor below what had been given to expect in "representations made by the agent of the Board" (Francis W. Gilmer) in Europe.[210] Dunglison cited a "circumstance" of two medical students leaving the University "from a fear that whatever might be the extent of their medical attainments, their knowledge of the Latin language although fully as respectable as that of the generality of the most eminent practising physicians of this country, might by the Professor of ancient languages be considered insufficient." Jefferson responded swiftly, acknowledging that the early enactment on diplomas had been "but little attended to" when it was composed, since "some time must elapse before it would be called for," before which they could count on "recieving the aid of the Professors, not then in place."[211] As rector of the University, he therefore referred the matter to the faculty with a request that they "propose such alterations as they may deem expedient." Accordingly, the question was brought before the entire faculty, and they agreed with Dunglison on a modification of the enactment related to graduation, which was adopted by the Board of Visitors. It was then determined that all efforts should be directed toward ensuring that every graduate of the University be thoroughly competent in reading and writing English.[212] Unlike other medical schools in nineteenth-century America, the University of Virginia would indulge no one unable to either speak or write his mother tongue with accuracy.[213]

During his term as chairman, Dunglison was quite pleased when the University of Virginia began writing diplomas in English so that they might be intelligible to everyone. At the time, virtually every medical school issued their diplomas in Latin, despite the fact that very few people in America could read that language, even including, as Dunglison wryly noted, many of those receiving the degrees. This could even lead to fraud, as one could with relative ease to pass off a lesser degree in a foreign language for a doctor's diploma.[214] In promoting a simple statement of competence in the vernacular, Dunglison quoted Joseph Chitty (1775–1841), who said "that perhaps a mouthful of nonsense sounds better in Latin, or other dead language, than in English."[215] The diploma awarded to meritorious students at the University of Virginia was an unembellished statement of fact. Dunglison said in this connection: "In the establishment of the University of Virginia, the venerable customs that had prevailed for ages were retained only when esteemed worthy of retention. Precedent was wholly disregarded."[216] Dunglison also used his position of influence as chairman of the faculty to herald the improving reputation of the school, which he accomplished by ensuring that the Proctor would make "a suitable advertisement" in "such newspapers in different portions of the United States – calculated to invite public attention to the University of Virginia."[217]

On July 9, 1831, Dunglison submitted a resolution at a faculty meeting urging the establishment of "an additional and higher degree with the title of the possessor of Master of Arts." This initiative grew out of a decision by the Board of Visitors on October 1, 1828, to appoint a committee on degrees, with Dunglison as a member, to investigate and report on "whether it might not be proper to adopt the ancient denominations of Bachelor, Master and Doctor; and whether it be not proper to prescribe what kind of proficiency in the learning of the several schools shall entitle a student to each degree."[218] Students could earn the new master's degree by receiving diplomas in five different schools—Ancient or Modern Languages, Mathematics, Natural Philosophy, Chemistry, and Moral Philosophy. In advocating this revolutionary addition,[219] Dunglison suggested that the proposed degree would (1) afford parents and guardians an important guide in the selection of studies; (2) enable the student to enter on professional or political life with every advantage; and would (3) keep the student longer at the University. Shortly after the Faculty expressed its unanimous support, the Board of Visitors authorized use of the new degree—not permanently, but "for the present." Between July 1832 and the outbreak of the Civil War, 144 students were awarded this prestigious honor.[220]

Dunglison's Departure from the University

Dunglison's fame as a teacher and writer in Virginia spread rapidly, and he soon began to receive offers for professorships elsewhere. On June 15, 1829, Dr. William Paul Crillon Barton offered him a post at Jefferson Medical College in Philadelphia, but he declined. In 1830, Dr. Daniel Drake (1785–1852), who was organizing the Miami Medical College in Cincinnati, invited him to join the proposed faculty, but this too he rejected because the school was situated too far inland to be convenient of access. Jefferson Medical College sought him again in 1831, but the inducements were still not strong enough, and Dunglison suspected that the school was founded in a spirit of opposition to the other colleges in Philadelphia and not as the result of any real demand for its creation in the urgent needs of the community.[221] In 1833, however, Dunglison accepted the chair of materia medica, therapeutics, hygiene and medical jurisprudence at the Medical College of Maryland,[222] feeling that the change from the rural Charlottesville environment to the city of Baltimore might improve the health of his wife, who was suffering from acute-on-chronic rheumatism, possibly with cardiac valve involvement. Ambition to exercise his teaching talents in a broader field than Charlottesville was probably also a factor, and the failure of the Board of Visitors to raise Dunglison's base salary could have contributed to his resignation.[223]

When Francis W. Gilmer was trying to entice foreign professors to Charlottesville in 1824, he optimistically estimated fees from students at $6,000 a year for at least one professor.[224] In reality, Dunglison's annual income from student fees never exceeded $1,200 during his eight years at the University of Virginia, and the prospects for much growth in student matriculates in his school were at best guarded. In contrast, income from student fees in some other departments of the university was disproportionately greater, by several thousand dollars, and this was the basis for Dunglison's request for a higher base salary. His rationale was straightforward—that his responsibilities, laborious service and experience were every bit the equal of those professors who received greater compensation.[225]

The historian Philip A. Bruce has also commented on Dunglison's exasperation at the lack of adequate building maintenance, and even suggested that his resignation might have been prompted, in part, by his inability on at least three occasions to get the University to fix a leaking roof.[226] Dunglison complained to the proctor of the University, "Will you be so kind to call in and examine our house, as we were up nearly all of last night in consequence of the rain soaking through on the floor and bed." Later, he added "Every part of the roof of my pavilion admits water like a sieve." Dunglison's friend and teaching colleague, John Patten Emmet, expressed similar exasperation when in the spring of 1832, he wrote that "Every member of my family, with the exception of the infant, is at present seriously indisposed by violent cold and fever taken immediately after the late rain. The room occupied by Mrs. Emmet dripped incessantly. I slept in the chamber with the children and felt the drops falling steadily on my pillow. I positively state to you my conviction that the complete prostration of my family is dependent on the leaking condition of the roof."[227] Leaking roofs were a widespread problem, possibly resulting from cost cutting, but more likely because Jefferson just loved flat roofs and seems to have been incapable of designing ones that did not leak. They leaked at Monticello, Poplar Forest, and throughout the University.

Taking all of these facts into consideration, Dunglison probably left the University not because he was dissatisfied there but rather for better remuneration and to give his many talents a broader scope.[228] He wrote himself that he found it attractive to join a staff of six professors in the Medical College of Maryland, who constituted "a corps of efficient teachers;'" and that Baltimore offered more extensive teaching facilities than even the eminent Philadelphia schools. One significant advantage was a ready supply of cadavers for dissection. The Maryland college boasted in its catalogues that it was actually able to export corpses to medical schools as distant as Maine.[229] Dunglison's departure from the University in 1833 was gradual and amicable. He announced his intention to resign a bit later than the school's regulations called for, but agreed to stay long enough for a successor to be found, and in departing he expressed much gratitude—both to the "enlightened" Board of Visitors "for their unvarying kindness" and to his faculty colleagues "for their goodness."[230]

Dunglison's farewell address to his students when he left Charlottesville rehearsed his philosophies of learning and understanding. The valedictory repeated one of Jefferson's most cherished medical beliefs, namely—that scientific advance would rid humanity of medieval mysticism and folly, and for this to occur, "one of the first things to be learned is to disinfect the mind of all bias."[231] In his speech, a small portion of which is reprinted below, Dunglison urged his students to avoid being wedded to any exclusive sect, scheme, or system, to watch the forward march of science carefully and, when in doubt, always to give the patient the benefit of doubt rather than risk safety by unproven treatment. His exordium also indicated a wide field of duties that Dunglison had cultivated in his students.

> It has been always my anxious endeavor to remove everything of mystery from the science which it is my line to teach; to separate fact from hypothesis, and to attempt to exhibit it, as far as it is capable of being exhibited, as a demonstrative science. I have ever recommended you, in deducing your therapeutical indications, to be guided by general principles; to avoid being wedded to any exclusive sect or system, – fondness for which has been and is a striking obstacle to the advancement of medicine; to watch philosophically and diligently the march of nature; to discard all blind empiricism, and where you are in doubt rather to give the patient the benefit of the doubt than to risk his safety by the rash administration of that which may be the bearer of good or evil; to cherish no arcana; and as a general principle to freely expose to your patient, if intelligent and if he desires it, the grounds on which you proceed in the management of his case. If you cannot do this, there will generally be good reason for supposing that your comprehension of the case is not as clear as it ought to be.[232]

During his eight years in Charlottesville, Dunglison did much to enhance the scientific reputation of his school. Shortly after departing his post, a number of letters and pamphlets attested to the high esteem in which the medical department of the University of Virginia was already held in the South and beyond. In one such writing, Dr. Robert Y. Conrad said that he "was told sometime time ago by a medical student in Philadelphia that the medical school [in Charlottesville] stood in high estimation, and that the students of one year from the University school almost invariably graduated in Philadelphia in the second year at the head of their classes, being much better prepared in the science than if they had attended the first year in Philadelphia."[233]

We can concdude that Robley Dunglison was not only the preternaturally energetic leader of a unique experiment in medical education, but also an adept administrative who, if not the architect of the University of Virginia, was its master builder, and its best example of academic professionalism in the early years. During the fifteen months that he and Jefferson worked together, Dunglison carried out the essentials of Jefferson's plans, especially the building and curating of an extraordinary library collection, a project that continued to be developed and refined even after the founder's death. While the elderly Jefferson stood on the mountaintop terrace at Monticello and peered through a telescope at the buildings taking shape below, he perceived a magnified image of the school from a distance. His protégé—and personal physician—experienced the University on site, confronting the day-to-day minutia attendant on an enormous number of obligations as he focused on lecturing, testing, and academic writing, as well as a panoply of meetings to chair and attend. As a respected physician whose services were in demand, Dunglison treated the illnesses of patients from presidents to enslaved laborers.

Dunglison's central contribution to the whole University community, however, lay less in his prodigious work ethic than in the way those efforts enabled the Medical Department to emerge on the national stage. By the time he left in 1833, his devotion brought the University beyond the pangs of birth to viability and even to reputable status.

The decisive interventions Dunglison was constrained to make regarding student infractions that verged on rebellion helped preserve the operations of the University in its earliest moments. Unlike Jefferson, he recognized that a university did indeed have to act *in loco parentis*. A typhoid epidemic brought a similar crisis to the University, and Dunglison acted decisively during its critical phases, averting tragedy by closing down the school, introducing quarantines and ordering disinfection, and thereby reducing the threat of both the disease itself and the rumors to which it gave rise. In recommending that the Latin requirement for graduation be jettisoned, Dunglison directly opposed one of Jefferson's ideals, because he astutely realized that the demands of acquiring high-level facility in Latin might interfere with attracting and retaining students whose primary objective was not literary studies.

In effect, Dunglison helped save the school. His intentions were not primarily founded on his own self–interest or that of his department or the faculty. Rather, as his correspondence and actions reveal, the status and reputation of the University as a whole, and the Medical Department in particular, most occupied his mind and attentions, and he realized that they needed active promotion. Dunglison readily defended the University against detractors but also anticipated objections that might arise due to its revolutionary structure. He understood that Jefferson's experiment, especially the study of medicine with its anomalously long semester and arduous examination schedule, was a project that had to be sold, given that it was new and unproven, with no network of graduates to advocate for it in the scientific and medical community. Dunglison's writing and teaching produced this first cadre of students and graduates, a small but increasing number, whose successes could convince sceptics of the medical curriculum's effectiveness.

The next chapter builds on this idea. How did Dunglison convey his and Jefferson's vision to other medical schools? And how did his former student James Lawrence Cabell and other professors continue to deepen it at the University of Virginia? What Dunglison and his colleagues in Charlottesville began grew to such an extent that many of the Medical Department's innovations came to be accepted as essential standards for the education of physicians nationwide.

Chapter 6

JEFFERSON'S LEGACY IN MEDICAL EDUCATION LIVES ON

If I have seen further it is by standing on the shoulders of giants.

Isaac Newton, 1675[1]

DUNGLISON'S MOVE to Maryland enabled him to propagate the ethos of Jefferson–inspired medical education to other schools. His transition also made room among the University of Virginia's medical faculty for the appointment of one of Dunglison's students, James L. Cabell, who over a fifty-two-year career would continue and deepen his mentor's reforms at Virginia and incorporate them into proposals for changing medical education throughout the United States.

This chapter clarifies the efforts of Dunglison and Cabell to foster a broader curriculum and more rigorous standards in all medical schools. Many of their proposals were clearly inspired by Jeffersonian ideas and rooted in what they had practiced at the University of Virginia. Their agenda was also formed from research they did into medical education in America, which, as the following section shows, had failed to evolve from its colonial foundations.

MEDICAL SCHOOLS IN ANTEBELLUM AMERICA

When Dunglison left Virginia in 1833, the United States was in the middle of Andrew Jackson's presidency, and in the decades leading up to the Civil War, the country was squarely in an "age of great retrogression,"

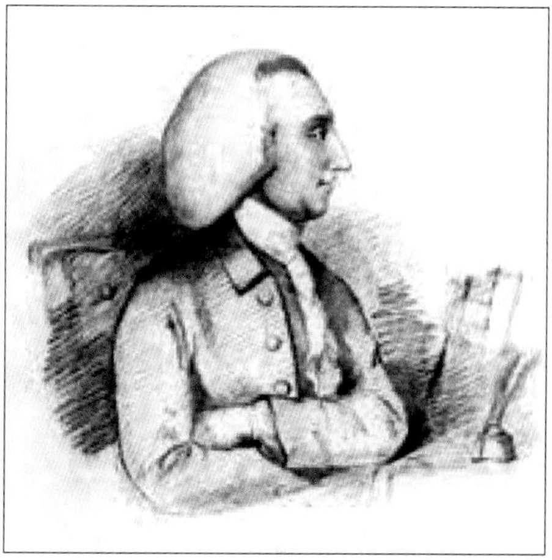

FIGURE 1. William Small (1734–1775), contemporary pencil sketch, by unknown artist. (Courtesy of William & Mary Special Collections Research Center)

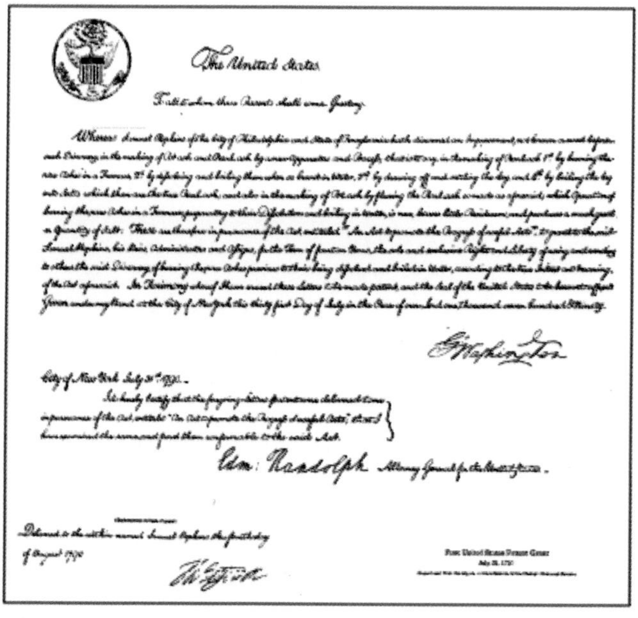

The United States

To all to whom these Presents shall come Greeting.

G Washington

Edm: Randolph

FIGURE 2. The first United States patent, granted to Samuel Hopkins of Philadelphia in July 1790, for a new process for making potash and pearl ash. The patent document was signed by President George Washington and Attorney General Edmond Randolph, and endorsed on the back by Thomas Jefferson, who was Secretary of State. Both potash and pearl ash were important ingredients in making glass, soap, fertilizer, and saltpeter, which in turn was an ingredient in gunpowder. The two chemicals were also used for the drying and shrinking of clothes. (Courtesy of U.S. Patent and Trademark Office and Chicago Historical Museum)

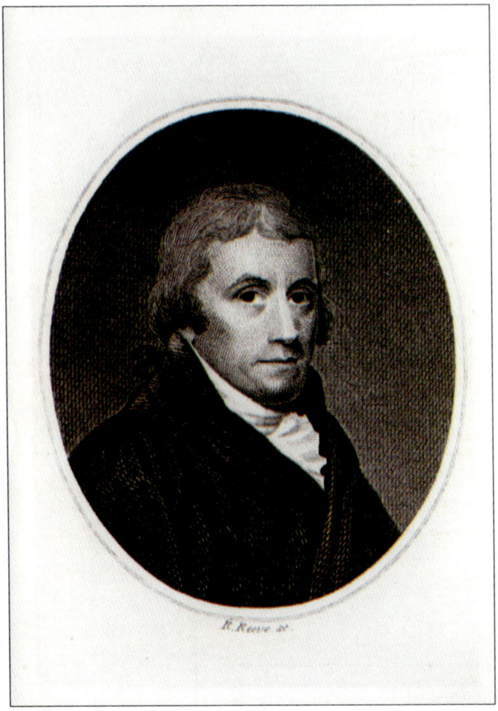

FIGURE 3. *Benjamin Waterhouse*, engraving by Richard Reeve, ca. 1801. (Courtesy of the Francis A. Countway Library, Harvard University)

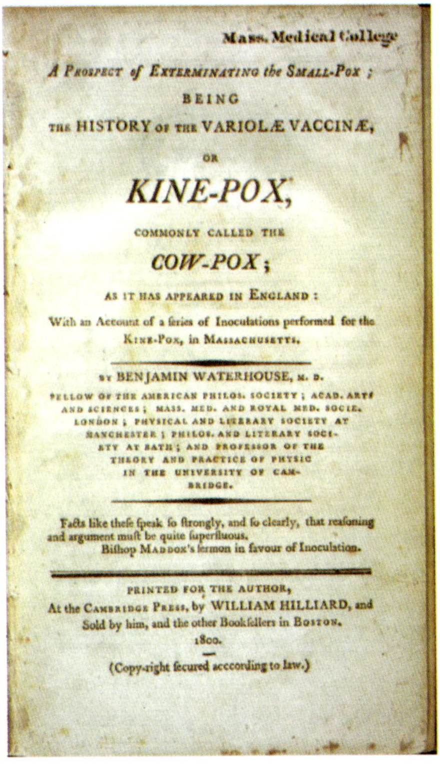

Mass. Medical College

A PROSPECT of EXTERMINATING the SMALL-POX;

BEING

THE HISTORY OF THE VARIOLÆ VACCINÆ,

OR

KINE-POX,

COMMONLY CALLED THE

COW-POX;

AS IT HAS APPEARED IN ENGLAND:

With an Account of a series of Inoculations performed for the KINE-POX, in MASSACHUSETTS.

BY BENJAMIN WATERHOUSE, M. D.

FELLOW OF THE AMERICAN PHILOS. SOCIETY; ACAD. ARTS AND SCIENCES; MASS. MED. AND ROYAL MED. SOCIE. LONDON; PHYSICAL AND LITERARY SOCIETY AT MANCHESTER; PHILOS. AND LITERARY SOCIETY AT BATH; AND PROFESSOR OF THE THEORY AND PRACTICE OF PHYSIC IN THE UNIVERSITY OF CAMBRIDGE.

Facts like these speak so strongly, and so clearly, that reasoning and argument must be quite superfluous.
Bishop MADDOX's sermon in favour of Inoculation.

PRINTED FOR THE AUTHOR,
At the CAMBRIDGE PRESS, by WILLIAM HILLIARD, and Sold by him, and the other Booksellers in BOSTON.
1800.

(Copy-right secured acccording to law.)

FIGURE 4. Title page of *A Prospect of Exterminating the Small-Pox* (1800), by Dr. Benjamin Waterhouse

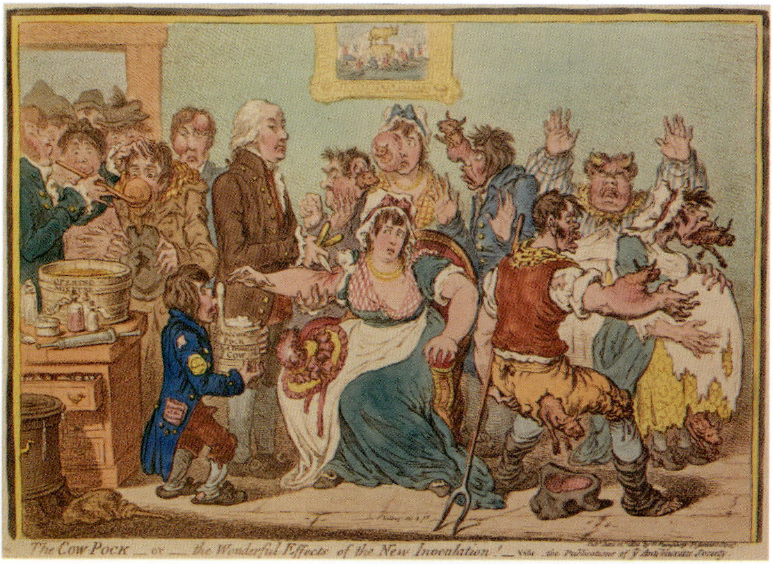
The Cow-Pock — or — the Wonderful Effects of the New Inoculation !

FIGURE 5. James Gillray's 1802 caricature of Edward Jenner vaccinating patients who feared it would make them sprout cow-like appendages. (Courtesy of The Morgan Library & Museum, New York)

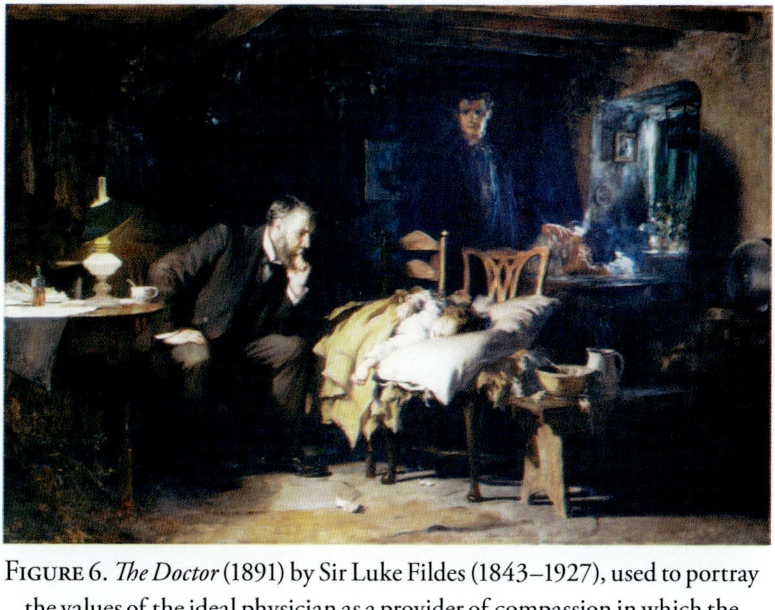

FIGURE 6. *The Doctor* (1891) by Sir Luke Fildes (1843–1927), used to portray the values of the ideal physician as a provider of compassion in which the patient is central, and the inadequacies of medical treatment for incurable infectious disease in the pre-antibiotic era. (Courtesy of Tate National Gallery, London)

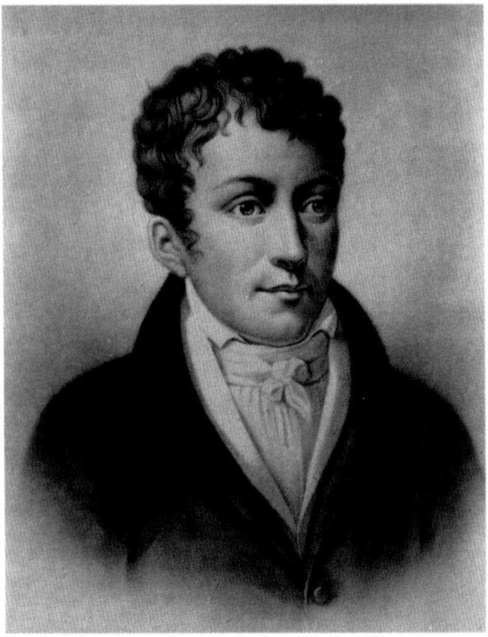

FIGURE 7. *Pierre Jean Georges Cabanis*, by Ambroise Tardieu. (Courtesy of National Library of Medicine)

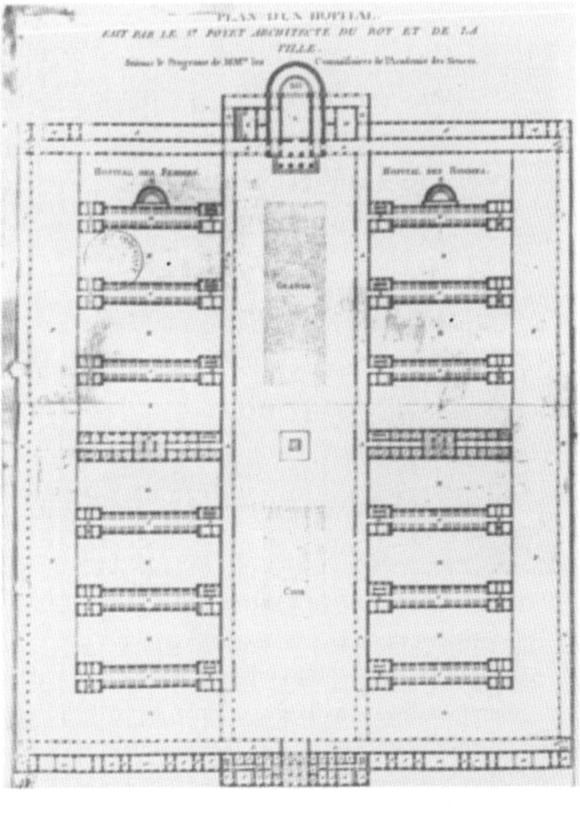

FIGURE 8. Pavilion hospital design from *Extrait des registres de l'Academie royales des Sciences du 12 mars* 1788

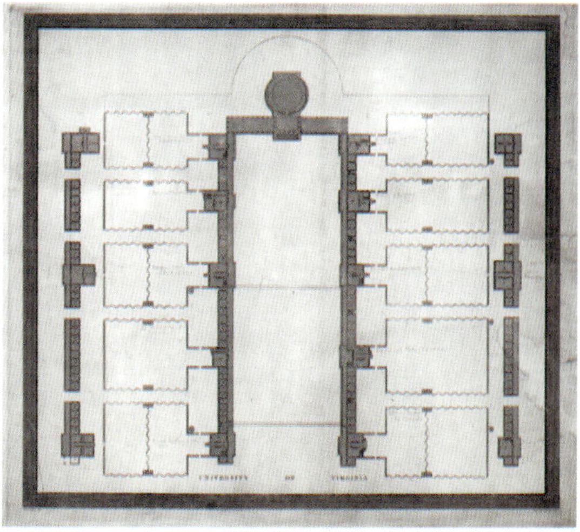

FIGURE 9. Jefferson's Ground Plan for the University of Virginia, John Neilson, draughtsman, Peter Maverick, engraver, 1822. (Courtesy of Albert and Shirley Small Special Collections Library, University of Virginia)

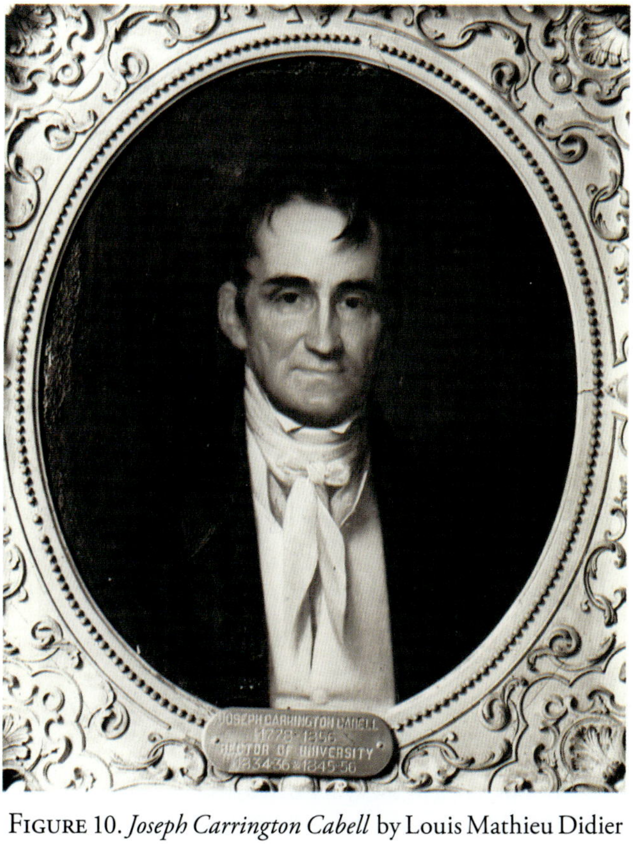

FIGURE 10. *Joseph Carrington Cabell* by Louis Mathieu Didier Guillaume (1816–1892). (Courtesy of Albert and Shirley Small Special Collections Library, University of Virginia)

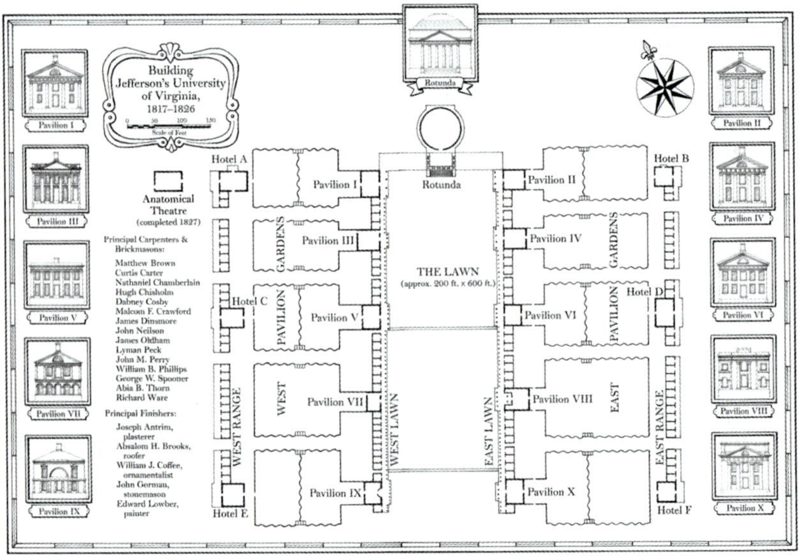

FIGURE 11. Building Jefferson's University of Virginia, 1817–1826. (Courtesy of the Thomas Jefferson Foundation at Monticello)

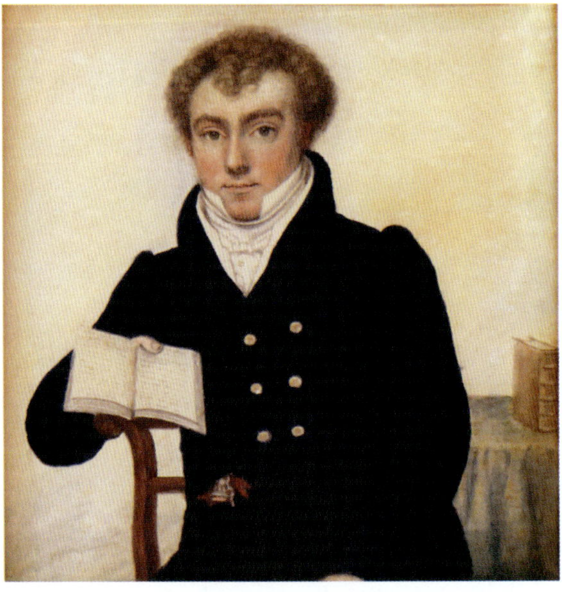

FIGURE 12. *Robley Dunglison*, painted in England by unknown in 1824, donated to the University of Virginia by his son, Richard J. Dunglison, in 1899. (Courtesy of Historical Collections, Claude Moore Health Sciences Library, University of Virginia)

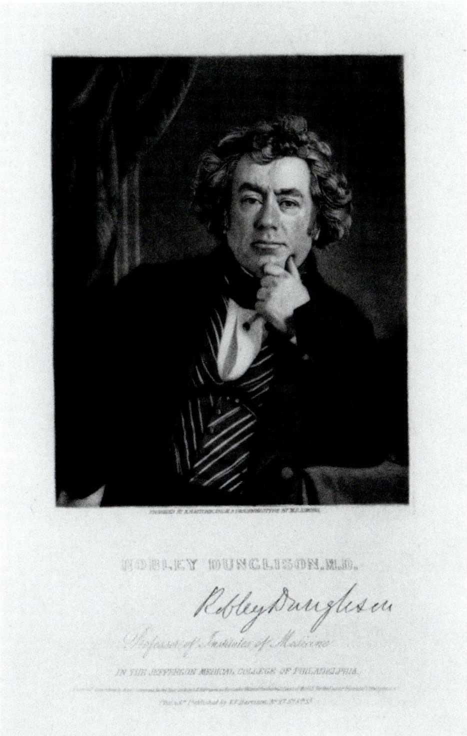
ROBLEY DUNGLISON, M.D.
Robley Dunglison
Professor of Institutes of Medicine
IN THE JEFFERSON MEDICAL COLLEGE OF PHILADELPHIA.

FIGURE 13. Dunglison in his prime, engraved by A. H. Ritchie, ca. 1846, from a daguerreotype by M. P. Simons. (Courtesy of the Library of Congress)

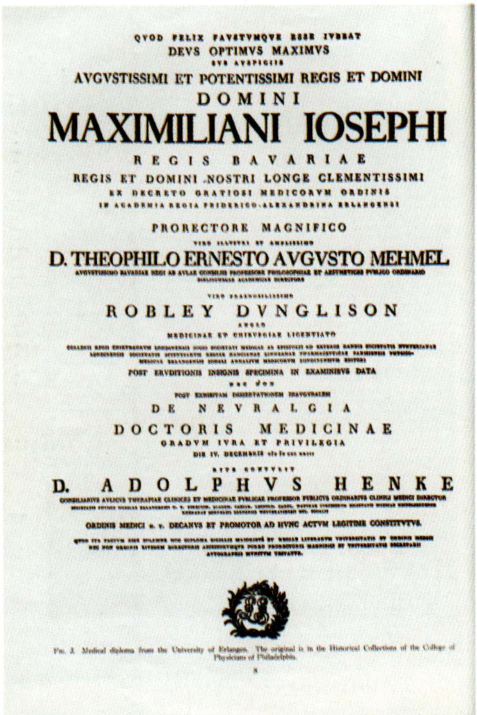

QVOD FELIX FAVSTVMQVE ESSE IVBEAT
DEVS OPTIMVS MAXIMVS
SVB AVSPICIIS
AVGVSTISSIMI ET POTENTISSIMI REGIS ET DOMINI
DOMINI
MAXIMILIANI IOSEPHI
REGIS BAVARIAE
REGIS ET DOMINI NOSTRI LONGE CLEMENTISSIMI
EX DECRETO GRATIOSI MEDICORVM ORDINIS
IN ACADEMIA REGIA FRIDERICO-ALEXANDRINA ERLANGENSI
PRORECTORE MAGNIFICO
VIRO ILLVSTRI ET AMPLISSIMO
D. THEOPHILO ERNESTO AVGVSTO MEHMEL
[illegible]
VIRO PRAENOBILISSIMO
ROBLEY DVNGLISON
ANGLO
MEDICINAE ET CHIRVRGIAE LICENTIATO
[illegible]
POST ERVDITIONIS INSIGNIS SPECIMINA IN EXAMINIBVS DATA
[illegible]
POST EXHIBITAM DISSERTATIONEM INAVGVRALEM
DE NEVRALGIA
DOCTORIS MEDICINAE
GRADVM IVRA ET PRIVILEGIA
DIE IV. DECEMBRIS [illegible]
RITE CONTVLIT
D. ADOLPHVS HENKE
[illegible]
ORDINIS MEDICI H. T. DECANVS ET PROMOTOR AD HVNC ACTVM LEGITIME CONSTITVTVS.
[illegible]

FIG. 3. Medical diploma from the University of Erlangen. The original is in the Historical Collections of the College of Physicians of Philadelphia.

8

FIGURE 14. Dunglison's medical diploma from the University of Erlanger in Bavaria. (Courtesy of Historical Collections of the College of Physicians of Philadelphia)

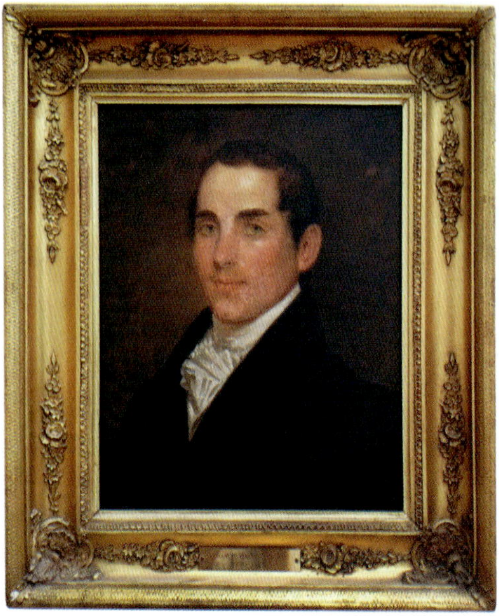

FIGURE 15. *Francis Walker Gilmer* (1790–1826), by unknown American artist, gift of Lucy A. Minor. (Courtesy of the Fralin Museum of Art, University of Virginia)

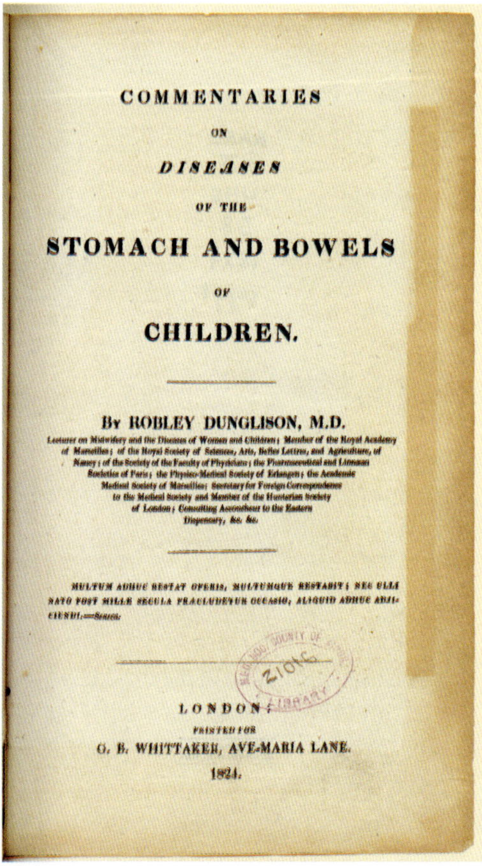

COMMENTARIES

ON

DISEASES

OF THE

STOMACH AND BOWELS

OF

CHILDREN.

BY ROBLEY DUNGLISON, M.D.

Lecturer on Midwifery and the Diseases of Women and Children; Member of the Royal Academy of Marseilles; of the Royal Society of Sciences, Arts, Belles Lettres, and Agriculture, of Nancy; of the Society of the Faculty of Physicians; the Pharmaceutical and Linnæan Societies of Paris; the Physico-Medical Society of Erlangen; the Academic Medical Society of Marseilles; Secretary for Foreign Correspondence to the Medical Society and Member of the Hunterian Society of London; Consulting Accoucheur to the Eastern Dispensary, &c. &c.

MULTUM ADHUC RESTAT OPERIS, MULTUMQUE RESTABIT; NEC ULLI NATO POST MILLE SECULA PRAECLUDETUR OCCASIO, ALIQUID ADHUC ADJICIENDI.—Seneca.

LONDON:

PRINTED FOR

G. B. WHITTAKER, AVE-MARIA LANE.

1824.

FIGURE 16. Title page of Dunglison's first textbook, 1824. (Courtesy of Historical Collections, Claude Moore Health Sciences Library, University of Virginia)

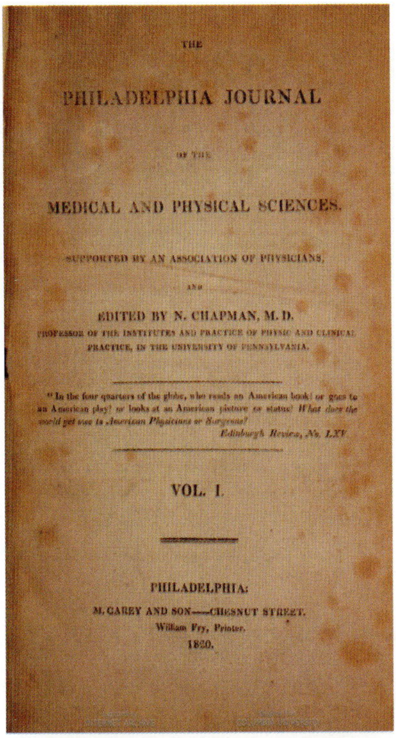

THE

PHILADELPHIA JOURNAL

OF THE

MEDICAL AND PHYSICAL SCIENCES.

SUPPORTED BY AN ASSOCIATION OF PHYSICIANS,

AND

EDITED BY N. CHAPMAN, M. D.

PROFESSOR OF THE INSTITUTES AND PRACTICE OF PHYSIC AND CLINICAL PRACTICE, IN THE UNIVERSITY OF PENNSYLVANIA.

"In the four quarters of the globe, who reads an American book? or goes to an American play? or looks at an American picture or statue? *What does the world yet owe to American Physicians or Surgeons?*

Edinburgh Review, No. LXV

VOL. I.

PHILADELPHIA:

M. CAREY AND SON——CHESNUT STREET.

William Fry, Printer.

1820.

FIGURE 17. Title page of the *Philadelphia Journal of the Medical and Physical Sciences*, 1820

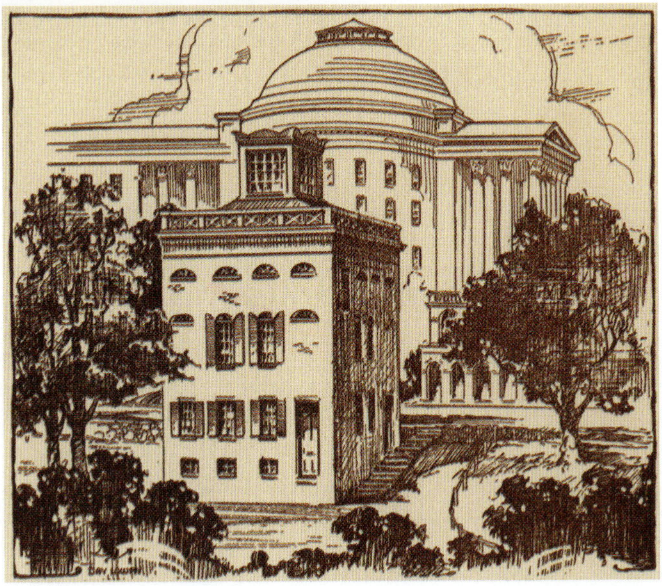

FIGURE 18. Anatomical Theater, next to Rotunda. (Courtesy of Albert and Shirley Small Special Collections Library, University of Virginia)

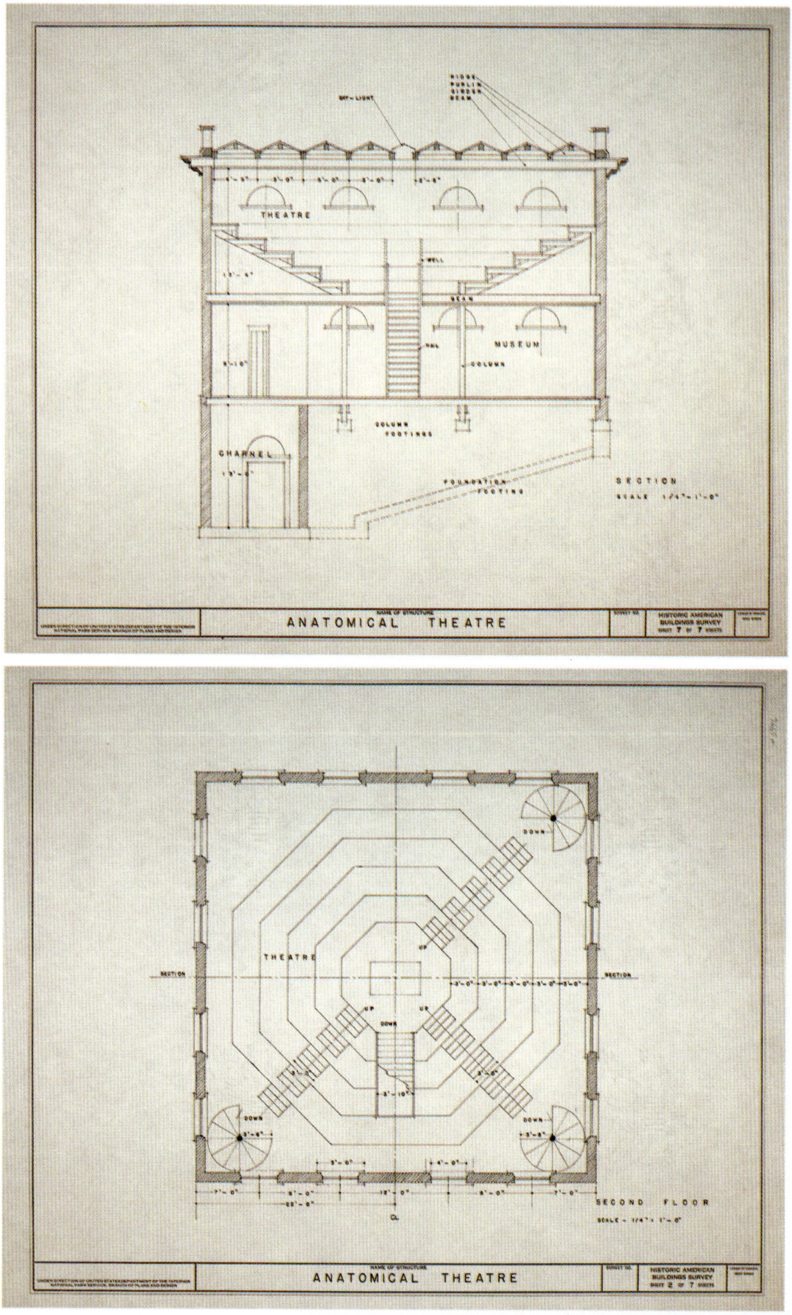

FIGURE 19. Measured drawings of Anatomical Theater based on Jefferson's plan, reconstructed by the Historical American Building Survey. (Courtesy of Albert and Shirley Small Special Collections Library, University of Virginia)

FIGURE 20. John Patten Emmet (1831), by James Westhall Ford, 1831. (Courtesy of Albert and Shirley Small Special Collections Library, University of Virginia)

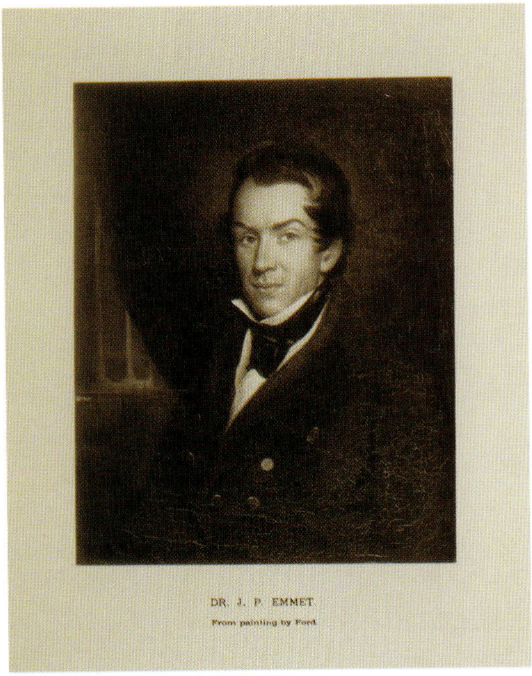

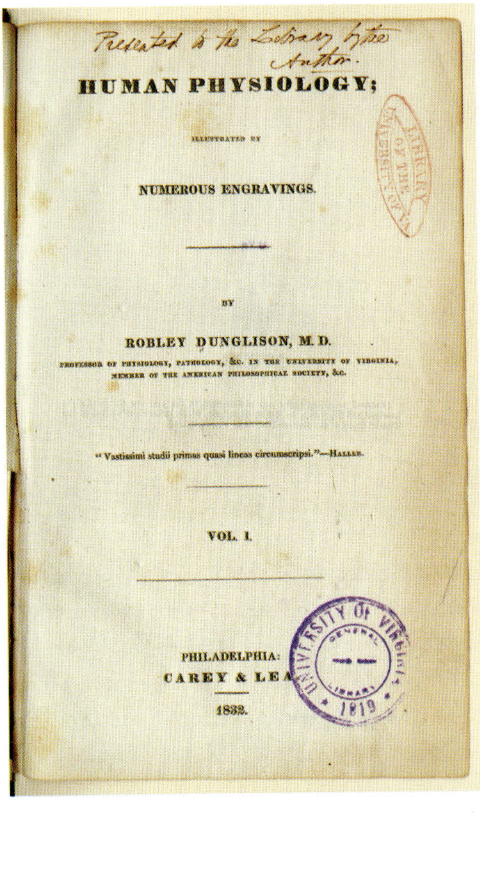
Presented to the Library by the Author.

HUMAN PHYSIOLOGY;

ILLUSTRATED BY

NUMEROUS ENGRAVINGS.

BY

ROBLEY DUNGLISON, M. D.

PROFESSOR OF PHYSIOLOGY, PATHOLOGY, &C. IN THE UNIVERSITY OF VIRGINIA, MEMBER OF THE AMERICAN PHILOSOPHICAL SOCIETY, &C.

"Vastissimi studii primas quasi lineas circumscripsi."—HALLER.

VOL. I.

PHILADELPHIA:
CAREY & LEA

1832.

FIGURE 21. Title page of Dunglison's *Human Physiology* textbook, 1832. (Courtesy of Historical Collections, Claude Moore Health Sciences Library, University of Virginia)

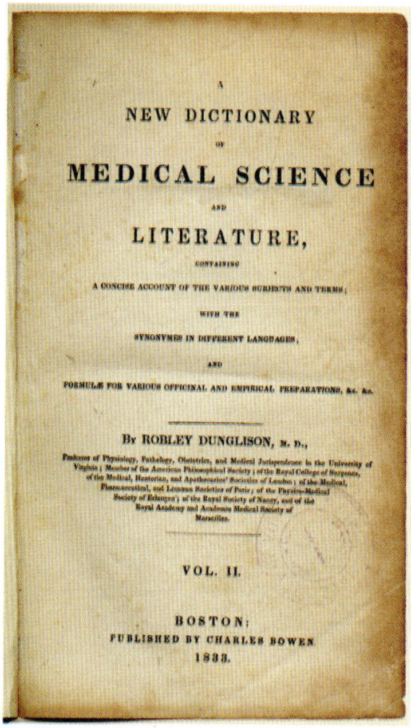

A
NEW DICTIONARY
OF
MEDICAL SCIENCE
AND
LITERATURE,
CONTAINING
A CONCISE ACCOUNT OF THE VARIOUS SUBJECTS AND TERMS;
WITH THE
SYNONYMES IN DIFFERENT LANGUAGES;
AND
FORMULÆ FOR VARIOUS OFFICINAL AND EMPIRICAL PREPARATIONS, &c. &c.

BY ROBLEY DUNGLISON, M. D.,

Professor of Physiology, Pathology, Obstetrics, and Medical Jurisprudence in the University of Virginia; Member of the American Philosophical Society; of the Royal College of Surgeons, of the Medical, Hunterian, and Apothecaries' Societies of London; of the Medical, Pharmaceutical, and Linnæan Societies of Paris; of the Physico-Medical Society of Erlangen; of the Royal Society of Nancy, and of the Royal Academy and Academic Medical Society of Marseilles.

VOL. II.

BOSTON:
PUBLISHED BY CHARLES BOWEN
1833.

FIGURE 22. Title page of Dunglison's *New Dictionary of Medical Science and Literature* textbook, 1833. (Courtesy of Historical Collections, Claude Moore Health Sciences Library, University of Virginia)

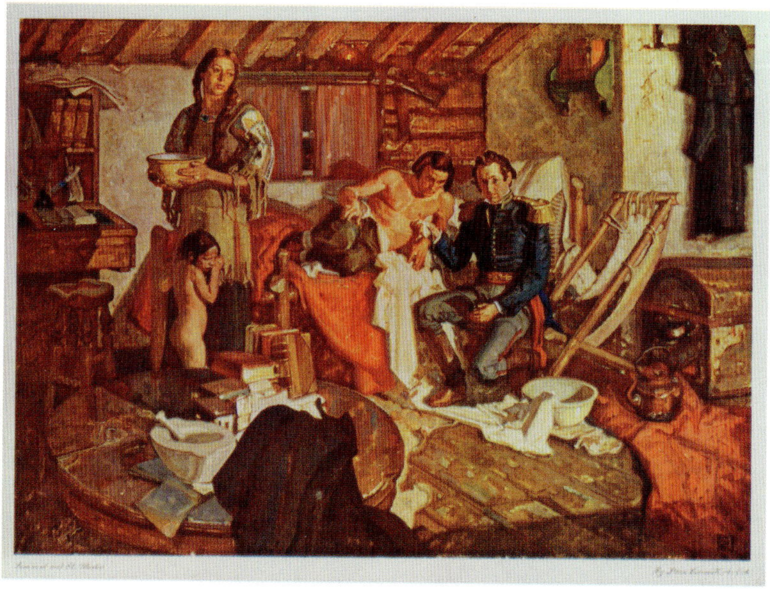

FIGURE 23. William Beaumont & Alexis St. Martin, by Dean Cornwell (1892–1960) showing the site of the fistulous tract into the stomach. The hole resulted from an accidental gunshot wound not fully healed, and it provided Beaumont with a unique window to collect gastric juice for his study into the process of digestion. (Courtesy of Library of Congress)

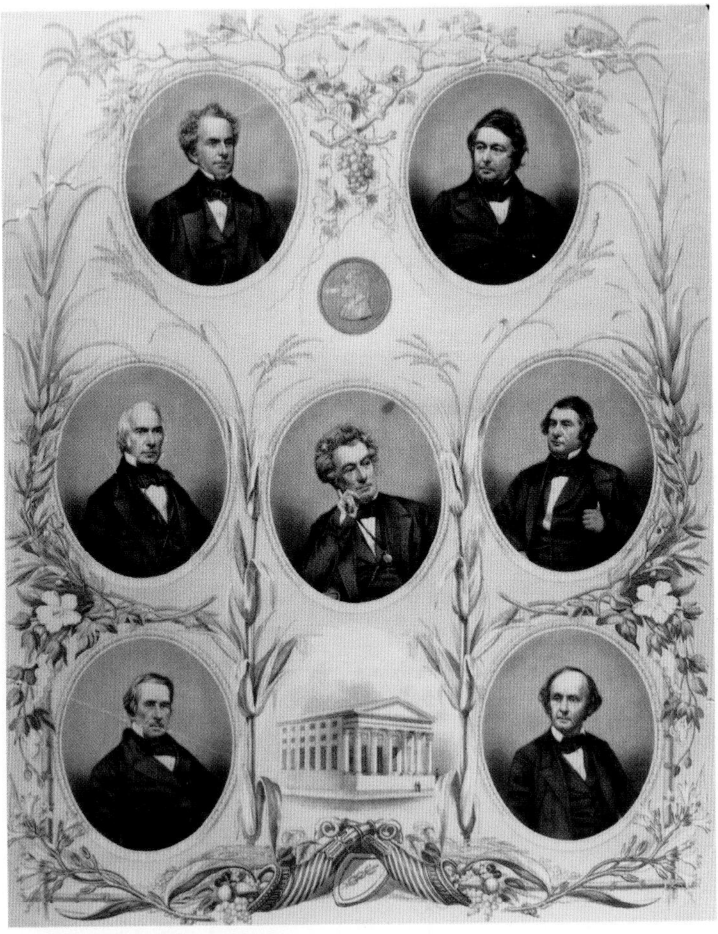

FIGURE 24. *The Famous Faculty of 1841*, engraved by R. Whitechurch and B. P. Newman, printed by Joseph M. Mason, 1855. Center portrait, Dunglison; from top left clockwise, Mutter, Pancoast, Mitchell, Meigs, Bache, and Huston. (Courtesy of Thomas Jefferson University Archives & Special Collections, Philadelphia, Penn.)

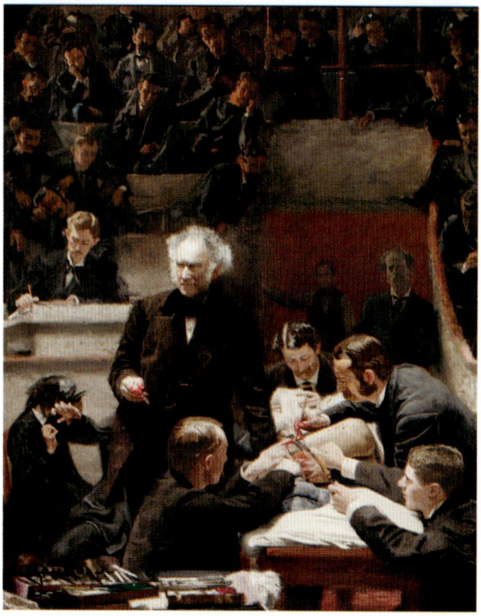

FIGURE 25. *The Gross Clinic*, Thomas Eakins, 1875, depicting Dr. Samuel D. Gross performing a surgical procedure on a patient in the surgical amphitheater at Philadelphia's Jefferson Medical College, while also demonstrating the surgeon's lack of aseptic technique. (Courtesy of the Philadelphia Museum of Art: Gift of the Alumni Association to Jefferson Medical College in 1878 and purchased by the Pennsylvania Academy of the Fine Arts and the Philadelphia Museum of Art in 2007 with the generous support of more than 3,600 donors)

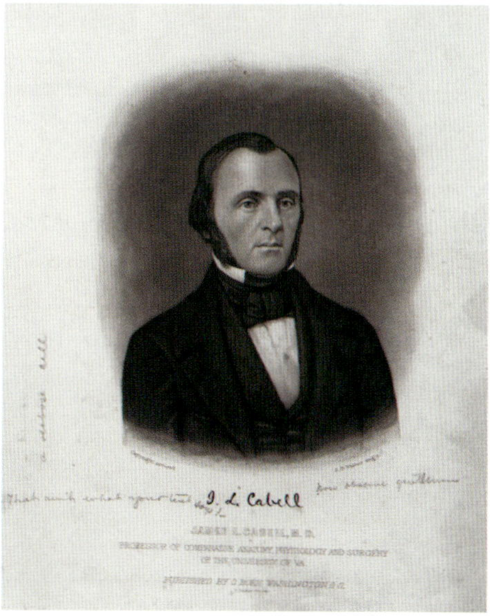

FIGURE 26. Engraving of young *James Lawrence Cabell*, by Adam B. Walter. (Courtesy of Albert and Shirley Small Special Collections Library, University of Virginia)

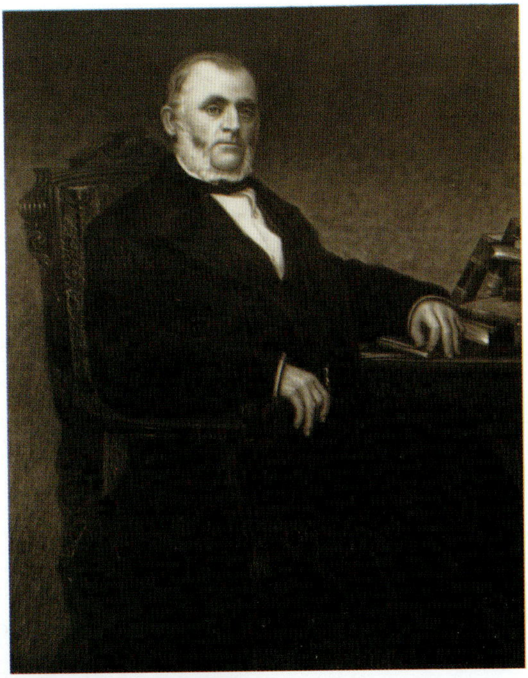

FIGURE 27. *James Lawrence Cabell*, in later life, by unknown artist. (Courtesy of Albert and Shirley Small Special Collections Library, University of Virginia)

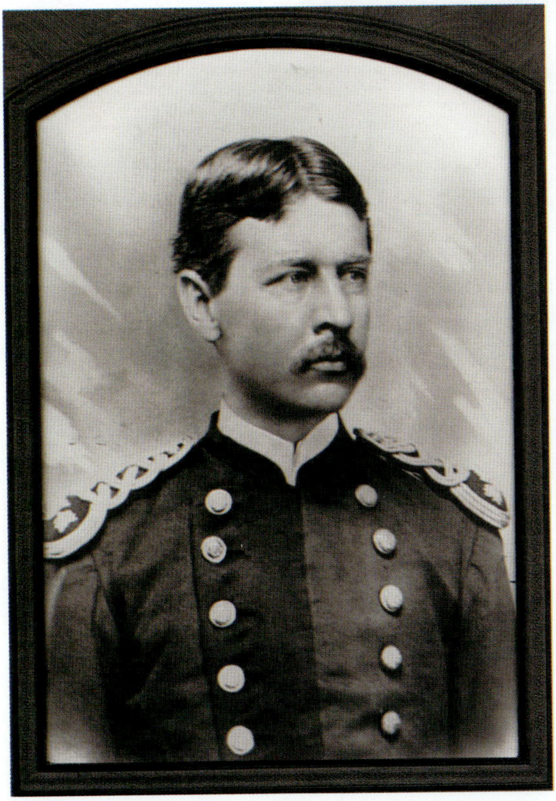

FIGURE 28. Portrait of Army Maj. (Dr.) Walter Reed, circa 1900, who, along with his team, showed that mosquitoes, specifically, the *Aedes aegypti* variety, were the transmission vector of yellow fever. (Courtesy of Claude Moore Health Sciences Library, Philip S. Hench Walter Reed Yellow Fever Collection, University of Virginia)

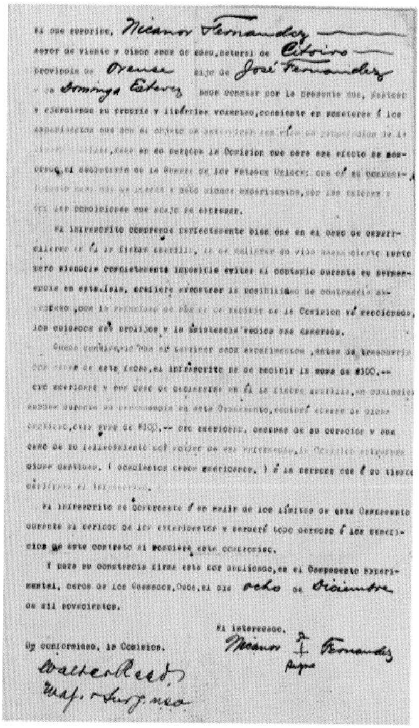

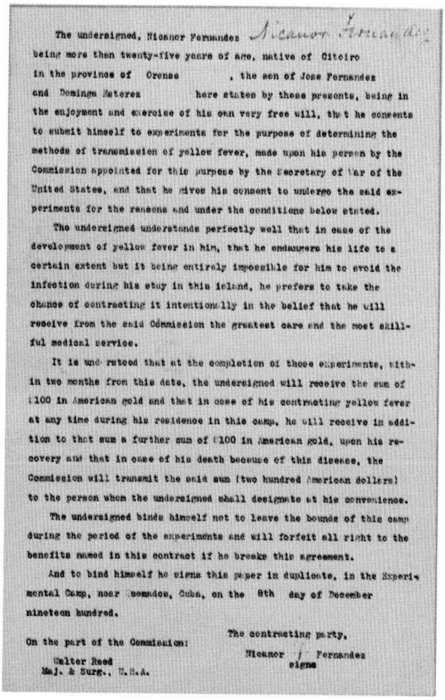

The undersigned, Nicanor Fernandez *Nicanor Fernandez*
being more than twenty-five years of age, native of Citeiro
in the province of Orense , the son of Jose Fernandez
and Dominga Esteres here states by these presents, being in the enjoyment and exercise of his own very free will, that he consents to submit himself to experiments for the purpose of determining the methods of transmission of yellow fever, made upon his person by the Commission appointed for this purpose by the Secretary of War of the United States, and that he gives his consent to undergo the said experiments for the reasons and under the conditions below stated.

The undersigned understands perfectly well that in case of the development of yellow fever in him, that he endangers his life to a certain extent but it being entirely impossible for him to avoid the infection during his stay in this island, he prefers to take the chance of contracting it intentionally in the belief that he will receive from the said Commission the greatest care and the most skillful medical service.

It is understood that at the completion of these experiments, within two months from this date, the undersigned will receive the sum of $100 in American gold and that in case of his contracting yellow fever at any time during his residence in this camp, he will receive in addition to that sum a further sum of $100 in American gold, upon his recovery and that in case of his death because of this disease, the Commission will transmit the said sum (two hundred American dollars) to the person whom the undersigned shall designate at his convenience.

The undersigned binds himself not to leave the bounds of this camp during the period of the experiments and will forfeit all right to the benefits named in this contract if he breaks this agreement.

And to bind himself he signs this paper in duplicate, in the Experimental Camp, near Quemados, Cuba, on the 8th day of December nineteen hundred.

On the part of the Commission:
Walter Reed
Maj. & Surg., U.S.A.

The contracting party,
Nicanor / Fernandez
signs

FIGURE 29. Contracts with experimental subject, Nicanor Fernandez. The original Spanish document along with the English translation, was developed by Major Walter Reed as part of his work leading the U.S. Army Yellow Fever Board. The forms seen here were signed by Reed and Fernandez. (Courtesy of Reeve Photograph Collection, Otis Historical Archives, National Museum of Health and Medicine)

with many institutions of higher education retreating from the values and rational emphasis of the Enlightenment.[2] The conduct of medical–school faculties was especially disappointing, resulting in a decline of educational standards, inadequate pedagogy, and severe intellectual paralysis. Only a small minority of practitioner-teachers engaged in scientifically focused medical writing, and even those who did often displayed a parochial bias. The worst consequences of rampant professional profit motives grew out of competition. When rivals threatened to undercut student enrollments, the invariable response was to lower requirements. Standards declined as medical schools defended market share. Moreover, the near universal repeal of state physician–licensing laws between 1830 and 1850 exacerbated the race to the bottom.[3]

A major reason for the worsening of medical education was the proliferation of new schools based on defective models. Medical schools, like colleges generally, were founded first in the Northeast (1765), then the South (1779) and eventually in the West (1817). From 1765 to the onset of the Civil War, a total of 110 medical schools, including 76 allopathic or orthodox schools, and 34 sectarian schools, were opened.[4] These medical schools were scattered throughout 25 States, from Maine to Georgia, westward to Louisiana and California, and north to Illinois and Michigan. The sectarian schools, often ignored by historians, are important for several reasons. They provided many practitioners in the middle and later decades of the 19th century. Unlike the allopathic schools, they accepted women; and, their rise, beginning in the 1840s, was a bellwether of increasing opposition to the "disastrous results of heroic medical practice."[5]

The routes by which 110 American medical schools came into being were diverse, and, with the exception of the University of Virginia, most were quite different from the more uniform system that prevailed in Europe. The impetus for medical–school development in the United States came not from colleges and universities intent on establishing and enforcing high academic standards for all students and professors, but from the medical community itself. Moreover, the educational qualifications of graduates were strikingly different because several determinative factors of sound pedagogical principles, such as *time* (duration of study), *curricular content* (learning what to do as a healer *and* why to do it as a scientifically prepared professional), and *proficiency* (robust performance requirements and examinations) were either ignored or abandoned in America.[6]

The antebellum era was a time of burgeoning laissez–faire capitalism spawned by the political forces of Jacksonian democracy that included hostility to elitism and occupational protectionism. Then and into the late

1800s, state governments were not interested in the content or duration of medical education nor the proficiency of training (competency to practice). The absence of legally binding regulations not only lowered educational standards but also encouraged the proliferation of competing sects. As more schools emerged and competition among the proprietors intensified, medical–school requirements were reduced even more.[7] The overwhelming majority of American medical schools continued the colonial model of physician–founded commercial ventures, owned and operated by the teaching faculty, who were not subject to stringent administrative oversight by collegiate officials, effective licensing laws, or watchdog boards at the state and national levels.

In fact, physician–licensing laws were weakened or abolished in the 1830s and 1840s. This encouraged medical sects and certainly contributed to the proliferation of second– and third–rate medical schools. Laws regulating medical practice were unpopular because: 1) they were considered class legislation; 2) demand for healers of all kinds was high during an age of large–scale immigration, territorial expansion, population shifts, wars, and economic change; and 3) the populace believed that every person had a right to choose his or her own medical attendant.[8] Success for medical schools was measured largely by profitability, which trumped educational achievement. Antebellum medical schools typically had an open–door admission policy, very short terms of study (3 to 4 months), reliance on part–time practitioner–teachers who rarely engaged in or promoted any element of enlightened scholarship, little or no personal contact between student and teacher (i.e., mentoring), inadequate clinical training, and lax graduation requirements. Due in part to the relatively high cost of medical education, a sizable proportion of aspiring doctors flocked to the medical schools that offered degrees in the shortest possible time with the least amount of academic labor and expense.[9]

One of the greatest challenges confronting all medical schools before the Civil War was substandard practice–based learning.[10] In contrast to German and French medical schools, those in America faced severe impediments to "learning by doing." The majority lacked proper laboratory facilities for teaching all students the practical aspects of anatomy, chemistry, and pharmaceutical science. Cadavers were difficult to obtain legally, and what dissection was done needed to be hurried due to a dearth of preservation or refrigeration facilities. No school included hospital training as a central part of the teaching program. Even in the large cities where urban hospitals existed, such as Philadelphia, New York and later Boston, the medical schools located in them did not require hands-on clinical experience because hospital managers opposed and defeated efforts to involve students personally in the direct care of patients. They were not permitted to examine patients or participate in treatment decisions. As a result, a substantial number of students graduated without ever touching a patient, attending a birth, or witnessing an operation.[11] While the New Orleans School of Medicine pioneered an authentic clinical clerkship experience for students in 1857, modeled on a similar plan in Vienna, the school fell victim to the Civil War and closed. Johns Hopkins in the 1890s finally established the clerkship as a permanent part of the curriculum.[12]

These systemic deficiencies, coupled with the unbridled pecuniary interests that dominated the medical profession throughout most of the nineteenth century and a general lack of public outcry, led to an enormous overproduction of poorly trained medical practitioners, even from the long–established Northeastern medical schools. The unfortunate consequences became abundantly clear with the outbreak of the Civil War. In this most lethal conflict in American history, disease accounted for nearly two–thirds of the 750,000 fatalities.[13] A medical as well as a societal tragedy, it highlighted the woeful deficiencies of mid-nineteenth-century American medical education. In the words of Kenneth Ludmerer, an acclaimed historian,

> The training and skills of the average doctor were hopelessly inadequate, even based on existing standards of the day. Elementary techniques of physical examination . . . [and] simple instruments were rarely employed by military practitioners, even though their use was already strongly advocated by the leading medical schools of Europe. Pain was frequently treated by the useless technique of applying opiate powders to wounds topically rather than by administering the drugs through hypodermic injections. Military physicians continued to purge their patients with dangerous doses of potent laxatives and emetics long after French medical scientists had convincingly demonstrated that these traditional "heroic" therapies were not only unbeneficial but often harmful. When a brave Union surgeon general, William Alexander Hammond, banned the use of two toxic drugs, calomel and tartar emetic, because of their severe side effects (profuse salivation and putrid gangrene of the gums, mouth, and face), he was court–martialed [fortunately without success] and condemned by the AMA.[14]

Dunglison at the Medical College of Maryland

Such was the state of medical education in 1833, when Dunglison went north to accept a teaching position at the Medical College of Maryland (1833–1836), and subsequently the Jefferson Medical College of Philadelphia (1836–1868).[15] Compared to the University of Virginia, these two urban schools were radically different in their originating sponsors, organizational structure and governance, and devotion to academic productivity.[16] Unlike his arrangement at Virginia, Dunglison received no salary or fringe benefits. Instead, his teaching income depended entirely on fees from students enrolled in his classes. Teaching from 120 to 500 or more students each year, with each student paying him $20 for the courses he taught, greatly increased his annual income. In Virginia, not counting income from book sales, Dunglison's annual compensation there never exceeded $3,000. His base salary was $1,500. He also received free housing valued at $350 and student fees, which peaked at $1,250 a year. In contrast, annual income from student fees in Baltimore and Philadelphia averaged more than $5,000, and the length of the teaching term was a mere 4 months, as compared to 10 months at UVA.[17]

The Medical College of Maryland was the sixth to open in the United States, preceded by the College of Philadelphia (1765, later the University of Pennsylvania); the Medical School of King's College (1767, later Columbia University College of Physicians and Surgeons); the Medical Department of William and Mary College (1779, closed permanently in 1782); the Medical School of Harvard College (1782); and the Medical Department of Dartmouth College (1797). Organized and incorporated by Baltimore doctors in 1807, it was a wholly independent proprietary school with no connection to an established college or university. As with the schools formed earlier, the course of instruction during the first session was incomplete and lectures were delivered at the houses of the professors. The number of matriculating students in the first three years of operations was seven, ten, and eighteen, respectively, and in 1810, degrees were conferred on five graduates. Eventually, a suitable building was acquired, after which enrollment steadily increased. However, in the 1820s, the school began a descent into schism, tumult, and lawsuits of the kind that plagued most urban proprietary medical schools.[18] With the opening in 1827 of a second medical school, the Washington Medical College of Baltimore, an acrimonious competition began.[19]

On October 31, 1833, Dunglison gave his inaugural lecture to a mixed assemblage of medical students, professors, and townspeople.[20] His main theme was the history of medicine, with a decided focus on the three branches of medical science that he was charged with teaching: general therapeutics and materia medica, medical jurisprudence, and preventive medicine or the "art of preserving health" through proper hygiene, added at Dunglison's insistence.[21] He began with a retrospective account of these subjects, replete with numerous exemplars, to show how former times were dominated by a plethora of irrational practices driven by ignorance, credulity, monstrous superstition and the machinery of magic and best exhibited by the "repulsive and ridiculous agents that were introduced or recommended by individuals, distinguished in their day." He then transitioned to more modern times, pointing out that immense progress had been made, especially in the European universities, after a long "period of defective observation and experience." He artfully and enthusiastically predicted that thereafter, "as the physical and moral sciences pursue their onward progress, and as the means of observation and experiment are augmented and facilitated, the science [of medical practice] may attain a pitch of perfection, of which at the present time we can form no adequate conception, shedding light where all is obscurity, and tending to dispel doubt and difficulty wherever existent." Dunglison's wonderful use of language, and precise argumentative logic was, throughout this lecture, vintage Jefferson. In it he quoted frequently from past and present charlatans and popular philosophers, including richly satirical writings and absurdly credulous anecdotes from Alexander Pope, William Shakespeare, John Dryden, John Webster, Sir Walter Scott, Samuel Butler, Hippocrates, Francis Bacon, Boyle, Celsus, Pliny the Elder, Cato the Censor, Samuel Johnson, Sir William Blackstone, Alexaner of Thales, Alexander of Tralles, Sir Theodore Turquet deMayerne, and Rosicruian teachings. Dunglison nonetheless expressed an optimistic faith in the perfectibility of the human intellect and race.[22] He spoke of the "precious fruit" that could emerge from "the tree of knowledge" if one were to "turn assiduously to the discovery and investigation of truth." Dunglison even called on his audience to imagine a future that might include a *Voyage to the Moon*, the turning of the desert into a paradise, and a far–off day when death might result only from extraordinary accidents.[23] The gist of the speech was that scientific principles that governed the empirical sciences and had begun to imbue medical practice in Europe were the only way that medicine and society in general could progress, even to the point where exploring the moon or seeing the lead-up to death as a controllable disease might be possible. In conveying such a message, Dunglison was acting as a kind of missionary of science to a field where its principles had yet to be applied in the classroom, the domestic sickroom, or the hospital.

Authorship of Textbooks

Dunglison continued to propose innovations in medical teaching. He wrote textbooks that expanded the scope of the medical–school curriculum by supporting new courses offered first by him and then by professors at other schools. For example, the course on preventive medicine and public health that he advocated for, organized, and taught at the Medical College of Maryland (1833–36) was arguably the first in America.[24]

Besides his duties to his students, Dunglison recognized his obligations to contribute, by way of scholarly writing, his quota to the stock of medical knowledge. Throughout his professional career, he fulfilled this obligation to such an extent that he became known as the "most voluminous writer of his day in the new world, and . . . in point of bulk the works of all his American contemporaries sink into insignificance besides his."[25] After leaving Virginia, Dunglison's major textbooks included: *Elements of Hygiene* (1835);[26] *General Therapeutics & Principles of Medical Practice, with tables of the chief remedial agents and their preparation, and of the different poisons and their antidotes* (1836); *The Medical Student: Aids to the Study of Medicine* (1837); *New Remedies: The Method of preparing and administering them, and their effects on the healthy and diseased economy* (1839); *The Practice of Medicine, or a Treatise on Special Pathology and Therapeutics* (1842); *A Dictionary for the Blind in tangible type* (1860); and *The History of Medicine from the Earliest Ages to the Commencement of the 19th Century* (published posthumously, 1872).

While in Baltimore, Dunglison completed work on the textbook on human health and hygiene. This project, first contemplated during his tenure at Virginia, grew out of his belief that the scientific aspects of hygiene "ought to form part of the curriculum of medical studies in every University; and that some knowledge of it would be most useful to the public generally, not only by enabling them to ward off attacks of disease, but to judge when the services of the professional adviser are needed."[27] It first appeared in print at the beginning of 1835, consisted of 514 pages, and was very favorably reviewed.[28] Although not nearly as popular as his work on *Human Physiology* or his *Medical Dictionary*, this book sold upwards of 3,000 copies in its first two printings, and its contents formed the basis of Dunglison's innovative course on public health and hygiene. Indeed, the principles he taught in person are all contained in his textbook, and today, the School of Medicine of the University of Maryland commemorates Dunglison's contributions in this area each year at commencement by conferring on a graduating student the Robley Dunglison Award for Excellence in Preventive Medicine.

The second major textbook Dunglison completed in Baltimore was, like his other works, written for the benefit of his medical students. The first edition of *General Therapeutics and Materia Medica*, published in 1836, was 1,322 pages in length and described by Dunglison as "the only one of the kind in the English language." It filled an important gap in that, as he later recalled, "whilst the properties and mode of administration of the various articles of the materia medica received ample attention, but little was paid to the great principles, that should guide the practitioner in prescribing them; and that the most crying defect, in practitioners in general, is their want of knowledge of general therapeutics. It is easy enough to prescribe, but not so easy to know when and what we ought to prescribe." The book, according to Dunglison, was "calculated to be of some service by inducing an inquiry into the *modus operandi* of remedial agents," and he heard that it exerted "a decided influence in modifying the heroic practice, which generally prevailed" then in Baltimore. Between 1836 and 1850, approximately 6,250 copies of the textbook were sold, and in a testimonial to its value, Dr. Henry Massie Bullitt (1817–80), who later founded the Louisville Medical College, credited the book with "having had great agency . . . in diminishing the destructive *calomelization* so universal in the west at the time." Another eminent physician, Dr. Jacob Bigelow (1787–1879) of Boston bestowed a similar accolade on Dunglison. A learned and accomplished educator at Harvard Medical College, Bigelow shared many of Dunglison's views, best exemplified in two of his more famous writings — on *Rational Medicine* and *Discourse on Self-Limited Disease.* Both of these mid-nineteenth-century publications had an important influence on moderating the treatment of disease in America. Fittingly, when Bigelow published a collected edition of his lectures in 1859, including *Nature in Disease*, he dedicated it to Dunglison for the principles he espoused in his *Medical Therapeutics*. Dunglison's textbook may also have had much to do with his appointment in 1840 as a delegate to the National Medical Council for the Revision of the Pharmacopoeia of the United States.[29]

In 1839 Dunglison published *New Remedies*, a book that nearly doubled in content by its 7th edition. The seed for this work was sown in 1822 when Dunglison, still in England, was editing the *Formulary of Magendie.* His book not only summarized instances of "modern introduction" to the materia medica, including formulae for their preparation and administration, but also described "certain older agents that have in recent times received novel applications."[30] The seven editions appearing between 1839 and 1856 sold more than 7,000 copies.

In 1842, Dunglison completed his work on the *Practice of Medicine.* It was dedicated "to the Gentlemen who have honored the author by their attendance on his lectures in the course of the last sixteen years." The two-volume work appeared in three editions. The last, in 1848, was upwards of 1,490 pages. Its contents emphasized that "The condition of a progressive Science" can inform current observations and that "the observations of *savans* of all periods — past and present" can lead to a picture that "must necessarily embody the collected wisdom of every age."[31] This text brought to fruition Dunglison's addition of the history of medicine to the curriculum.

Dunglison's unflagging commitment to literary usefulness led one associate to remark at his death that "In a science so rapidly progressive as that of medicine, even the best books speedily grow out of date, but Dunglson's industry kept his works on a level with the advance of knowledge, and most of them in repeated editions maintained their positions for a period far longer that is generally allotted to the life of a scientific book."[32] Dunglison was pleased that his textbooks won wide acceptance in many medical schools in America, and even some European universities, and that they provided a valuable source of postgraduate education for practicing physicians. He also surmised, perhaps naively given their cost and complexity, that his textbooks would "enable the well–educated individual [layperson] to form some judgment of the qualifications of the medical practitioner; to distinguish the ignorant pretender from the man of science; and, of consequence, to cleave to the one, whilst he eschews the other."[33] Regardless of this aspiration, an effect of Dunglison's literary diligence was to expand the ambit of medical expertise, that is, the scope of knowledge a well–rounded physician must master during training.

Dunglison as Journal Author and Editor

Dunglison wrote for his peers, as well as for students, and like Jefferson, he established links between American and European scholars. While in Baltimore, he wrote various articles for the *Baltimore Medical and Surgical Journal* and its successor, the *North American Archives of Medical and Surgical Science,* and he continued as a collaborating editor of the *American Journal of Medical Science.*[34]

Later, after moving to Philadelphia, Dunglison edited the *American Medical Library and Intelligencer*, a monthly journal, from 1837 to 1842.[35] In Philadelphia, he solidified his reputation as a prolific author, prompting a colleague to write after his death, "He was a reformer of the prejudices of his age, and powerfully aided not only in emancipating the professional mind from the errors of false observation, so common in our day, but also laying a solid and enduring foundation of a medical literature, destined to exalt the national character, and to rival at no distant period, in depth and vigor, that of the Old World."[36]

Dunglison's forays into scholarly publishing were not limited to the United States. In 1835 he partnered with Sir John Forbes (1787–1861) of London as a founding editor of the *British and Foreign Medical Review,* a new journal intent on "promoting the general progress of medical science" in England, Europe, and America, by providing "Reviews of all the *good books* [and journal articles] published in *every* country, where there is a Medical press;" "*Annual Reports* of the state of medicine in them during the preceding year, noticing the discoveries and improvements, the new theories and practices, the books published, and the obituaries of eminent men;" and "an account of the Medical Schools, Hospitals, Medical Societies, State of the Medical Press, Lists of Journals, Transactions of Societies, Etc., general character of the profession, mode of remuneration, grades etc." In 1836 Dunglison submitted an article containing "An Account of the Medical Colleges" in the United States, as regarded their history, organization, professors, opportunities for instruction and fees. The following year, he communicated an article on the "Medical Associations for the Regulation of Practice" and another on the "Remuneration of the Medical Profession," with a comparative table of the prevailing medical, surgical and other fees of New York, Baltimore, and Charleston, and yet another on the "Charges for Medicine supplied by the Druggists" of New York and Charleston.[37] These articles illustrate Dunglison's research into the conditions of American medicine at the levels of training, oversight, and professional compensation, specifically the length of study it took to become a physician, how organizations might supervise the profession, and how doctors and druggists were paid. These articles, as well as his editing of news about medical science around the world, demonstrate that Dunglison's efforts to improve medical pedagogy stemmed from and were informed by data describing professional practice and advances from a startling variety of venues. Moreover, Dunglison's international collaboration achieved some success in neutralizing the scorn of American scientists by their European counterparts.

Upgrades in Clinical Training

Dunglison's instructional agenda was not confined to writing textbooks and giving lectures. He also practiced and taught in one of the earliest medical-school hospitals in the United States, the Baltimore Infirmary, also called "University Hospital," which was erected in 1823 and modeled after the Edinburgh Infirmary in name and function. It was the first in America to be built and controlled by a medical-school faculty.[38] Unlike Charlottesville, the city of Baltimore, with a population of 80,000, offered many clinical opportunities for medical students, including the Baltimore Almshouse, with over 2,000 inmates, and the Baltimore General Dispensary, built in 1801. This fact prompted at least one of Dunglison's Virginia students, James Lawrence Cabell, to follow him to Baltimore to complete his undergraduate medical studies. Their teacher-student relationship proved fruitful for the field of medicine as a whole, as will be seen below.

Influences on Fellow Faculty in Maryland

Dunglison came to view his fellow teachers during his three years in Baltimore as "a corps of efficient instructors." Admittedly he also judged that "the members of the Faculty of the University of Maryland were by no means equal as teachers, or in their general or professional qualifications," as his former colleagues in the Old Dominion, although he thought highly of two colleagues, Drs. Nathan Ryno Smith and Eli Geddings.[39] The Baltimore faculty were not as well read or zealous in the pursuit of scholarship, and they seemed to focus more on the clinical, as opposed to the scientific, aspects of medicine—perhaps because the facilities afforded so much opportunity for students to witness sickness at the bedside and to prosecute their anatomical studies given the ample material for dissection, admittedly often obtained for them illicitly through grave robbing from potters' fields and even in some cases from victims murdered so that their corpses could be sold.[40] In his memoirs, Dunglison observed that "Amongst the Faculty themselves, there were elements of discord, which threatened its destruction." He was pleased that "the conciliating course I always pursued" earned him, "during my residence in Baltimore, the reputation of being "a peacemaker."[41] The odious conduct of faculty members toward each other was not confined to the Maryland school. Behavior toward professional brethren and competing institutions that was disparaging, bordering on defamatory, was common in virtually all medical schools with a proprietary structure, likely born out of jealousy, and unscrupulous fighting for greater income from student fees. Dunglison's pacific intentions and diplomatic skills were also to be tested during his next professorship in Philadelphia.

Jefferson Medical College and Philadelphia

In September of 1836, Dunglison moved to Philadelphia to take the chair in institutes of medicine and medical jurisprudence at Jefferson Medical College, which included the teaching of physiological science, and he held this position until his death in 1869. He was attracted to the city as what he called "the great center for medical education in the United States." Other reasons for leaving Baltimore included a lack of harmonious cooperation between Maryland faculty and its Board of Trustees and doubts regarding the future prosperity of the medical school and a suspicion that it would likely not become "a permanently large" institution of higher education.[42] The medical college was the seventeenth to open in America and the second in Philadelphia. It came into being in 1824 when a local practitioner, Dr. George McClellan (1796–1847), secured an affiliation agreement with a small college located in Canonsburg, Pennsylvania, 310 miles west of Philadelphia. After receiving his M.D. in 1819 from the University of Pennsylvania, McClellan had opened a private anatomy school and then campaigned to found a new medical school in Philadelphia, much to the consternation of his alma mater. The Canonsburg Academy's name was changed to Jefferson College in 1802 in honor of the newly elected president. In 1838, Jefferson Medical College gained its own independent charter and severed its ties with the college.[43]

The newly organized medical college was similar to the proprietary schools of the time. In return for authority to grant degrees, the medical branch in the city would have no claims on the funds of the foster-mother institution in Canonsburg. The financial and scholastic success of Jefferson Medical College was entirely up to its faculty, which controlled its administrative affairs, including the nomination of professors, the establishment of educational standards such as curricular content and graduation requirements, and the setting, collection, and distribution of student fees. It remained a proprietary institution until 1895, when it became a nonprofit corporation with a single board of trustees responsible for the complete management of the college and hospital.[44] When the medical school began classroom instruction in November 1825, at nearly the same time as the University of Virginia, 107 students were enrolled compared to 440 at its cross-town rival, the University of Pennsylvania. In April 1826, fewer than six months later, inaugural degrees were awarded to twenty men.[45]

Throughout the antebellum history of the Jefferson Medical College, Philadelphia's population grew exponentially and considerable rivalry, at times acrimonious, existed between the college, the University of Pennsylvania, and some of the nine other medical schools, mostly short-lived, that opened in the city. The competitors included a mix of allopathic and sectarian schools: Medical Department of Pennsylvania College (1840–61), Philadelphia College of Medicine (1847–1859), Franklin Medical College (1846–48), Homeopathic Medical College of Pennsylvania (1848), Female Medical College of Pennsylvania (1850), American College of Medicine (1853–54), Eclectic Medical College of Pennsylvania (1851), Pennsylvania Medical University of Philadelphia (1853), and the Eclectic Medical College of Philadelphia (1856).

Intercollegiate bitterness led to fractiousness among Jefferson's professors, to which Dunglison, as a newly appointed professor, took steps to subdue, soon after taking up his new post. With two quarreling factions, Dunglison took a neutral stand and became the mediating tiebreaker. His pacifying policy eventually resulted not only in harmony among the Jefferson faculty, but a cordial and productive relationship with the University of Pennsylvania. Within a year of Dunglison's arrival in Philadelphia, all the professors of the University of Pennsylvania had called on him except Nathaniel Chapman, who disliked him both as a foreigner and a rival.[46]

By 1837 Dunglison was being hailed by most of his cross–town colleagues as "a scholar, a profound physician, and an enlightened physiologist of the highest rank," in America and Europe, and as "an elegant and popular lecturer who had no superior." He presented himself as an optimist who believed it possible to "feel and act – not as bitter rivals endeavouring to injure or destroy each other, but as energetic and devoted members of a <u>profession</u>... competing with each other as to which can render the greatest amount of benefit to mankind."[47] This attitude surely helped weed out the dissenting troublemakers in his own institution, some of whom engaged in open warfare with the University of Pennsylvania. By 1841 Dunglison had reconfigured the entire staff. The new faculty, carefully engineered by Dunglison, resulted in durable stability and peace at Jefferson Medical College, as well as enhanced opportunities for supervised clinical instruction. He saw to it that the two great seats of clinical teaching, the Philadelphia General Hospital and the Pennsylvania Hospital, were represented on the faculty, thus providing students access to a vast amount of clinical teaching material at the two oldest hospitals in the United States, and he also placed a faculty member on staff at the Philadelphia Dispensary, established in 1786 to serve the poor.[48] The revamped corps of professors included, in addition to Dunglison, Robert Mendenhall Huston (materia medica and therapeutics), Joseph Pancoast (anatomy), John Kearsley Mitchell (practice of medicine), Thomas Dent Mutter (practice of surgery), Charles Delucena Meigs (obstetrics and diseases of women & children), Franklin Bache (chemistry), all medical graduates of the University of Pennsylvania (see Figure 24). Dunglison later added Samuel David Gross, an early graduate of Jefferson Medical College, who went on to found the American Surgical Association. These like-minded men, all scholars in their own right, taught at the Jefferson Medical College for a combined total of 186 years and accounted for several seminal advancements in surgical technique—for example, the Mutter Flap used to treat burn victims—were the first to use ethyl ether anesthesia in Philadelphia, received much acclaim for their collection and cataloguing of thousands of medical specimens, especially oddities, and authored many important textbooks and essays, such as Bache's *Dispensatory*. Dunglison praised them as "possessing congenial sentiments, ample qualifications, untiring industry, and . . . honorable and upright deportment."[49]

In 1844, Dunglison proclaimed the success of his faculty reorganization as measured by the steady increase in the size of the classes. In his time, the number of students attracted to a medical school was a popular measure of success, and in the three years between 1841 and 1844, the Jefferson Medical College more than doubled its enrollment. Within five years, the classes grew so large that the school's building had to be enlarged in order to accommodate the hosts of young men attracted to its classrooms. The impressive numbers of matriculates and graduates are shown in the following Table:[50]

Session	**Class Size**	**Graduates (from VA)**
1839–1840	145	56 (12)
1840–1841	163	52 (11)
1841–1842	209	59 (13)
1842–1843	229	47 (12)
1843–1844	341	117 (15)
1844–1845	409	116 (20)
1845–1846	469	170 (41)
1846–1847	493	181 (47)
1847–1848	480	178 (46)

1848–1849	477	188 (62)
1849–1850	516	211 (63)
1850–1851	504	227 (55)
1851–1852	506	213 (62)
1852–1853	556	223 (54)
1853–1854	627	270 (46)
1854–1855	565	256 (49)
1855–1856	510	215 (36)
1856–1857	488	211 (33)
1857–1858	501	209 (46)
1858–1859	630	256 (47)

Jefferson Medical College attracted students from every state in the Union, as well as from nineteen foreign countries or principalities.[51] Students from the South accounted for a surprising 51 percent of all graduates (1,776 of 3,455) during the period between 1840 and 1859, and 43 percent of the graduates from southern states were from Virginia (770 of 1,776). Overall, as the Table shows, 22 percent of Jefferson graduates were Virginians. This remarkable migration of southern students to Philadelphia occurred despite the fact that many influential southern physicians argued strongly for both "cultural" and "educational separatism," based on their belief that diseases and treatments in the South were fundamentally different from those elsewhere, especially when compared to northeastern practices, and thus required that doctors intent on serving the medical needs of this region, including the "singularly" distinct Black population, must be trained in southern schools. Southern students nonetheless kept coming to Philadelphia for clinical experience, the quality and reputation of the teaching faculties, the city elite's prosouthern sympathies, the presence of numerous southerners on the faculties, and the potential for acquiring social status along with a medical degree.[52] The faculty changes Dunglison helped orchestrate, the clinical opportunities he expanded, and his textbook authorship most likely also played a role in the popularity of Jefferson Medical College.

Although enrollment and graduation numbers fell dramatically in the 1860s, virtually all of the decline resulted from the rising sectional tension between North and South, the Civil War itself, and its aftermath. The eventual exodus of Southern medical students from Philadelphia was mostly a political act by students driven by a desire to be removed from "immoral" abolitionist rhetoric. Immediately after secession, two Philadelphia medical teachers from Virginia, Drs. Hunter Holmes McGuire and Francis E. Luckett, helped convince 198 southern students to leave the city and travel to Richmond, where many enrolled in the Medical College of Virginia. This migration had nothing to do with medical education or criteria designed to serve educational excellence.[53]

Dunglison: the Quintessential Academic

Dunglison served as dean of Jefferson Medical College for much of his time in Philadelphia, and he continued to teach and mentor students while fulfilling his responsibilities as an academic scholar and change agent. His devotion to teaching and the betterment of students was evinced in a book that first appeared in 1837, *The Medical Student: Aids to the Study of Medicine*, in which Dunglison presented his refined views on medical education. Its content was highly regarded, being described as a work "of inestimable value to the medical neophyte in the development of proper conduct and medical etiquette." The four chapters included a set of standards with enlightened commentary on preliminary education; medical education prior to attendance on lectures; medical education during the period of attendance on lectures; and medical education after graduation. An exquisitely composed annotated bibliography was appended with notice of 195 important works for students to digest, and the volume concluded with a historical account of and comments on existing conditions at the twenty-three allopathic medical colleges in the United States. The book as a whole dealt with medicine as taught in America, and its purpose was to inform young medical aspirants as to "the best method of study for one about to enter upon professional life, as well as for one engaged in its prosecution."[54] While it was a handbook for new students, it also revealed Dunglison's continuing research into medical education throughout the country, previously manifested in his journal articles enumerating defects in American medical education, such as "College Instruction and Discipline" (1831) and "An Account of the Medical Colleges in the United States" (1836, modified in 1837).

Dunglison's counsel embraced ethical as well as professional standards. During his career at Jefferson Medical College, he expanded his previous counsel to students and to everyone engaged in the practice of medicine, arguing that the discipline needs to be governed by principles of right and wrong, thus stressing that a profession is defined not by technical expertise alone but by adherence to ethical codes, concepts shared with Jefferson.

Throughout his academic life, in Charlottesville, Baltimore or Philadelphia, Dunglison promoted the importance of humility, compassion, sympathy for suffering, justice and benevolence, gentleness and equanimity, temperance and sobriety, obligation to discretion and honor, charity and good will to all, disdain for all artifice, therapeutic appropriateness and restraint when evidence is lacking, avoiding the fallacy of individual experience that lacked an understanding of the accumulated wisdom of the ages, the sanative power of nature, and the inestimable value of health preservation for individuals and the community at large.[55] He also encouraged students to read the works of John Gregory *(Lectures on the Duties and Qualifications of a Physician*, 1772) and Thomas Percival *(Medical Ethics or, a Code of Institutes and Precepts, adapted to the Professional Conduct of Physicians and Surgeons*, 1827).[56]

By the time he retired as a professor, Dunglison had signed the diplomas of more than five thousand medical students.[57] The passage that follows, from his valedictory address at Jefferson Medical College, illustrates his life's credo. This speech, like the one that Dunglison gave in 1833 to the graduating class of the University of Virginia, shows his desire to waken in each student the precious qualities of human sympathy, benevolence, and charity to all:

> Unflinching devotion to your profession; conduct humane, charitable, and without reproach; a gentle sympathizing demeanor; entire freedom from envy, hatred and malice, and all uncharitableness towards your fellow man; and especially towards your professional brethren; and a rigid observance of the heaven–desired invocation of 'peace and goodwill toward men', can scarcely fail to lead you to distinction; but should inevitable circumstances prevent this desirable consummation you will have the heart–felt consolation of knowing that you have done all in your power to merit it; and to be regarded, at the close of it, I trust, a long life, as the skillful, upright, benevolent, conscientious and beloved physician.[58]

Dunglison exemplified these principles of generosity as much in civil society as in his teaching.[59] While in Philadelphia, he was a founder and long-time president of the Musical Fund Society of Philadelphia. Dunglison also took up the plight of the less fortunate members of society. He chaired the Committee of Instruction of the Pennsylvania Institution of the Blind and was quite successful in promoting the development of a tactile mode of communication similar to braille. With William Chapin (1802–88), he prepared a three-volume *Dictionary for the Blind,* set in raised type, based on Joseph Emerson Worcester's English Dictionary. In the early 1840s, Dunglison served as director and vice president of the Pennsylvania Training School for Idiotic and Feeble–Minded Children, and with Dorothea Dix he helped promote legislation leading to the construction of the Pennsylvania Asylum for the Insane Poor. He also wrote several valuable articles on the importance of providing the insane poor with suitable institutional care.[60]

Dunglison's Final Years

During his last decades, Dunglison was an invalid. Gout made him lame, gallbladder disease resulted in recurrent episodes of abdominal pain, at times severe, and heart disease made him dyspneic and edematous. Yet despite these progressive infirmities, he soldiered on "with manly courage. If he could not stand to lecture, Dunglison sat, and he wrote lengthy articles in bed while propped up on pillows." Finally, in 1868, worsening congestive heart failure forced him to retire despite continued intellectual vigor, and he died at his home on April 1, 1869. True to his belief in the value of postmortem examination, Dunglison gave over his own body to science for anatomical dissection, as he had done with those of his daughter and wife—both of whom died of rheumatic endopericarditis. His autopsy revealed "an astonishing amount" of pathological cardiovascular disease.[61] Dunglison was buried at the Laurel Hill Cemetery in Philadelphia, by the side of his beloved wife and daughter.

Encomia from Dunglison's Peers

His contemporaries and many later medical leaders held Dunglison in high esteem. In 1856 Hugh Blair Grigsby (1806–81), the leading Virginian historian of his generation, described him to Henry Stephen Randall, Jefferson's New York biographer, as "a gentleman in every aspect of the term, eminently learned, liberal, courteous, and full of that chivalry of literature which leads him to think that the greater wealth he can bestow upon his literary compeers the richer he is himself."[62] Dr. William Osler of the Johns Hopkins School of Medicine, one of the leading figures of late nineteenth and early twentieth-century medicine, stated that "Dunglison had all of the wisdom of his day combined with a colossal industry," that he was "a warm friend to generations of American medical students," and that "Thomas Jefferson did a good work when he imported him from London."[63] In his memorials, Dr. Samuel D. Gross, a famous professor of surgery at Jefferson Medical College (see Figure 25), recalled that,

> Of all the colleagues—nearly forty in number, Robley Dunglison was by far the most learned. His range of knowledge was almost encyclopedic. With his vast acquisitions he combined remarkable clearness of intellect and soundness of judgment... He was a medical philosopher, a savant, rather than a physician......who never wrote an unkind paragraph against any human being in or outside the profession... As a husband, father, brother, neighbor and friend, there was never a kinder or better man. In all of his relations of life he was a model. As a profound medical scholar, ages will probably elapse before the profession will have another Dunglison... He had little faith in active or heroic medication, and had a firm conviction that Nature, assisted by rest, abstinence, and good nursing, was fully competent in ordinary cases to dislodge disease and restore the sick to health...He despised meddlesome medication, and was unsparing in his denunciation of it.[64]

The last several sentences attest to the conviction of his fellow physicians that Dunglison practiced professionally what Jefferson had preached: nature left alone can be a competent healer; heroic medical intervention may cause more harm than good; and unproven pills and potions should be neither ingested nor prescribed.

Not all comments about Dunglison were as laudatory. While conceding that he was "in many ways a remarkable man" and praising him for his industry and his influence as an author and educator, Russell H. Chettenden in the *Dictionary of American Biography* suggested that Dunglison "was not, however, a, profound thinker, and his knowledge of disease came mainly from reading the work of others rather than from personal observation or research."[65]

Dunglison's skill as a writer was certainly held in high regard, and probably no contemporary American scientific author was more prolific. An estimated 155,000 copies of Dunglison's major textbooks circulated during the nineteenth century in America and Europe.[66] He also wrote forty-four chapters for other authors' textbooks, provided more than seventy original essays or other contributions to the scientific literature, and edited numerous medical journals. His writings encompassed many nonmedical disciplines, including ancient history, anthropology, etymological history (e.g., sanscript language), geography, mathematics, meteorology, music, spaceflight, statistics, penitentiary discipline, and popular superstitions. He belonged to and actively participated in a huge number of civic and academic organizations, and his society memberships stretched from London and Edinburgh, to Paris, Marseilles, and Nancy, to Erlanger and Hamburg, to Brussels and Canton, China (Medical Missionary Society of China), to Toronto and Montreal, and in the United States as far west as Missouri and Iowa.

Dunglison's forty-five-year career spanned a trying period for American medicine, and his notes and recollections provide excellent insight into early American medical education.[67] Lacking any understanding of pathologic organisms, the medical profession often found itself at a loss in dealing with the great epidemic diseases and lapsed into bitter debate around a host of exotic medical theories, and treatments that ranged from the highly intrusive and harmful, to a plethora of sectarian alternatives, some of which were characterized as "cultic quackery."[68] Without a strong professional organization, with only a poorly developed concept of professional ethics, and to a large extent isolated from European advances, American doctors openly and acrimoniously aired their dirty linen. Dunglison's account of the most notorious public feuds, particularly that between Drs. Richard Harlan and William Gibson, clearly illustrates how the quarrels within the profession contributed to public distrust of physicians. During this dark age of American medicine, Dunglison came to be known as "a beacon of light."[69]

Much more than a trainer and mentor of physicians, Dunglison recognized that since antiquity, a liberal-arts curriculum has formed the basis for educating society's leaders, and he was himself a good example of this. At the University of Virginia in its early days, he reveled in the idea that medical students could attend lectures in the humanities, social sciences, physical and human science, and mathematics, not just to acquire intellectual understanding, but to learn to think critically, to speak and argue effectively, and to appreciate and analyze a multiplicity of viewpoints. In 1963, the University of Virginia School of Medicine established the Robley Dunglison Award for Teaching Excellence, bestowed annually by the graduating medical school class on a member of the medical faculty "in recognition of outstanding teaching efforts and personal contributions towards arousing academic interests and inspiring the endeavors of students." Such commitments to a broad and deep premedical as well as medical education were carried on at University of Virginia by Dunglison's student, James Cabell.

James Lawrence Cabell

Public health service should be as fully organized and as universally incorporated into our governmental system as is public education. The returns are a thousand fold in economic benefits, and infinitely more in reduction of suffering and promotion of human happiness.[70]

In many respects, the education and academic career of James Lawrence Cabell (1813–89) (see Figure 26 and 27) epitomized Jefferson's aspiration that the University of Virginia produce a professionally trained class of socially aware men who, because its members had pursued learning to the highest level, might be entrusted with the highest offices and responsibilities in society. To Jefferson, the consummate academic in medicine should promote both individual and community health, exert moral leadership locally and nationally, act as an agent to elevate the standards of education in America while promoting those characteristics that gave legitimacy and authority to scientific endeavor. Cabell exemplified these ideals in Virginia and beyond.

Cabell's Ancestry and Education

James L. Cabell was the youngest of five children of Dr. George Cabell Jr. (1774–1827) and Susanna Wyatt Cabell. From his birth in Nelson County, Virginia, on August 26, 1813, he was raised in a family whose genealogy was intimately intertwined with the history of the Commonwealth of Virginia, including the founding of its public university in Charlottesville. As outlined by the genealogist, Alexander Brown, the Cabell family in the American colonies could trace its origins to the arrival of Dr. William Cabell in 1723.[71] His descendants provided the South with prominent soldiers during the American Revolution and the Civil War, as well as prestigious lawyers, legislators, and statesmen. A former surgeon in the British Royal Navy and a practicing physician himself,[72] the original patriarch's descendants also included numerous medical practitioners. Three received their medical education from the University of Pennsylvania, all before 1800, including James Lawrence's father, Dr. George Cabell, Jr. After the University of Virginia opened its doors in 1825, the Cabell family switched its educational allegiance from Philadelphia to Charlottesville. Between 1826 and 1860, no fewer than twenty-eight Cabells attended classes in the various schools of the University of Virginia.[73]

From an early age, James L. Cabell displayed several "conspicuous capacities" of an academically minded young man. He often spoke of becoming an eminent professor at an influential institution of higher education. While attending the private secondary schools of Richmond, he was described by Judge William H. Cabell, his uncle and a former governor of the state, as, "The finest boy I ever saw…In returning home from parties, I have frequently found him at his studies at twelve or one o'clock. I think he bids fair to be one of the cleverest men in the country."[74]

In 1829, at the age of sixteen, James L. Cabell began his collegiate study of Latin, Greek, natural philosophy, and mathematics at the University of Virginia. Between 1829 and 1833, he took classes in every one of the University's eight schools, in the latter year becoming one the first students to earn the coveted master of arts degree by earning graduate diplomas in five different schools: ancient languages, chemistry, mathematics, moral philosophy and natural philosophy. During his four years at the University, he also took Dunglison's courses in medicine. When Dunglison left Charlottesville for Baltimore to take up the position of professor of materia medica & therapeutics, medical jurisprudence and hygiene at the Medical College of Maryland, Cabell quickly followed and enrolled in the Baltimore school. He was not to be disappointed. Dunglison proved to be a wonderful mentor, personally examining him twice a week in all of his subjects, in marked contrast to some other professors. In the spring of 1834, Cabell finished the medical requirements and was awarded an M.D. degree from the Maryland medical college. Over the next eighteen months, he completed a postgraduate course of study that combined proctored anatomical dissection and clinical instruction under Dunglison at the Baltimore infirmary with work as a "resident pupil" at the Baltimore Almshouse, a position that Dunglison helped him obtain. There he "pursued his medical studies in a hospital . . . which enjoyed the distinction of being the only one in America in which students were permitted to perform the surgical operations." In February of 1835 he performed his first surgical operation—a leg amputation on a patient with a non–healing ulcer. Such experience proved most valuable. The young practitioner noted that "I shall probably see almost every variety of disease which the climate and season present," and "the house is now crowded with the sick and every moment of my time will be engaged until I become more ready and expert in practice."[75]

Even with these postgraduate experiences, the young Cabell yearned for even more supervised education and began lobbying his uncle-guardian to help fund additional study in Baltimore or, better yet, in Paris.[76] Behind this maneuver was Cabell's resolve to seek a path toward professional distinction, which he surmised would be best achieved with a course of "intensive study" in a French "clinical school." Just as it had been early in the nineteenth-century, Paris was still not only a cultural mecca but also the home of the world's best-organized hospitals, and thus the place to go for those seeking the ultimate in clinical instruction.[77] Cabell's aspiration was not immediately embraced by his uncle, who instead arranged for some practical experience for him in an established practice in Richmond.

In the summer of 1836, Cabell settled in Richmond to begin practicing his art, but he quickly grew dissatisfied with the professional lethargy there, insisting that medicine in Richmond was a "mere trade." In letters to his uncle in October 1836, he lamented that "I have no means of continuing the study of my profession and no means of making myself eminent in the profession." Cabell correctly recognized the importance of what today is called application scholarship when he said, "For the practice of medicine is not to be learned by books alone; the first principles of the science may indeed, but no man can keep pace with its improvements who has not the means of testing [constantly] the truth or fallacy of what he reads." Of Richmond, he wrote "we have no large hospitals, no professional intercourse between the physicians, each moving in their own separate sphere and knowing nothing of the practice of a brother physician. The only chance I have of acquiring eminence [in my field] is to throw myself prominently before the profession in a large city where the facilities for study and of making oneself an author are greater than in Richmond."[78]

Cabell's persistence paid off. His uncle finally relented, and he left New York for Paris in December 1836. In France, Cabell focused on internal medicine and seemingly took advantage of every learning opportunity. In underscoring the advantages of the trip to his uncle, he wrote that "I am still more convinced by the reports of one or two young men whom I have just seen and who spent a year or more in Paris. The mere fact, generally known, that they studied in France… gained them more distinction than other men would acquire in double the time [if all training occurred in America], and this coupled with the information obtained there will give a standing which would require years of labor to obtain." Cabell quenched his thirst for broad clinical experience in several creative ways. Because all of the medical professors in the various hospitals of Paris made their teaching rounds on the wards at the same hour of the morning, he skipped "from place to place" to see cases of interest – at one hospital, heart cases, at another those of the lungs, and at other hospitals, midwifery or cases of the eyes or skin." Cabell also arranged with an intern or medical assistant to admit him to the hospital wards at hours when students were typically shut out. Joining these evening rounds "on payment of 30 francs per month" allowed for small-group clinical instruction and the opportunity to examine patients personally, which was generally not possible during morning rounds with the professor because of the "large size of the crowd."[79]

John Harley Warner, a noted historian of nineteenth-century medical education and practice, includes Dr. Cabell in a "professional elite" of American doctors, numbering several hundred, who went to Paris because of the rich opportunities for experiential learning in its hospitals and dissecting rooms. Warner asserts that the migration of young graduates to Paris had less to do with being on the forefront of medical science than the opportunity it offered students to "closely observe and touch sickness at the bedside and to dissect an endless supply of cadavers."[80] In France at the time, unlike America, revolutionary morality had displaced the religious qualms that might otherwise have blocked postmortem examinations, and public funding had opened access to Parisian hospital clinics to foreign medical students at nominal cost. Although Cabell praised the knowledge produced by the Paris clinical schools, he, like many American physicians, had very little confidence that French discoveries would lead to improved therapeutics. While they were ardent in their desire to understand disease, French physicians seemed apathetic in their efforts to cure or even treat it. One critic went so far as to declare that they were more interested in performing autopsies than preventing them.[81] Much as it had Jefferson, this attitude distressed Cabell.

Contributions to the Medical School and University at Large

Dr. James L Cabell was offered the professorship at the University of Virginia in the winter of 1837. Only twenty-four years old and lacking the experience of a seasoned academic, some viewed him as a mere student, albeit one very advanced in his study of medicine. Several faculty members attributed the selection to the lobbying by his uncle Joseph C. Cabell, a prominent member of the Board of Visitors, implying that it was based on nepotism rather than meritorious academic accomplishment. However, Cabell soon proved himself to be one of the most gifted and useful instructors on the faculty, thus fully justifying his uncle's endorsement.[82]

In December of 1837, Cabell was duly appointed professor of anatomy, physiology and surgery of the University of Virginia, replacing Dr. Augustus L. Warner (1807–47). Warner had resigned to help organize a new medical school in Richmond, the Medical Department of Hampden-Sydney

College, which would later become the Medical College of Virginia. Cabell quickly demonstrated an indomitable energy and penchant for innovative action. Within a year of joining the medical faculty, he initiated improvements in the curriculum, rearranging courses on physiology and surgery, while announcing to the delight of students that surgical operations would be performed upon a cadaver *a capite ad calcem* ("from head to heel"). This early adaptation of a European method of teaching surgery was later replicated in practically every American medical school. A full prospectus of his courses was penned in time to be incorporated into the 1837–38 catalogue of the University. In it, Cabell insisted that all medical–school matriculates have a thorough "preliminary knowledge of English," evidently one of the earliest mentions of an entrance requirement anywhere in American medical education. He also organized and taught a course in comparative anatomy, another possible first in American medical schools.[83] Cabell requested and received funds from the Board of Visitors to buy color anatomical plates for use in his anatomy and surgery instruction. He secured additional money for the purchase of more cadavers, anatomical material for the museum, textbooks and medical periodicals, and was instrumental in arranging for necessary interior modifications in the University's Anatomical Theater, such as expansion of and improved heating and lighting for the lecture room; an apartment for reception of fresh cadavers; additions of an "unequaled collection" of anatomical plates and color drawings to the museum that were "executed with exquisite truth to nature, making them invaluable"; and the addition of a suitable dissecting room.[84] Thus, in addition to changing the character of the curriculum and the way in which medical instruction was given, Cabell's actions emphasized the importance of a robust medical-school physical plant, replete with suitable laboratory facilities, a museum and sundry appliances for proper teaching expositions, and an up-to-date medical library, the museum and medical library having languished since Dunglison's departure. In sum, Cabell provided the technologies for students to carry out the hands-on anatomical training he had himself experienced in Paris.

During most of his tenure at the University of Virginia, Dr. Cabell lived in Pavilion II on the Lawn (see Figure 11). He consistently followed one of Jefferson's original requirements of the faculty of his "academical village" by having dinner with the students at least once a week.[85] Cabell understood the importance of bringing "himself into such living contact with each pupil so that he could better appreciate [their] difficulties," and in turn, "give him necessary and timely aid."[86]

The Infirmary: a First in Student Health Services

Dunglison had attended to the medical needs of students and Charlottesville residents. Cabell went farther by helping to create the University's first Board of Health in 1849 and convincing the Visitors to adopt more stringent guidelines for sanitation on campus. In 1857 he persuaded University officials to appropriate $7,500 for the erection of a student infirmary. The need of such an establishment had been evident to the medical professors for many years. Besides routine bouts of sickness, the university suffered through many epidemics. During Cabell's tenure, a typhoid outbreak in 1857–58 took nineteen lives, and another in 1875 took five more. In some cases medical faculty members had brought dangerously ill students to their own pavilions to care for them, but doing so as a matter of course would endanger their families.[87] Under rules created by Cabell and fellow medical-faculty member Dr. John Staige Davis (1824–85),[88] at matriculation each student paid a five-dollar "infirmary fee" which, in the case of sickness, entitled him to free prescriptions at the infirmary, lodging and board under its roof if he was confined to bed, and the attendance of a nurse and physician without further charge. A medical teacher who was designated the health officer of the day cared in rotation for the sick, but the ill student was always at liberty to summon a doctor from beyond the precincts at his own expense. Following a suggestion by Cabell, University officials also decided that when faculty treated patients in the infirmary, medical students were allowed to go on rounds with the attending physician. This arrangement gave students valuable experience with local disease.

Historians of American college health services, and preservation architects, regard the University of Virginia Infirmary as one of the first buildings dedicated to the provision of health care to students on a university campus, and it is certainly one of the oldest surviving infirmary buildings in the United States.[89] Moreover, the design that Cabell and Davis implemented when the building opened in the fall of 1858 was an engineering marvel. It was equipped with a state-of-the-art central heating system, which was a very new innovation, and it had a sophisticated ventilating system with masonry ducts and retractable, specially louvered windows that assured improved ventilation in warm weather. Rainwater runoff was collected in attic cisterns from which fresh water was piped to the bathrooms. The building had twelve large rooms on two floors, with bathrooms on each floor. The basement was given over to service space, not used for patients. Its six rooms included a kitchen to prepare hot meals for sick students.

Cabell's Efforts to Broaden and Protect Student Experiences

As hard as Cabell worked to limit the spread of communicable disease, he worked still harder to care for the spiritual needs of students at the University, a commitment he associated with religion. He led a weekly bible study session, "with the door open to all," worked to establish a parsonage at the University for the school's chaplain and was the leader of a movement to build a chapel on grounds. According to Henry Gamble, professor emeritus of religious studies, Cabell along with two other faculty members "brought about an enormous increase in religious zeal in the University, laboring to strengthen the presence of Christianity among the student body and within the University as an institution."[90] In recognition of his efforts to raise the funds for the chapel, a stained-glass window honoring Cabell was placed behind its dais, proclaiming that one of "the ennobling features of his character was his deep and abiding religious faith."[91]

Although these endeavors were arguably compatible, at some level, with Jefferson's ideal that mental, or broadly, spiritual well-being was a condition of physical health, the University's founder would most definitely not have approved of officially sanctioned religious services on-campus. Under his influence no clergyman was initially employed on the university faculty, but in 1845 the Reverend William Holmes McGuffey, a Presbyterian, joined the teaching staff as professor of moral philosophy. He held this position until his death in 1873 and won renown for his series of eight textbooks that became the standard reading texts for most schools across the United States during the mid- to late-nineteenth century. Evidently aided by McGuffey's appointment and Cabell's initiatives, student enrollment began to climb significantly and reached Jefferson's original projections, quite possibly because the image of the university as an "infidel institution" had finally been overcome, making it a much more appealing place for the sons of devout families.[92]

Whatever his religious enthusiasms, throughout his career at the University, Cabell, like Dunglison before him, was admired first and foremost in the eyes of his students "as a teacher, unexcelled." He knew how to "explain the most abstruse and complex questions in terms comprehensible to all of his class… with a kindling enthusiasm that awakened in the dullest intellect a responsive activity," wrote one of his students, adding that Cabell constantly searched for new discoveries and was at pains to "recast his lectures from year to year" so that his class would be on the forefront of the latest developments of science. As one example, a former student recalled of Cabell's presentation on Sir Joseph Lister's antiseptic method of operating and treating wounds, that "With characteristic sagacity Dr. Cabell appreciated the value of this new discovery, and with enthusiastic ardor advocated its claims to his pupils," doing so "at a time when the vast majority of surgeons, in this country, showed a marked reserve or else took ground against it."[93] Indeed, as will be discussed further below, Cabell's often-criticized endorsement of Lister's theories of hygiene as applied to surgery was one of his key contributions to American medicine.

Cabell possessed a refined concept of what it means to be an academic, and his devotion to his students, faculty colleagues, and the university was demonstrated in action. As a physician, he was deemed to be skillful and sympathetic, always ready to relieve suffering. On the faculty he developed a reputation as a wise and weighty counsel, fair and firm in judgment. The faculty attested to his extraordinary depth and breadth of knowledge by nominating him in 1845 for the vacant chair of moral philosophy and ethics, a position soon filled by the Reverend McGuffey. When McGuffey died in 1873, Dr. Cabell, in association with the University chaplain, the Reverend Thomas Dwight Witherspoon (1836–98), filled the post until a successor could be chosen. The growing admiration for Cabell was also revealed by his election as chairman of the faculty in 1846. A year later the Medical College of Virginia in Richmond vigorously recruited him for a professorship. Fortunately, he was persuaded to withdraw his resignation and remain in Charlottesville, where he flourished up to, during, and after the Civil War.

Cabell was severely tested as he and other professors tried to continue medical education during the Civil War. Like his teacher, Cabell helped save his school, albeit under much more dire conditions than Dunglison ever faced. Indeed, he led efforts that kept Jefferson's institution from closing down. Deprived by war of students and funding, only two of the nineteen medical schools in states that seceded from the Union, that at the University of Virginia and the Medical College of Virginia, remained open throughout the war. The five medical professors at the University, Cabell, John Staige Davis, Benjamin W. Allen, Henry Howard, and Socrates Maupin, made significant contributions to the Confederate war effort, including daily work in the Charlottesville General Hospital, where faculty members cared for more than twenty-one thousand wounded and sick soldiers, all while continuing to deliver lectures, prepare various demonstration exercises, and administer examinations. Furthermore, unlike the Richmond school, which had to lower its standards during the Civil War, the Charlottesville school did not alter its curriculum, daily teaching schedule, tests and examinations, nor shorten the academic term of nine months, nor weaken its rigorous graduation requirements. When it was suggested that it close down or relax its standards, the faculty on November 6, 1863, "Resolved that in the opinion of the Faculty it is impractical by any change in the scheme of lectures or plan of instructions to fulfill the conditions coupled with the proposition for shortening the session and that the same is inexpedient in view of the obligations we owe to our students and the future welfare of the institution." Throughout the war, one might have supposed from the language in the University's newspaper advertisements for upcoming academic sessions that the war had not touched Charlottesville.[94] Due to rampant inflation throughout Confederacy, the faculty also granted "every reasonable indulgence to students in regard to the payment of tuition fees," such that by the last year of the war, nearly 40 percent of them attended classes without paying fees. Combined with huge reductions in salaries, the loss of income from student fees led to near insolvency among professors, whose annual salaries dropped from more than $1,000 in gold in 1861 to the equivalent of barely $30 four years later.[95] One student from the class of 1864 expressed nothing but praise for the faculty, writing, "These noble men staid at their posts of duty during all of that dark and gloomy period, just because they felt it to be their duty to do so, and because of their love for the University. They met their classes promptly on the hour each day and did their work as faithfully, as efficiently and as conscientiously as if all around them had been prosperous and serene."[96] In the professors' eyes, the depredations of war never offset duty to the University or medical training. Perhaps the teaching mission was preserved in part by the fact that the school, under Cabell's tutelage, devoted its energies to supporting a military hospital and convalescent center.

Innovative Contributions to Military Medicine During the Civil War

When the Civil War broke out, Dr. Cabell, as professor of physiology and surgery at the University of Virginia, did not take up arms against the Union. Instead, he helped establish, maintain and staff one of the largest hospital systems in the rural south in Charlottesville. The Confederate government selected the town as a site for a military hospital for several reasons. With most of the coast soon falling under Union control, Confederate casualties were transported primarily by rail, and towns situated along railways were natural choices for hospitals.[97] Conveniently, both the Virginia Central and the Orange and Alexandria railway lines passed through Charlottesville, and the town was far enough removed from the front lines to be an appropriate place to organize the care of the sick and wounded soldiers.[98] Furthermore, the buildings of the University of Virginia were suitable for the housing of patients, and the Confederate government planned to draw on the faculty and students of the medical school to staff the hospital, a plan facilitated when student dormitories and other university buildings suddenly became available in the spring of 1861 when a large number of students left to join the Confederate cause, as shown in the following Table. More than two thousand alumni joined them, and by 1865, five hundred men associated with the university had died in the war.

Effect of Civil War on Student Enrollment[99]

Academic Session	Total Enrollment	Medical School Size
1858–1859	625	99
1859–1860	606	99
1860–1861	604	96
1861–1862	66	12
1862–1863	46	14
1863–1864	50	14
1864–1865	55	12
1865–1866	258	36
1866–1867	490	81
1867–1868	475	78

The hospital system contained about five hundred beds and was designated as the Charlottesville General Hospital, with the care of the patients dispersed among the facilities of the University and satellite locations nearby. Cabell and his staff of talented surgeons, joined by approximately three hundred townspeople, cared for more than twenty-one thousand soldiers between July 1861 and March 1865, with capacities severely strained after most of the major battles in the Virginia Theater.[100] During almost four years as surgeon-in-charge or chief surgeon in Charlottesville, Cabell displayed both professional and administrative expertise, implementing a team-based approach to cleanliness, proper sanitation, isolation of patients with potentially contagious disease, and uniform and nondiscriminatory treatment of all patients and their problems. Confederate and captured Union soldiers received the same respect and salubrious care, in contrast to the massive Chimborazo hospital in Richmond.[101] Cabell also hired a chaplain to address the spiritual welfare of patients. The care provided in this hospital system was truly remarkable for the times. Only 5 percent of those who were treated there died, a mortality rate much lower than at other hospitals in the South, including those that comprised the enormous hospital systems in Richmond.[102] As many as fifty practitioners at a time worked under Cabell's auspices. One of them was Dr. Oriana Moon of Charlottesville, who was one of the first two women from the South to graduate from medical school, and the only female physician to serve in the Confederate medical corps, albeit as a nurse.[103] Cabell also exhibited farsightedness in the daily operational routine of the hospital. This included setting up a hierarchical system whereby the university-trained medical staff provided supervision, education on best prescribing practices, and decision support regarding when to perform surgery—for example, limb amputation—and by whom. Many of the elite practitioners taught less-trained staff members that old-style heroic remedies should be avoided, that less drugging was usually better than more, and that prescribing a course of therapy that strengthened the body's own "healing power of nature" afforded the best outcomes in medical care. They also encouraged the use of quinine, both as a preventive for and treatment of malaria, and research on plant botanicals when standard remedies were unavailable.[104] Oversight was partially exercised by establishing "the morning report," during which ward teams presented updates to the medical leaders each morning, a tradition still in evidence today in many American teaching hospitals.[105] Cabell also started a hospital statistical service, which was charged with classifying gunshot wounds and non–combat–related sickness and summarizing the care being provided on a daily, weekly and monthly basis.

On September 5, 1863, Dr. Joseph Jones inspected the Charlottesville General Hospital in a visit authorized by the surgeon general of the Confederacy. According to the historian James O. Breeden, Jones was highly pleased with the "organized system of investigation" and its "skillful management." He asserted that despite having "received more than its just proportion of seriously sick and seriously wounded," the Charlottesville General Hospital "was one of the best, if not the very best… in the Southern Confederacy." Similarly favorable testimonials came from staff members, UVA medical students, and patients.[106] Jones's statistics, completed after the war, reveal much about the care that was delivered by Cabell's dedicated team (see following Table). Of particular note is the 4.9

percent mortality among the 5,339 men with gunshot wounds, a figure well below the 14 percent wartime average of the Union army.[107]

Medical Statistics for Charlottesville General Hospital, July 1861—March 1865[108]

Primary Diagnosis	Number of Cases	Deaths (% of Cases)
Typhoid Fever	1,429	357 (24.9%)
Malaria	850	1 (0.1%)
Diarrhea & Dysentery	2,172	77 (3.5%)
Measles	1,137	19 (0.2%)
Pneumonia	851	250 (29.4%)
Gunshot Wounds	5,337	263 (4.9%)
All Other Diseases	9,764	156 (0.2%)
Totals	**21,540**	**1,123 (5.2%)**

The work done by university faculty amounted to volunteer service. They were said to have deposited any payments they received from the Confederate government in the University's treasury.[109]

In the postwar period, Cabell and several other prominent surgeons published papers describing their wartime experience at the various Confederate military hospitals in Virginia.[110] As a result, their peers came to class these men with the most influential surgeons of the period. In the rebuilding South, Cabell and his associates did much to bring surgical acclaim to the Commonwealth of Virginia. As Wyndham B. Blanton comments, "After the war surgical advance was chiefly due to Hunter McGuire, James L. Cabell, John Syng Dorsey Cullen, Francis Deane Cunningham, and George Ben Johnston, a group of unusual and brilliant men whose influence still lingers in the position that surgery attained through them in the state."[111] Robert E. Lee also demonstrated postwar esteem for Cabell by seeking his medical advice.[112]

In 1867, just as the University was recovering from the Civil War, Cabell was instrumental in defeating a covert legislative action to uproot the medical school in Charlottesville and move it to Richmond. This attempted "amalgamation" with the Medical College of Virginia, whose enrollment and financial viability had plummeted after the war, followed four previous unsuccessful efforts instigated by its professors, mostly for financial reasons. Cabell and his faculty colleague, John Staige Davis, spearheaded a vigorous campaign against the proposed merger, using the press, an open letter to the General Assembly, and a massive letter-writing campaign to state officials from University alumni. The ensuing outpouring of support for Jefferson's university and the unique features of its medical curriculum in Charlottesville was uniformly positive and effective. Given the choice between the University of Virginia and the Medical College of Virginia, the state's populace overwhelmingly trusted Jefferson's creation more than a hodgepodge of medical professors in Richmond. The Medical College's reputation both as a "monopoly operated [by the faculty] for personal gain and aggrandizement" and a "diploma mill" also hurt its case for amalgamation among Virginians.[113] Thereafter, no further threats to modify the University by removing its medical department were attempted until 1921.

Cabell's Role in Reforming Medical Education Nationwide

By the mid-nineteenth century, the practice of medicine in America was widely dismissed as a mere trade, largely unscientific, and infested with mercenary quacks. At the first meeting of the American Medical Association in Philadelphia in 1847, Nathaniel Chapman complained that "The profession to which we belong... has become corrupt, and degenerate, to the forfeiture of its social position and with it, of the homage it formerly received spontaneously and universally."[114] This situation dismayed Cabell and other members of the academic elite. To them, the culprit was clear—a defective system of medical education. In advocating for reform, these men showed a certain courage in their rhetoric, not sparing the organized medical schools of the day from scrutiny and criticism nor failing to recommend potential changes in the educational system that might aid in rectifying problems. In Cabell's words, "If it is true that the profession has ceased to be an educated class, and no longer occupies that elevated position in public confidence which was once accorded to it, we conceive it to be more important to indicate the probable sources of this deplorable degradation, and the means of real and effectual reform, than to inquire what the schools are willing to do, in an emergency which they have been largely instrumental in producing."[115] As will be seen below, by "educated class," Cabell meant a group that had received a diploma from a college and studied subjects beyond those required of an apprentice or tradesman.

The Cabell Report to the AMA

Cabell used his professional association as a founder of the American Medical Association (AMA) to promote medical-education reform on a national stage. At the 1854 meeting of the AMA, Cabell, who was then chair of its Committee on Medical Education, delivered a paper outlining his views on the topic.[116] Using data from previous inquiries to thirty-six American medical institutions and numerous practitioners throughout the country, Cabell and his committee concluded that "the most judicious, safe, and practicable means for remedying the evil" was to recapitulate and extend public discussion of the major defects that had attracted the most "unfavorable criticism," and encourage "removing or lessening" them via local licensure. In the report, Cabell supported "a divorce between the teaching and the licensing powers" and called on all states to require as a legal condition of practice serious proof of proficiency exhibited by "the possession of a license from an extra–collegiate board of examiners."[117] These boards should adopt "a uniform standard [of testing] throughout the Union, or throughout the limits of each of those States in which such a board may be appointed." Despite these recommendations, many years elapsed before "the establishment of boards of examination, distinct from the faculties of the schools," came into favor. Indeed, only in the 1883–84 session of the Virginia General Assembly was a state examination board created.[118] Virginia was one of the last southern states to establish a board of examiners, trailing North Carolina (1859), Texas (1876), Alabama (1877), Georgia and South Carolina (1881), and Mississippi and Louisiana (1882).

In the 1854 report, Cabell used survey-based data to demonstrate almost all of the deficiencies in American medical education. More importantly, his report contained a series of corrective action steps. These included: (1) the need to establish and enforce a uniform standard of preliminary education for all wishing to study medicine, either under a private preceptor or in collegiate classes. As prerequisites this background was to include "A good English education; a knowledge of natural philosophy, and the elementary mathematical sciences, including geometry and algebra, and such an acquaintance, at least, with the Latin and Greek languages, as will enable the students to appreciate the technical language of medicine, and read and write prescriptions;" (2) a call to abandon the largely unregulated apprenticeship model as the prevailing teaching strategy, and to promote instead training that includes attendance at lectures on "fundamental branches of medical science" in a good college or university; (3) the need for a significant lengthening, in all organized medical schools, of the annual term of medical lectures from the customary 13 to 16 week range to a minimum of 8 months, thereby eliminating "the very obvious evil of crowding six or seven lectures into the compass of a single day" – a situation that did not allow adequate time for reflective learning by students; (4) elimination of the "most flagrant and mischievous of all the defects," namely, the absence of proof of proficiency, evidenced by "numerous and rigid examinations"; (5) approval of the establishment of "private schools" to supplement medical–school lectures by "giving that species of instruction which consists 'in demonstrations' and other practical exercises" undertaken by the student himself but supervised by a suitably qualified professor, "embracing the whole circle of clinical observation and practice" including laboratory work; and finally, (6) recognition that "to insure the efficient and beneficial operation of the proposed measures of reform," the AMA should strongly endorse a national, "uniform system of examining candidates for admission to the ranks of the medical profession, *in addition to the collegiate examinations for degrees.*"

Throughout the 1854 report, Cabell promoted his own institution and the Jeffersonian ideals on which it had been founded. Indeed, many of the changes he endorsed had already been part of the University of Virginia's Medical Department for over a quarter century. In particular, he advocated a long and arduous basic-science curriculum that would "enable the student to appreciate the force of the evidence upon which the modern doctrines of physiology mainly rest," and the demonstration of proficiency by repeated examination before clinical instruction commenced, inasmuch as "the fundamental branches of medical science" are the foundation "on which the whole superstructure of professional education must rest." At the time the report was delivered, students at the University of Virginia, as has been noted previously, were required to attend medical lectures throughout an unusually long academic term, to demonstrate satisfactory preparation based on the results of daily oral examinations in all the classes, and to pass a set of seven final examinations, one for each of the seven courses of lectures, all written and proctored by a committee of professors and enforced by a strict honor code, with the tests "occupying each the greater part of a day," in an effort to "require the most positive and unmistakable evidence of attainments, rather than a specific number of course of lectures, as a condition of graduation." Cabell stated that, "The rigor of these examinations [at the University of Virginia] and the high degree of the standard exacted from the graduates, may be inferred from the fact that, while all the matriculates are permitted to become candidates, and about five–sixths do usually announce themselves as such at the commencement of the session, the number of actual graduates is far smaller than in any other American school, being between a sixth and a fifth of the class."[119]

In his report, Cabell admonished medical-school professors and private preceptors not to rush their students into practical exercises before they had acquired a thorough familiarity with the anatomy, physiology and pathology of every organ, as well as whole-body comparative anatomy, basic and practical chemistry, and medical jurisprudence or forensic medicine—the latter to inculcate the principles of a defensible evidentiary argument. To do otherwise would promote the production of simple empirics rather than scientific thinkers. In his criticism of other medical schools, Cabell used Jefferson's university as a model, with its uniquely high standards. Just two years after the Cabell report appeared, the April 1856 edition of the *Southern Literary Messenger* pointed out that graduates of the Virginia school were required to demonstrate distinction in their fields of study, asserting that "the standards of examination must be higher than at any other College in the Union." Comparing the University of Virginia to Harvard and Yale, the *Messenger* concluded that "it is not that a young man may not be a scholar at Yale or Cambridge, but that he need not be."[120]

Like Dunglison, Cabell recognized the woeful inadequacy of clinical instruction that characterized most American medical schools. The vast majority of medical schools did not require it, and, fewer than 10 percent of those educated before 1850 had hospital training. Even one of the most respected physicians of the era, William Wood Gerhart (1809–72), expressed ambivalence about the value of clinical instruction.[121] With the benefit of his postgraduate medical experiences in Baltimore and Paris, Cabell in his report articulated a refined understanding of the role of both the clinical preceptor and his pupils in promoting genuine practice-based learning:

> But the most important agent in this work is the clinical teacher, under whose superintendence each pupil should be required, to observe cases; keep a record of the observed phenomena; announce his diagnosis and the grounds upon which it is based; indicate the course of treatment which might appear to be applicable upon a rational consideration of the known pathology of the disease, or which an enlightened and reliable empiricism had proved to be efficacious in similar cases; and, finally, to analyze a large number of cases, whether perceived by himself or recorded by trustworthy observers, with a view of enlarging his acquaintance with those general truths that might escape notice in the contemplation of

> isolated facts. The first crude performance of the tyro should be kindly but faithfully criticised, models of excellence should be held up before him to study, and such incentives to earnest and patient labor should be employed as might appear to promise benefit.[122]

The Cabell report of 1854 was remarkably comprehensive in scope. The committee's proposals addressed virtually all of the trappings of American medical education, calling for: the imposition of reasonably robust conditions of matriculation, sufficient to ensure proper mental and moral culture for all students commencing the study of medicine; satisfactory completion of a graded basic medical-science curriculum before clinical instruction; extension of the academic term of study so as to relieve the onerous overcrowding of the curriculum and promote active learning by students; and, most importantly, the need for uncompromising, rigorous requirements for graduation. Moreover, the report touched on the fundamental pedagogic issues of what subjects should be taught and when and how they should be taught, during both the basic science and clinical years of training. Finally, Cabell recognized the emerging importance of laboratory instruction by advocating greater use of the microscope, proper anatomical dissection, the chemistry laboratory, and other "appliances" necessary for practical exposition of factual material. At the completion of training, the report recommended extra collegiate licensing as a legal condition of practice.

While Cabell was not at the meeting to present the report in person, it was presumably read widely in the published transactions. Unfortunately, it fell on deaf ears. Cabell's effort and those of others had little visible effect, in part because of disabling internecine squabbles within the AMA and the medical profession at large. Lacking any legal incentives, reform-minded men could only seek change by moral suasion. Medical schools were simply unwilling to consider any change for the better.[123] Not until almost half a century later did a small but influential cadre of newly appointed college and university presidents begin demanding the establishment and enforcement of uniformly high standards in all school departments within their control. These enlightened leaders, all of whom had a cogent reform agenda, included Frederick A. P. Barnard of Columbia (term 1864–89), James McCosh of Princeton (term 1868–88), Charles Eliot of Harvard (term 1869–1909), Noah Porter of Yale (term 1871–86), Andrew Dickson White of Cornell (term 1866–85), James Burrill Angell of Michigan (term 1871–1909) and Daniel Coit Gillman of the Johns Hopkins University (term 1876–1901). In addition, the four founding physicians of the Johns Hopkins School of Medicine, pathologist William H. Welch, surgeon William S. Halsted, internist William Osler, and gynecologist Howard Kelly, deserve considerable credit in creating and promoting a gold-standard academic model that led the way toward correcting all of the major deficiencies of antebellum medical education. Other contributing factors included the proliferation of progressive era ideology, accreditation requirements established by the Council on Medical Education of the AMA and the American Association of Medical Colleges, licensing laws imposed by the states, the publication of the 1910 Flexner Report, scientific advances in America and Europe (especially Germany), societal pressures, and economic exigencies that included the force of philanthropy.[124]

Cabell's Work on Evolution, Race, and Religion

While Cabell was well known as an educator, his activity as an author was more limited than, and by no means comparable to, that of his prolific mentor, Dr. Robley Dunglison. Nevertheless, several of his works remain important testaments to his scholarly ambitions, theoretical sophistication, and participation in politically weighted scientific controversy. Cabell's role was most significant in discussions of the nature and ancestry of humans that had been percolating for decades and would continue into the 20th century. In 1859, the same year that Charles Darwin's work *On the Origin of Species* appeared, Cabell published a lengthy treatise, *The Testimony of Modern Science to the Unity of Mankind*,[125] a manuscript he had been working on for many years.[126] Encouraged to take on the task by members of the religious community, he sought to refute the positions of George R. Gliddon, Dr. Josiah Clarke Nott, Louis Agassiz, and others regarding the origin of the human species. Cabell's book had its origins in his earlier, scathing review of Nott and Gliddon's *Types of Mankind*, where he wrote that "A failure at any one step is fatal, and, as we have seen, they fail everywhere."[127] In their writings, these men promoted a theory intended to serve a social and political doctrine justifying racial inequality, the gist of which was that the human races they regarded as inferior (for example, Negroes) had evolved from distinctly separate lineages.[128] The theory of multiple origins, also called polygenism, caused considerable concern among many religious leaders of the day, as it denied the ancestry of man as laid out in the Book of Genesis.

Although a deeply religious man, Cabell made it a point to "set aside for the present the testimony of Scripture, and treat the whole question as one of pure science."[129] Instead of invoking a theologically based scriptural position, he marshaled the biological and anthropological knowledge of the day to argue that sound scientific inquiry and reasoning could prove that all varieties of humankind did, indeed, descend from a single ancestral pair (monogenism) and that modern men [and women] in all of their varieties "are of one blood,"[130] a position that Darwin's findings soon reinforced. In considering the significance of Cabell's work, one must recognize that he was engaging a range of opponents who also used science to defend political, as well as theological, positions. Many southern slave owners in antebellum America defended the institution by appealing to polygenism, which at the time was a hypothesis still defended by reputable scientists. Proponents of slavery argued that the slave population stemmed from a separate species, which was genetically inferior "in rank of mind and even in moral features," compared to their white masters.[131] This could imply that enslaving individuals of such lesser species was not an abuse of "true" human beings.

In tracing the lineage of white and black races back to a common ancestry, thus perceiving unity in diversity, Cabell presented a scientific theory that was anathema to entrenched "protohereditarian" dogma, briefly discussed in Chapter 1. The term hereditarian, which did not come into common usage until 1881, refers to those who believe that differences between individuals or groups, including moral and intellectual attributes, are predominantly determined by genetic factors, and thus that one's destiny is fixed at birth. This has sometimes been used as a synonym for biological determinism, the first traces of which were suggested in Aristotle's *Politics* when he proclaimed that, "there are species in which a distinction is already marked, immediately at birth, between those of its members who are intended to be ruled and those who are intended to rule." When Carl Linnaeus (1707–78), a Swedish scientist, published his *Systema Naturae* in 1735, this line of thinking began to take hold. Using what would prove to be a faulty scientific approach, he was the first to divide the human race into four distinct categories (red, yellow, white, and black). Some scholars have traced the origins of scientific racism (the pseudoscience of categorizing humans by racial types and hierarchies) back to Linnaeus.[132]

Drawing on his vast knowledge of physiology, psychology, comparative anatomy, zoology, and historical antecedents, Cabell constructed a cogent argument for monogenism, as well as a theory of evolutionary biology that came close to the conception of natural selection proposed by Darwin.[133] Cabell also speculated that spontaneous mutations could give rise to new varieties of mankind, fully forty-three years before the "Mutation Theory" would be advanced by Hugo de Vries.[134]

In his treatise, Cabell demonstrated an exceptional command of the extant scholarship on matters of racial differences and social separation. In constructing his argument, he examined the published writings of more than seventy different authors, including all of the leading figures who participated in the Unitarian-Pluralist debate. Cabell then "clearly and brilliantly set forth his insights," which provided "a foundation for modern biological thought."[135] Using his encyclopedic knowledge of natural and physical science, including ethnological research, he supported his evolutionary argument with keen observations from the historical record of plant and animal husbandry. In particular, he noted the importance of such environmental factors as climate, altitude, food, lifestyle, and other external conditions, contending that "by carefully changing the food and other agents of vital stimulation, we may modify, to an extent sometimes quite considerable, the outward structural character of many plants and low animal organisms; and these newly acquired characters may then be perpetuated by hereditary transmission, under the influence of the law of assimilation between parent and offspring, even though the causes which originally determined the variation from the primitive type have ceased to operate."[136] This position was similar to Lamarck's notion, also accepted by Darwin, that traits acquired during an organism's lifetime could be transmitted genetically.

Although Darwin's work largely overshadowed Cabell's *Testimony*, his original goal for the book was rather convincingly achieved. Gliddon, Nott, and other polygenists of the period relied heavily on the archaeological monuments of Egypt to substantiate their arguments for separate lineages of the races. These individuals based their theory of polygenic evolution primarily on paintings and art found by archaeologists and traceable to the reigns of the pharaohs.[137] They argued that since these artistic works from an ancient civilization clearly depicted individuals of different skin color and appearance in subordinate positions, the various races must have evolved along separate lines. Such archaeological inferences were used to validate the ownership of slaves by perceiving blacks to be as already a separate and inferior lineage in antiquity. Cabell, however, refuted the foundation of these claims by identifying a fundamental fallacy: "We refer to the use made by them of the fact, that the Negro and three other leading types of men were accurately delineated on the monuments of Egypt several thousand years ago. But as we have already had occasion to remark, the famous 'monumental history of man' throws no light at all upon the obscure question of the origin of the different leading human types. Whatever date be assigned to these inscriptions, there must have been an antecedent period quite long enough to have given origin to any number of types."[138] Where proslavery apologists sought support from the Hebrew Scriptures and thus avoided the need to be governed by scientific evidence, Cabell recognized that eons were required to evolve human differences and that these millennia must have transpired long before historical depictions of putatively different types or classes of mankind.

Proponents of the monogenist school usually insisted on the equality of mankind. Alexander von Humboldt was a particularly forceful advocate, arguing at length against the ranking of humans on mental or aesthetic grounds in his five–volume *Cosmos* (1849). He maintained the unity of the human species, while at the same time rejecting the depressing assumption of superior and inferior races of man.[139] This viewpoint was especially widespread in the northern states, where it was often assumed that the biological uniformity of the species as a whole entailed a claim to equal rights for all. Cabell, however, did not go this far. Descended from a long line of Southern gentry, he did not inherit a proclivity to an Enlightenment natural-rights egalitarianism. Indeed, several historians maintain that Cabell "defended slavery," albeit "as a temporary expedient designed by God to preserve the Negro," since any perceived "inferiority was only a temporary state, and that colored people would soon achieve equality with the whites."[140] This analysis, however, does not provide a complete picture of Cabell's beliefs, especially when his classroom teaching is taken into account. In his lectures to students at the University of Virginia, he said that all races share a common physiology, and that despite differences in aesthetic or somatic appearances, they have "the same intuitive convictions, the same primary faculties of the mind, the same kind of susceptibility to improvement, though, perhaps, not always equal in degree, and the same feelings of fear or hope in reference to a future state of existence beyond the grave."[141] Accordingly, Cabell most likely considered backwardness among blacks to be mostly cultural, rather than genetic, and that it could be eradicated by "vital stimulation," meaning perhaps that further cultivation, such as education, might elevate their social status. Similarly, Cabell's mentor, Robley Dunglison, acknowledged that "great intelligence [of some] in the Negro [race] was not unique, and it exhibits what may be expected from him under favorable circumstances."[142]

In the years leading up to Cabell's controversial publication in 1859, many of his faculty colleagues, and some influential alumni, of the University of Virginia were firmly entrenched in promoting Southern Nationalism and proslavery thought on campus and in "developing an extensive body of scholarship" that defended a chattel slave society based on constitutional, commercial, and natural-law principles, as well as misguided biblical interpretations. Among the most notable exponents and proponents of proslavery views with connections to the university were former students and plantation owners: Robert Toombs, law student and senator from Georgia; Robert Mercer Taliaferro Hunter, law student, U.S. congressman, Speaker of the House, and senator from Virginia; and Muscoe Russel Hunter Garnett, law student and U.S. congressman from Virginia. Proslavery faculty members included: James Philemon Holcombe, a law professor who gave three incendiary speeches at UVA in the 1850s and whose proslavery writings were widely circulated; Henry St. George Tucker, a professor of law who maintained in his lectures that slavery was consistent with natural law; George Frederick Holmes, professor of history and literature who wrote in support of Aristotle's thesis that some men were born to be masters and others to be slaves; and Albert Taylor Bledsoe, a professor of mathematics who in 1856 composed an *Essay on Liberty and Slavery,* in which he argued that slavery was a positive good. These professors, imbued with formidable prejudices and fueled by sectional pride that had grown into overt animosity, surely advanced these theories in the classroom.[143]

Yet not all individuals affiliated with the University accepted this attitude of white supremacy. Those who criticized the University as a hub of proslavery thought and secessionist thinking included former faculty members Charles B. Shaw and George Tucker; alumni such as Henry Winter Davis, Gessner Harrison, and Henry Tutwiler, a distinguished professor and former president at the University of Alabama; and student advocates of emancipation who published editorials in university literary magazines. Tucker, professor of moral philosophy from 1825 to 1845, wrote extensively on the subject of negro slavery, expressing "doubts about the inferiority of the colored race." In his *Letters from Virginia* (1816), he attributed the cause of racial differences solely to "time and circumstance." Shortly after joining the faculty in 1825, he published a three–volume antislavery novel, *The Valley of Shenandoah: or Memoirs of the Graysons.* In 1832, Tucker was one of only two faculty members who supported a highly controversial public speech, given by a student, Merritt Robinson, on the immorality of slavery. Robinson argued for the immediate emancipation of Virginia slaves, and supported his convictions by quoting opinions which had been expressed by George Washington and Thomas Jefferson. Tutwiler, a staunch abolitionist, called slavery the source of "almost all moral and political evil in the state." As secession approached, a sizable minority of students supported calls for "a patient and conciliatory attitude" when "the causes of controversy between the two great divisions of the Union" were being debated on Grounds and urged "that, however much we may differ in our views of the peculiar institution, we are still brethren of one family, the people of one nation, with one hope, one destiny, and one common love for the starry ensign of freedom, and the whole country over which it floats." The most outspoken antislavery voice was that of Charles B. Shaw, a Virginian and adjunct engineering professor in the mid-1850s. In his provocative pamphlet *Is Slavery a Blessing?* published anonymously in 1857, Shaw argued that slavery was not fit for progressive thinkers and that its benefits did not offset its enormous human costs. He held that slaves should be taught to read and write for the sake of humanity, that human nature could and should be improved, not simply restrained in the South by its intolerant "slaveocracy." And he added that "gradually, a funeral pall has been drawn over any rational discussion of the slavery question, and if there be any now here who hold the sentiments once openly expressed, they are only whispered in confidence...No person can safely reside in the South who is suspected of liberal views on the subject of slavery."[144]

Recently, it has been shown that at least sixty-eight UVA students, alumni, and faculty members served in the Union military, and dozens more supported the Union cause as citizens. The story of UVA's Unionism also includes John Barbee Minor who headed the School of Law from 1845 to 1895. In the years leading up to the Civil War, he was described as a "conditional" Unionist. However, he did much in post-war years to repurpose his school's curriculum—as an "incubator of Lost-Cause ideology, Jim Crow segregation," and patriarchy.[145]

Proponent of Antisepsis

Cabell also became an active participant in several national debates regarding healthcare quality.[146] One of the best examples came in his address on antisepsis given in 1882 at the behest of the first president of the recently founded American Surgical Association, Dr. Samuel D. Gross of the Jefferson Medical College of Philadelphia. Most of the leading surgeons of the day attended this meeting. In his controversial speech, Cabell presented the arguments for and against the principles of antisepsis espoused by Dr. Joseph Lister of the University of Glasgow.[147] Cabell's presentation was reportedly given in an "impartial spirit," but though "the weight of evidence was decidedly in favor of the advocates of antiseptic surgery," his address excited intense opposition, even "unbounded ridicule." One participant declared, with great vehemence, "that prejudice was stamped on every page [of the speech] and that the author had regulated his statistics to sustain his theory."[148]

Though considerably past the age of sixty years at which it was said that very few medical men grow old gracefully,[149] Cabell embraced the new method as best practice, doing so "with an intelligent enthusiasm which characterizes a noble nature, a genuine lover of the truths of science, and a mind trained to the critical investigation of an abstruse problem." Instead of rejecting the remarkable revelation of Lister "as absurd and unworthy of investigation, these truths found in his mind a congenial soil, prepared not only to receive them, but to give them full opportunity for development." The use of antiseptic methods in wound care led to the germ–free aseptic doctrine that was advanced by German scientists and surgeons and eventually came to be widely accepted.[150]

Pioneer in Public Health at the State and National Level

Like Jefferson, Cabell was a staunch advocate for both individual health and community or public health. His experience organizing what was in effect a community hospital rekindled his interest in public hygiene, which dated back to his establishment of the first Board of Health at the University of Virginia. Cabell began to endorse the tenets of sanitary science, including the belief that animal and other wastes can cause disease, and to initiate structural reforms at the state and national level.[151] He also recognized the importance of building a coalition of committed sanitarians that included men from both the South and North who were intent on improving public health throughout the United States. In fact, his closest associates and allies at the national level were Northern men of principle who had played a large role in the Union medical corps and thereafter most notably Drs. Stephen Smith (1823–1922) and John Shaw Billings (1838–1913). By way of contrast, Cabell's quest to establish reliable sanitary practices met with considerable opposition from southerners like Dr. Joseph Jones of New Orleans, who repeatedly appealed to states' rights and vehemently opposed any mandate by the federal government.[152]

At the second postwar meeting of the Medical Society of Virginia, Cabell spearheaded a successful effort in 1872 to lobby the state legislature to create the Virginia Board of Health. Named its first President, he immediately commenced work to secure an annual appropriation of funds. On account of a treasury hampered by wartime debt and a general refusal to address problems proactively, all such efforts met with failure despite repeated attempts by Cabell. Only after his death, when cholera threatened Virginia in the spring of 1893, did the state legislature allocate funds for a state board of health.

Undaunted by this early setback, Cabell continued to work to raise awareness about issues of public health and sanitation. At the 1874 meeting of the Medical Society of Virginia, he presented the results from a "circular letter of inquiry" regarding sanitation, which he had distributed to municipal authorities in all 101 counties in Virginia. This paper called attention to the hazards of defective sanitary conditions, notably their contribution to the proliferation throughout the state of malaria and other endemic diseases.[153] In recognition for his effort, the society elected him chairman of its section on State Medicine and Public Hygiene, commissioning him to report periodically on the interplay between environmental factors and disease. Aided by Cabell's connections with the American Medical Association, his ideas about sanitation, expressed in his many reports and presentations, achieved national notice and did much to show how scientific advances could reveal the causes of communicable disease.[154]

Dr. Stephen Smith, who had been leading similar efforts in the state of New York, recognized the need for a national health authority—a coordinated network of well-trained professionals who would engage in and promote sanitary science through research, enlighten the public on how to improve community health, and ignite civic support for public–health initiatives throughout the country. His efforts led to the formation of the American Public Health Association (APHA), and Drs. Smith and Cabell both served as president of the organization in the 1870s.[155] Its constitution gave the objectives of the APHA as the "advancement of sanitary science and the promotion of organizations and measures for the practical application of public hygiene." Its members would be, the constitution said, "selected on their acknowledged interest in, and devotion to, sanitary studies and allied sciences, and to the practical application of the same."[156] As president of the APHA and chairman of its Committee on Legislation, Cabell played a "conspicuous part" in securing congressional authorization on March 3, 1879, for a National Board of Health (NBH), which gave the United States its first central health authority.[157] The new agency was staffed by men who had all served in the Civil War and shared a common point of view about the value of public hygiene and the power of disinfectants. Cabell served as president of the NBH from 1879–1883, during which he helped usher in a new era of ship sanitation that revolutionized quarantine regulations, as well as a set of interstate standards for the transport of goods from diseased areas. He also helped develop four "refuge stations" on the southern coast of the United States, intended to diminish invasions of foreign pestilences, and he promoted the first grant–in–aid program that channeled federal dollars to colleges and universities for medical research, an important predecessor to the current grant system of the National Institutes of Health.[158] A particular focus of the National Board of Health was yellow fever, and this emphasis led to the formation of the Havana Yellow Fever Commission. Eventually headed by one of Cabell's former students, Dr. Walter Reed (see Figure 28), this group famously confirmed that yellow fever was transmitted by mosquitos, and it also produced what may be a first–of–its–kind informed–consent form to be signed by all human research subjects (see Figure 29). The work executed by Reed and his colleagues, including the aggressive mosquito–eradication procedures, involving the control of larvae and water–breeding spots greatly diminished the incidence of yellow fever in Cuba, and a few years later, in Panama, where more than 40,000 laborers were building the canal. Of note, an 1870 graduate of the University of Virginia, Henry Rose Carter (1852–1925) may have set the stage for the Walter Reed successes in Cuba by discovering the "extrinsic incubation" period of yellow fever. Another graduate, Major Jefferson Randolph Kean (1860–1950, medical class of 1883) as Chief Sanitary Officer of Havana ensured that the Commission findings were put immediately into practice. He led the government's entire command on the eradication of the Aedes aegypti mosquito and worked tirelessly to accord public recognition of mosquito-borne disease.

To inform health-care providers throughout the United States of advances in public-health science, the National Board of Health also began publishing a weekly on public-health issues called *The National Board of Health Bulletin*, arguably an early progenitor of the *Morbidity and Mortality Weekly Reports* currently published by the Centers for Disease Control and Prevention.[159] The work of Drs. Cabell and Smith, and perhaps even most importantly that of Dr. John Shaw Billings, led eventually to the development of the National Library of Medicine, and Index Medicus.[160] Other students of Dr. Cabell besides Walter Reed attained national prominence in public health, including two surgeon generals and two assistant surgeon generals of the U.S. Public Health Service. In the decades preceding the outbreak of the World War, former University of Virginia students and trainees held between 14 and 30 percent of all commissions in the U.S. Public Health Service, possibly because Virginia graduates outperformed all other "seats of learning" in tests of admission for Federal service in the Army, Navy, and Marine Hospital System.[161] Most of these public-health-service officers were influenced directly or indirectly by Dr. Cabell and his emphasis on scientific advance leading to effective policy decisions.

Neither was Cabell's promotion of public health confined to the continental United States. During his term as president of the National Board of Health, and in concert with the National Academy of Science, he was instrumental in organizing an International Sanitary Conference that was worthy of the name. Of nineteen such conferences held between 1851 and 1938, this was the only one held in the Western Hemisphere, and evidently the most internationally representative of all of the nineteenth-century conferences, with participation for the first time not only by the U.S.A. but by seven Latin American countries, fourteen European nations, and Haiti, Hawaii, China, Japan, and Liberia. Dr. Carlos Finlay, one of the delegates sent by Spain, represented the interests of Cuba and Puerto Rico and argued presciently that some intermediate host must transmit yellow fever from the sick to the healthy. The conference opened on January 5, 1881, and lasted nearly two months. The sole objective of the United States in convening the conference was obtaining international cooperation for a piece of domestic legislation that would otherwise have been unenforceable. Congress had approved an Act "to prevent the introduction of contagious or infectious diseases into the United States." This act, which had become law on June 26, 1879, clarified and strengthened the NBH's authority and gave it wide quarantine powers, albeit with an expectation that the NBH would collaborate with city and state health officers. The difficulty in implementing it grew out of its requirement that any vessel arriving at an American port produce a certificate from a United States consular official "setting forth the sanitary history of the said vessel." Moreover, this official was expected to satisfy himself as to the truth of the facts stated on the certificate, and the only practical way of doing this was to inspect the ship. The statute therefore implied that no ship could leave its home port for the United States before it had been boarded, inspected, and given a satisfactory bill of health by an agent of a foreign maritime power. Although Cabell did his best to convince delegates to create and monitor an effective "international system of notification," his efforts failed, largely because of concern that approval of such "onerous restrictions" would have a disastrous effect on international commerce. Indeed, the discussions at this international conference and many that followed "show that all hopes of international agreement on preventive measures against epidemic disease" would have to wait for decades, until there was "scientific proof of the real etiology and epidemiology" of the common pathogens. Once these issues were unraveled, particularly for cholera and yellow fever, "the pace of international health cooperation quickened, leading to the foundation, one after another, of the Pan American Sanitary Bureau, the

Office international d 'hygiène publique, the Health Organization of the League of Nations and, finally, the World Health Organization, which incorporated all its predecessors."[162]

Close of Life and Eulogies

Because of failing health, Cabell gave up teaching in July 1889. He died at his adopted daughter's summer residence in Albemarle County on August 13 of that year and was buried in the University of Virginia Cemetery.[163] A tribute by one of Dr. Cabell's colleagues, addressing a meeting of the Medical Society of Virginia in 1889, summarizes the sentiment of virtually all who knew him: "A luminous star in the constellation of eminent physicians and scholars has been extinguished. Science has sustained a loss which she will long deplore. The seat of learning, which owed so much to the ripe wisdom and sound judgement of James L. Cabell, will, for many a day, lament the departure of one of its most illustrious sons. And, throughout this great land, his friends and admirers will feel that so long as they are able to appreciate what is noble and excellent in human character, his name shall not be allowed to sink into oblivion."[164] At a university ceremony commemorating Dr. Cabell's life and accomplishments, one of his former students said of him, "He was a man of the highest sense of honor; a man who had the courage of a lion and the tenderness of a women…a man full of sympathy for all suffering; indignant and haughty in the presence of tyranny… a man made and ordained by nature to be a leader of men. The great qualities which he possessed and which chiefly attracted our love and admiration, can never perish. They will dwell in the memories of his friends for years, and will live always in the records of his fame."[165] Another former student at the same ceremony described how Dr. Cabell had appeared to him in life: "There was never an effort at pose, but a composed dignity of mien was as natural to him as the toga to a Roman Senator. The whole appearance of the man betokened earnestness of soul, self-confidence, strength of character, and marked him as one fully equipped to battle with the difficulties and perplexities of human existence in general, and, in especial, of those belonging to the academical teacher."[166]

Conclusion

Dunglison and his student, Cabell, strove to extend the innovations at the University of Virginia to medical education outside of the state. In this they were motivated by Jefferson's ideal that education, particularly at a university, was the principle medium for individual and societal betterment. Their paths to reforming medical education were, as this chapter has demonstrated, differentiated by their talents and professional positions. After his achievements as head of the Medical Department at the University of Virginia, documented in Chapter 5, Dunglison found his way to Philadelphia, arguably the center of American medical education, where he assembled one of the most outstanding medical-school faculties in the city and brokered peace with rival schools, while continuing to expand the boundaries of the medical–school curriculum through his textbooks. Yet, for all his erudition and administrative acumen, Dunglison did not live to see a widespread adoption of what he and Jefferson had created on a more limited scale.

This was in some way also the case for his protégé, Cabell, whose propagation of a more rigorous curriculum based on what Jefferson and Dunglison had implemented encountered indifference, if not resistance. However, perhaps even more than his mentor, Cabell realized the ideals of a Jeffersonian activist and scholar. At the state and national level, he developed public-health organizations that promoted prevention and probed empirically plausible causes of disease outbreaks. Just as Jefferson was an early adopter of Jenner's system of smallpox vaccination, so Cabell urged adoption of Lister's techniques of wound hygiene. Cabell lobbied for legal licensing of physician competence, really a community acknowledgment of what the passing of rigorous exams had verified at the academic level. Finally, he marshaled scientific, philosophical, and historical discoveries to engage the most pressing questions of the day: human evolution and the legitimacy of slavery, the intellectual questions reflective of Jefferson's researches into the nature of man and the foundations of human rights.

Still, while Jefferson revolutionized the government of a nation, Dunglison and Cabell were at best able only to recommend a national revolution in medical education. While their influence went far beyond the local and was buoyed by an emerging self-consciousness of medicine as a medical profession that laid a claim to national uniformity, as articulated by groups like the American Medical Association and the American Surgical Association, the application of the ideas and ideals of Jefferson's University to other medical schools was, at best, halting. Neither the intellectual climate nor the economic culture of United States medical education in the mid-nineteenth century were sufficiently advanced to embrace the scientific rigor both men exemplified, the public supervision and legal standards they lobbied for, and the university-based model of preparing individuals to become, students first, and only after that, students of medicine. Later generations, however, followed the lead of Dunglison and Cabell and brought Jefferson's vision to fruition.

Notes

Chapter 1

1. Jefferson to Jeudy de l'Hommande, 9 August 1787, in Thomas Jefferson, *The Papers of Thomas Jefferson,* (hereafter cited as *PTJ*), ed. Julian P. Boyd and others (Princeton, N.J.: Princeton University Press, 1950–), 12:11.
2. From welcoming remarks by President Kennedy, 29 April 1962, at a dinner honoring Nobel Prize winners, as cited in Arthur M. Schlesinger, Jr., *A Thousand Days: John F. Kennedy in the White House* (Boston: Houghton Mifflin, Co. and the Riverside Press, 1965), 773.
3. Jefferson to Oliver Evans, 2 May 1807, Library of Congress, *The Thomas Jefferson Papers,* https://www.loc.gov/item/mtjbib017171/; Jefferson to Isaac McPherson, 13 August 1813, in *The Papers of Thomas Jefferson: Retirement Series* (hereafter cited as *PTJRS*), ed. J. Jefferson Looney and others (Princeton, N.J.: Princeton University Press, 2005–), 6:379–86; Jefferson to Hutchins G. Burton and Samuel Brown, 28 September 1821, *PTJRS,* 17:520–522; and Keith Thomson, *Jefferson's Shadow: The Story of his Science* (New Haven: Yale University Press, 2012), 4.
4. Jock Murray, "Thomas Jefferson and Medicine," *Journal of Medical Biography* 5 (1997), 146.
5. Oscar A. Thorup, "Thomas Jefferson: Founder of Two Medical Schools," *Transactions of the American Clinical and Climatological Association* 92 (1980):16–22 and T. C. Moore and J. A. Shield, "Medical Education at America's First University," *Journal of Medical Education* 44 (1969): 241–248. See also "Jefferson's Notes on his Early Career (the so–called Autobiography)," 6 January–29 July 1821 (hereafter cited as "Jefferson's Early Career") *PTJRS,* 17:328–29; and Roy J. Honeywell, *The Educational Work of Thomas Jefferson* (Cambridge: Harvard University Press, 1931), 55–56.
6. Silvio A. Bedini, *Thomas Jefferson: Statesman of Science* (New York: Macmillan Publishing Co., 1990).
7. Technically he went over as a trade commissioner and then became minister to France.
8. Thomas Jefferson to Harry Inness, 7 March 1791, *PTJ,* 19:521–522. See also Jefferson to Giovanni Fabbroni, 8 June 1778, *PTJ,* 2:195–196; Jefferson to Lafayette,

4 August 1781, *PTJ*, 6:111–112; Jefferson to Thomas Mann Randolph, 1 May 1791, *PTJ*, 20:341; Jefferson to Martha Jefferson Randolph, 11 February 1800, *PTJ*, 31:365–366; Thomas Jefferson to John Adams, 21 January 1812, *PTJRS*, 4:428–430; Randall, *The Life of Thomas Jefferson*, 1:6–7; Gerald Holton, *Science and Anti–Science* (Cambridge: Harvard University Press, 1993), 109–25.

9. Jefferson to Pierre Samuel Du Pont de Nemours, 2 March 1809, in Gilbert Chinard, ed., *The Correspondence of Jefferson and Du Pont de Nemours* (Baltimore: The Johns Hopkins University Press, 1931, reprint 1979), 144–145; Jefferson to Dr. Benjamin Rush, 16 January 1811, *PTJRS*, 3:304–308.
10. Scholarly works that well describe Jefferson's scientific philosophy, interests, and accomplishments include Edwin T. Martin, *Thomas Jefferson: Scientist* (New York: Henry Schuman, 1952); C. Randolph Benson, *Thomas Jefferson as Social Scientist* (Cranberry, N.J.: Fairleigh Dickinson University Press, 1971); John C. Greene, *American Science in the Age of Jefferson* (Ames, Iowa: Iowa State University Press, 1984): Silvio A. Bedini, *Thomas Jefferson: Statesman of Science* (New York: Macmillan, 1990); I. Bernard Cohen, *Science and the Founding Fathers: Science in the Political Thought of Jefferson, Franklin, Adams and Madison*, (New York: W. W. Norton & Co., 1995); and Thomson, *Jefferson's Shadow: The Story of his Science.*
11. "Jefferson's Early Career," *PTJRS*, 17:309–310; Jefferson to John Brazier, 24 August 1819, *PTJRS*, 14:629–631; James Maury, "A Dissertation on Education in the Form of a letter from James Maury to Robert Jackson, July 17, 1762, edited and with an Introduction by Helen D. Bullock," *The Magazine of Albemarle County History* 2 (1942): 36–60; Keith Thomson, *A Passion for Nature: Thomas Jefferson and Natural History* (Chapel Hill: University of North Carolina Press, 2008), 10–11. For Jefferson's early life, see Marie Kimball, *Jefferson, the Road to Glory, 1743–1776* (New York: Coward–McCann, 1943); Harold Hellenbrand, "Mentors and Affectionate Friends," in *The Unfinished Revolution: Education and Politics in the Thoughts of Thomas Jefferson* (Newark, DE: University of Delaware Press, 1990), 21–37; Susan Kern, *The Jeffersons at Shadwell* (New Haven: Yale University Press, 2010); and Kevin J. Hays, *The Road to Monticello: The Life and Mind of Thomas Jefferson* (New York: Oxford University Press, 2008), chapters 3–5.
12. James Maury, "To Christians of Every Denomination among Us, Especially Those of the Established Church, An Address" (Annapolis Md., 1771), as cited in Thomas Buckley, *Seeing Jefferson Anew: In His Time and Ours* (Charlottesville: University of Virginia Press, 2010), 133.
13. Thomson, *Jefferson's Shadow*, 25.
14. Herbert L. Ganter, "William Small, Jefferson's Beloved Teacher," *The William and Mary Quarterly* 4, no. 4 (1947): 505–11; Dumas Malone, *Jefferson and His Time*, vol. 1, *Jefferson the Virginian* (Boston: Little, Brown and Co., 1948), 49–74; Hellenbrand, *The Unfinished Revolution*, 26–27, 29–30, 35, 89, 133; Bedini, *Statesman of Science*, 26; Mark Wenger, "Thomas Jefferson, the College of William and Mary, and the University of Virginia," *Virginia Magazine of History and Biography* 103, no. 3 (1995): 340; and Martin Clagett, "William Small, 1734–1775: Teacher, Mentor and Scientist" (PhD thesis, Virginia Commonwealth University, 2002).
15. Jefferson, "A Bill for Amending the Constitution of the College of William and Mary, and Substituting More Certain Revenues for its Support," *PTJ*, 2:535–543.
16. Sarah N. Randolph, *The Domestic Life of Thomas Jefferson, compiled from Family Letters and Reminiscences* (New York: Harper & Brothers Co., 1871), 15; "Jefferson's Early Career," *PTJRS*, 17:310. Jefferson to William Small, 7 May 1775, *PTJ*,

1:165–167; John D. Burk et al., *History of Virginia from Its First Settlement to the Present Day* (Petersburg, Va.: Dickson and Pescud, 1804–1816), 3:399; Jack E. Morpurgo, *The Majesties Royal Colleges: The College of William and Mary in the Seventeenth and Eighteenth Centuries* (Washington, D.C.: Hennage Creative Printers, 1976), 125; Dumas Malone, *Jefferson and His Time*, vol. 1, *Jefferson the Virginian*, 55–56; Kimball, *Jefferson, the Road to Glory*, 48; Clagett, "William Small," 153.

17. Endrina Tay, "Thomas Jefferson and Books," *Encyclopedia Virginia* (accessed 23 February 2021). https://encyclopediavirginia.org/entries/Jefferson–thomas-and-books.
18. Jefferson to Louis H. Girardin, 15 January 1815, *PTJRS*, 8:200–201; Dumas Malone, "Jefferson Goes to School in Williamsburg," *Virginia Quarterly Review* 33 (1957): 483–491; and John Peter Carey, "Influences on Thomas Jefferson's Theory and Practice of Higher Education" (PhD diss., University of Michigan, 1969), 205–220; Clagett, *William Small*, 153–154.
19. "Jefferson's Early Career," *PTJRS*, 17:310.
20. Jefferson to Thomas Jefferson Randolph, 24 November 1808, Library of Congress, *The Thomas Jefferson Papers*, https://www.loc.gov/item/mtjbib019337/. Jefferson also relied on George Wythe and Peyton Randolph as guides when he felt temptations.
21. Jefferson to Thomas Jefferson Randolph, 24 November 1808, Library of Congress, *The Thomas Jefferson Papers*, http://hdl.loc.gov/loc.mss/mtj.mtjbib019337 and Jefferson to Louis H. Girardin, 15 January 1815, *PTJRS*, 8:200–201.
22. Fairfax Harrison, "A Portrait of Governor Fauquier," *Fauquier Historical Society Bulletin* no. 4 (1924): 346, 348; Bedini, *Statesman of Science*, 26–32, 43–44; Malone, *Jefferson and His Time*, vol. 1, *Jefferson the Virginian*, 49–61, 75–77; Richard Bevier Kirkland, *George Wythe: Lawyer, Revolutionary and Judge* (New York: Garland, 1986); and Thomson, *Jefferson's Shadow*, 32, 35.
23. "Jefferson's Notes for a Biography of George Wythe, ca. 31 August 1820," *PTJRS*, 16:229–232.
24. Jefferson to Rev. James Madison, 19 July 1788, *PTJ*, 13: 380–381 and Livia Kohn and Stephen Jackewicz, *Health and Long–Life, The Chinese Way* (Three Pines Press, 2005).
25. M. Andrew Holowchak, "The Diffusion of Light: Jefferson's Philosophy of Education," *Democracy and Education* 21, no. 2 (2012): 2, 10; Karl Lehmann, *Thomas Jefferson, American Humanist* (New York: The Macmillan Co., 1947), 201–202; Malone, *Jefferson Goes to School in Williamsburg*, 492; *PTJ*, Introduction, 1:viii; and Bedini, *Statesman of Science*, 486.
26. Randolph, *The Domestic Life of Thomas Jefferson*, 34; L. Degrasse, "Thomas Jefferson as a Collector of Books," *AB Brookman's Weekly* 86 (1990): 121–123.
27. Jefferson to John Adams, 17 May 1818, *PTJRS*, 13:48–49; Jurretta Jordan Heckscher, "At All Times His Chosen Companion: Some Notes on What Books Meant to Thomas Jefferson," in *The Founding of Mr. Jefferson's University*, eds. John Ragosta, Peter S. Onuf, and Andrew J. O'Shaughnessy (Charlottesville: University of Virginia Press, 2019), 190–201.
28. Jefferson to John Adams, 10 June 1815, *PTJRS*, 8:522–523 and to Richard Rush, 22 June 1819, *PTJRS*, 14:452–453.
29. Jefferson to John Brazier, 24 August 1819, *PTJRS*, 14:1629–1631.
30. Jefferson to John Adams, 17 May 1818, *PTJRS*, 13:48–49.
31. Keven J. Hayes, "The Libraries of Thomas Jefferson," in Francis D. Cogliano, ed.,

A Companion to Thomas Jefferson, (Malden, Mass.: Wiley-Blackwell, 2012), 333; Endrina Tay, "Forming the Body of a Library. Based on the 'Illimitable Freedom of the Human Mind,'" in *The Founding of Thomas Jefferson's University*, eds. John Ragosta, Peter S. Onuf, and Andrew J. O'Shaughnessy (Charlottesville: University of Virginia Press, 2019), 208–223.

32. William H. Peden, "Thomas Jefferson: Book Collector" (PhD diss., University of Virginia, 1942), 2–18.
33. Thomas E. Keys, "The Colonial Libraries and the Development of Sectional Differences in the Colonies," *The Library Quarterly* 8 (1933): 382.
34. Peden, "Jefferson: Book Collector," 17.
35. Tay, "Thomas Jefferson and Books"; Jefferson's letters to Thomas Cooper, 16 January 1814, *PTJRS*, 7:124–131; to Samuel Harrison Smith, 21 September 1814, *PTJRS*, 7:681–684; and to James Madison, 24 September 1814, *PTJRS*, 7:691–693.
36. Jefferson to John Page, 21 February 1770, *PTJ*, 1:34–37.
37. Thomas Jefferson, *Jefferson's Memorandum Book: Accounts with Legal Records and Miscellany, 1767–1826,* James A Bear Jr. and Lucia C. Stanton eds. (Princeton: Princeton University Press, 1997), 1:332.; Jefferson, *1783 Catalogue of Books*, Coolidge Collection of Thomas Jefferson's Manuscripts, Massachusetts Historical Society, Boston, Massachusetts, 5.
38. Jefferson to Samuel Harrison Smith, 21 September 1814, *PTJRS*, 7:681–684.
39. According to Bedini, Jefferson paid more than $50,000 at the time of purchase for these 6,500 books. Bedini, *Statesman of Science*, 440 and Endrina Tay, "Forming the Body of a Library," 215.
40. Tay, "Jefferson, Thomas and Books"; Jefferson to George Watterston, 7 May 1815, *PTJRS*, 8:473–475 and 2 March 1816, *PTJRS*, 9:531–532; William H. Peden, *1828 Catalogue of the Library of the University of Virginia* (Charlottesville: Alderman Library, University of Virginia, 1945), v; James Gilbreath and Douglas L. Wilson, eds. *Thomas Jefferson's Library: A Catalogue with Entries in His Own Order* (Washington: Library of Congress, 1989), 3; William Dawson Johnston, *History of the Library of Congress: 1800–1864* (Washington: Government Printing Office, 1904), 142–147.
41. Thomson, *Jefferson's Shadow: The Story of His Science*, 14–22.
42. Clagett, *Scientific Jefferson: Revealed*, 115–116, deriving the estimate from the Nicholas Trist catalogue of 1823 and Millicent Sowerby's multi-volume catalogue published between 1952 and 1959.
43. Jefferson's explanatory note in his 1783 library catalogue, MHi, https://www.masshist.org/thomasjeffersonpapers/doc?id=catalog1783_11&mode=lgImg (http://tjlibraries.monticello.org/transcripts/March1783/March1783.html).
44. Jefferson to George F. Hopkins, 5 September 1822, *PTJRS*, 18:625–626. See also Jefferson to Sheldon Clark, 5 December 1825, http://hdl.loc.gov/loc.mss/mtj.mtj.mtjbib025588.
45. Jefferson to John Adams, 14 October 1816, *PTJRS*, 10:458–461; Jefferson's prospectus for Destutt de Tracy's *Treatise on Political Economy*, [ca. 6 April 1816], *PTJRS*, 9:630–633; E. Millicent Sowerby, *Catalogue of the Library of Thomas Jefferson* (Washington: The Library of Congress, 1952–59), 2:1–3; Adrienne Koch, *The Philosophy of Thomas Jefferson* (New York: Columbia University Press, 1943), 66–72; Hellenbrand, *The Unfinished Revolution:* 150, 152–153, 159–163 and John Peter Carey, "Influences on Thomas Jefferson's Theory and Practice of Higher Education" (PhD diss., University of Michigan, 1969), 168–169.

46. These lists or "syllabi" are discussed in William Peden, *Some Aspects of Jefferson's Bibliography* (Lexington, Va.: Journalism Laboratory Press, Washington and Lee University, 1941); Peden,"Some Notes Concerning Thomas Jefferson's Libraries," 266–272; and Douglas L. Wilson, *Jefferson's Books* (Charlottesville: Thomas Jefferson Memorial Foundation, 1996), 50.
47. Jefferson to Nathaniel Burwell, 14 March 1818, *PTJRS*, 12:532–535.
48. Lucia C. Stanton, *Those Who Labor for My Happiness: Slavery at Thomas Jefferson's Monticello* (Charlottesville: University of Virginia Press, 2012), 164–166.
49. Jefferson to John Wyche, 19 May 1809, *PTJRS*, 1:205.
50. Jefferson to Walter Jones, 2 January 1814, *PTJRS*, 7:100–104 and Jefferson to John Norvell, 11 June 1807, Library of Congress, *The Thomas Jefferson Papers*, https://www.loc.gov/item/mtjbib017268/.
51. Jon Meacham, *In the Hands of the People* (New York: Random House, 2020), 17. For optimistic views on a free press, see Jefferson to Edward Carrington, 6 January 1787, *PTJ*, 11:48–50; Jefferson to Archibald Stuart, 14 May 1799, *PTJ*, 31:109–111; Jefferson to Charles Yancey, 6 January 1816, *PTJRS*, 9:328–331; and Jefferson to the Marquis de Lafayette, 4 November 1823, in Gilbert Chinard, ed., *The Letters of Lafayette and Jefferson,* 1929, reprint 1979, 414–416.
52. Jefferson to Nicolas G. Dufief, 19 April 1814, *PTJRS*, 7: 303–305.
53. Jefferson's Bill for Establishing a Public Library, 18 June 1779, *PTJ*, 2:544–545.
54. Examples include Jefferson to Robert Skipwith, 3 August 1771, *PTJ*, 1:76–81; Jefferson to Bernard Moore, circa 1773, contained in the letter to John Minor, 30 August 1814, *PTJRS*, 7:625–631; Jefferson to Peter Carr, 19 August 1785 and 10 August 1787, *PTJ*, 8:405–408 and 12:14–19; Jefferson to Walker Maury, 19 August 1785, *PTJ*, 8:409–412; Jefferson to Thomas Mann Randolph, 27 August 1786, *PTJ*, 10:305–309 and 6 July 1787, *PTJ*, 11:556–559; Jefferson to John Garland Jefferson, 11 June 1790, *PTJ*, 16:480–482; Jefferson to William G. Munford, 5 December 1798, *PTJ*, 30:594–597 and 18 June 1799, *PTJ*, 31:126–130; and Jefferson to Samuel R. Demaree, 4 October 1809, *PTJRS*, 1:575–576.
55. Alan Taylor, "The Virtue of an Educated Voter," *American Scholar* 85 (autumn 2016): 18–27; Jefferson to Charles Yancey, 6 January 1816, *PTJRS*, 9:328–331.
56. Jefferson's Bill to Promote the Progress of the Useful Arts, 1 December 1791, *PTJ*, 22:361; Editorial Note on Campaign to Abolish Tariffs on Books, [30 November 1821], *PTJRS*, 17:655–659.
57. Tay, "Forming the Body of a Library," 208–223. Editorial Note on The Sale of Thomas Jefferson's Library to Congress, [21 September 1814], *PTJRS*, 7:670–684. THOMAS (http://thomas.loc.gov/) now redirects to Congress.gov, which provides searchable access to many government documents.
58. Hume to Franklin, 10 May 1762, in Leonard W. Labaree et al., eds. *The Papers of Benjamin Franklin*, 1959–, 10:80–82.
59. Jefferson to Noah Webster, 4 December 1790, *PTJ*, 18:131–135; Jefferson to John Hollins, 19 February 1809, Library of Congress, *The Thomas Jefferson Papers*, https://www.loc.gov/item/mtjbib019768/; Douglas Wilson, "Jefferson and the Republic of Letters," in Peter S. Onuf, ed., *Jeffersonian Legacies* (Charlottesville: University of Virginia Press, 1993), 50–76.
60. Thomas Jefferson, *Notes on the State of Virginia*, William Peden, ed. (New York: W. W. Norton & Co., 1954) (hereafter cited as Peden, *Notes*); and Bedini, *Statesman of Science*.
61. Examples include James E. McClellan, *Science Reorganized: Scientific Societies in the*

Eighteenth Century (New York: Columbia University Press, 1985).
62. Patrick Spero, "The Other Presidency: Thomas Jefferson and the American Philosophical Society," *Proceedings of the American Philosophical Society* 162, no. 4 (2018): 321–360; Gilbert Chinard, "Jefferson and the American Philosophical Society," *Proceedings of the American Philosophical Society*, 87, no. 3 (1943): 263–276;
63. Edward C. Carter, "Jefferson's American Philosophical Society Leadership and Heritage," in *The Most Flattering Incident of my Life: Essays Celebrating the Bicentennial of Thomas Jefferson's American Philosophical Society Presidency* (Philadelphia: Friends of the American Philosophical Society Library, 1997), 9–15.
64. Jefferson to Thomas Mann Randolph, 1 May 1791, *PTJ*, 20:341–342, "APS Circular on the Hessian Fly," 17 April 1792, *PTJ*, 23:430–433, "Jefferson's Notes on the Hessian Fly," 1–15 June 1792, *PTJ*, 24:11–14; and "Editorial Notes on Report of Weights and Measures," 4 July 1790, *PTJ*, 16:602–675.
65. Jefferson to Dugald Stewart, 2 June 1797, *PTJ*, 29:415; "Editorial Note on Jefferson and André Michaux's Proposed Western Expedition," 22 January 1793, *PTJ*, 25:75–84; and Jefferson to Caspar Wistar, 16 December 1800, *PTJ*, 32:311. See also Spero, "The Other Presidency," 349.
66. Personal communication from Patrick Spero, PhD, Librarian of the APS.
67. Jefferson to John Adams, 15 June 1813, *PTJRS*, 6:193–194; 5 July1814, *PTJRS*, 7:451–455; 14 March 1820, *PTJRS*, 15:469–470, Adams to Jefferson, 16 July 1814, *PTJRS*, 7:476–482; 20 June 1815, *PTJRS*, 8:552–554; 21 February 1820, *PTJRS*, 15:410–411. Jefferson to William G. Munford, 18 June 1799, *PTJ*, 31:126–130; Jefferson to Joseph Priestley, 21 March 1801, *PTJ*, 33:393–395; and Jefferson to Pierre Samuel Du Pont de Nemours, 24 April 1816, *PTJRS*, 9:699–702.
68. John Adams, "An Essay on Man's Lust for Power," 29 August1763, in John Adams, *Papers of John Adams*, Robert J. Taylor et al., eds. (Cambridge, Mass.: The Belknap Press of Harvard University Press, 1977–), 1:81–84; Adams to Jefferson, 17 April 1826, in John Adams, *The Adams–Jefferson Correspondence: The Complete Correspondence Between Thomas Jefferson & Abigail & John Adams,* Lester J. Cappon, ed. (Chapel Hill, NC: The University of North Carolina Press, 1959), 2:614; Gordon S. Wood, *The Creation of the American Republic: 1776–1787* (Chapel Hill: University of North Carolina Press, 1969), 181, 569; John Ferling, *John Adams: A Life* (New York: Oxford University Press, 1992), 289, 452; David McCullough, *John Adams* (New York: Simon and Schuster, 2001), 589.
69. John Adams to Thomas Jefferson, 21 February 1820, *PTJRS*, 15:410–411; Jefferson to Joseph Priestley, 21 March 1801, *PTJ*, 33:393–395.
70. Daniel N. Robinson, "Jefferson and Adams on the Mind–Body Problem," *History of Psychology* 6, no. 3 (2003): 228.
71. John Adams to Thomas Jefferson, 21 February 1820, *PTJRS*, 15:410–411; Darren Staloff, *Ideology, Empiricism, and Politics: The Philosophical Exchanges of Thomas Jefferson and John Adams*, Paper presented at the 2017 SAR Annual Conference on the American Revolution, Quincy, Mass. (9 June 2017), 24–25. See also Jefferson to Adams, 15 June 1813, *PTJRS*, 6:193–195.
72. Martin, *Thomas Jefferson: Scientist*, 31.
73. Dumas Malone, *Jefferson in His Time,* vol. 6, *The Sage of Monticello* (Boston: Little Brown, 1981).
74. Jefferson to James Madison, 20 December 1787, *PTJ*, 12:434–443; Jefferson to John Breckinridge, 29 January 1800, *PTJ*, 31: 344–345; Jefferson to Bishop

James Madison, 31 January 1800, *PTJ*, 31:349–352; Jefferson to John Dickinson, 6 March 1801, *PTJ*, 33:196–197, Jefferson to Joseph Priestley, 21 March 1801, *PTJ*, 33:393–395; Jefferson to Caesar A. Rodney, 10 February 1810, *PTJRS*, 2:209–210; Jefferson to John Adams, 1 August 1816, *PTJRS*, 10:284–286; Jefferson to Benjamin Waterhouse, 3 March 1818, *PTJRS*, 12:517–519; John Adams to Thomas Jefferson, 21 February 1820, *PTJRS*, 15:410–411; and Jefferson to William Ludlow, 6 September 1824, Library of Congress, *The Thomas Jefferson Papers*, https://www.loc.gov/item/mtjbib025119/. See also Wood, *Creation of the American Republic*, 121.

75. Thomson, *Jefferson's Shadow*, 235–236.
76. Jefferson to William G. Munford, 18 June 1799, *PTJ*, 31:126–130.
77. John Adams to Jefferson, 20 June 1815, *PTJRS*, 8:552–554; Linda Kerber, *Federalists in Dissent: Imagery and Ideology in Jeffersonian America* (Ithaca: Cornel University Press, 1970), 74–76, 91–92, 134.
78. Jefferson to Adams, 15 June 1813, *PTJRS*, 6:193–195.
79. Jefferson to John Trumbull, 15 February 1789, *PTJ*, 14:561 and Jefferson to Benjamin Rush, 16 January 1811, *PTJRS*, 3:304–308.
80. Jefferson to Robert Fulton, 16 April 1810, *PTJRS* 2:332–333; Bedini, *Statesman of Science*, 488.
81. Jefferson to Rev. James Madison, 19 July 1788, *PTJ*, 13:379–383; Jefferson to Charles Thomson, 20 September 1787, *PTJ*, 12:159–161; Jefferson to James Maury, 16 June 1815, *PTJRS*, 8:542–545; Jefferson to George Fleming, 29 December 1815, *PTJRS*, 9:302–304. See also Jefferson to John Rutledge, 9 September 1788, *PTJ*, 13:593–594; Jefferson to George Washington, 30 July 1791, *PTJ*, 20:704–705; and Jefferson to John Adams, March 14, 1820, *PTJRS*, 14:469–470.
82. Jefferson's draft of the 1818 Rockfish Gap Report of the University of Virginia Commissioners, *PTJRS*, 13:189–208. See also Jefferson to Francis Eppes, 21 May 1816, *PTJRS*, 10:72–73; "Editorial Note on Campaign to Abolish Tariffs on Books, November 30, 1821," *PTJRS* 17:655–659; Jefferson to Cornelius Camden Blatchly, 21 October 1822, Library of Congress, *The Thomas Jefferson Papers*, https://www.loc.gov/item/mtjbib024471/.
83. Jefferson to George Washington, 14 August 1787, *PTJ*, 12:36–38; Jefferson to David Williams, 14 November 1803, *PTJ*, 41:726–728; Jefferson to John Jay, 23 August 1785, *PTJ*, 8:426–428; Lewis C. Gray, "History of Agriculture in the Southern United States to 1860," *Carnegie Institute* (Washington) 2 (1933): 612, 779; and Ronald L. Numbers and Todd L. Savitt, eds., *Science and Medicine in the Old South* (Baton Rouge, LA:, Louisiana State University Press, 1989), 104.
84. Jefferson's Notes on Arthur Young's letter to George Washington, *PTJ*, 24:95–99; Jefferson to George Washington, 28 June 1793, *PTJ*, 26:396–398; Jefferson to Thomas Mann Randolph, Jr., 30 June 1793, *PTJ*, 26:422–424; Jefferson to John Taylor, 29 December 1794, *PTJ*, 28: 230–234, and Jefferson to Charles Willson Peale, 17 April 1813, *PTJRS*, 6:68–70. See also August C. Miller, "Jefferson as an Agriculturist," *Agricultural History* (1942): 65–78; Silvio Bedini, *Jefferson and Science* (Thomas Jefferson Foundation and University of North Carolina Press, 2002), 92–99; Clagett, *Scientific Jefferson Revealed*, 1–14; and Richard L. Bushman, *The American Farmer in the Eighteenth Century: A Social and Cultural History* (New Haven: Yale University Press, 2018).
85. Mark Sturges, "Founding Farmers: Jefferson, Washington and the Rhetoric of Agricultural Reform," *Early American Literature* 50, no. 3 (2015): 681–709 and

Charles A. Miller, *Jefferson and Nature: An Interpretation* (Baltimore: Johns Hopkins University Press, 1988), 59–63, 223, 257.

86. Henry A. Wallace, "Keynote Address," *Proceedings of the Association of Land-Grant Colleges and Universities* 51 (1937): 336–346.
87. William A. Koelsch, "Thomas Jefferson, American Geographers, and the Uses of Geography," *Geographical Review* 98 (2008): 260–279, as cited in Thomson, *Jefferson's Shadow*, 180; and Peden, *Notes*, Query VII, 73–81.
88. Peden, *Notes*, Query VII, 73–81; Jefferson to the Marquis de Chastellux, 2 September 1785, *PTJ*, 8:467–470; Jefferson to Jean Baptiste Le Roy, 13 November 1786, *PTJ*, 10:524–530; Jefferson to Thomas Mann Randolph, 18 April 1790, *PTJ*, 16:351–352; Jefferson to Nathaniel Chapman, 11 December 1809, *PTJRS*, 2:70–72; Jefferson's "Analysis of his Weather Memorandum Book, January 1817," *PTJRS*, 11:33–41; Jefferson to George F. Hopkins, 5 September 1822, *PTJRS*, 18:625–626; and Jefferson to Lewis C. Beck, 16 July 1824, Library of Congress, *The Thomas Jefferson Papers*, https://www.loc.gov/item/mtjbib025071/. Jefferson Weather and Climate Records, https://jefferson–weather–records.org/ is a splendid website. See also Keith Thomson, "The Question of Climatic Stability in America before 1900," *Climate Change* 3 (1981): 224–241 and Bedini, *Statesman of Science*, 467–468.
89. For Jefferson's role in the infant science of paleontology, his mistakes, as well as his contributions, see "Jefferson's Memoir on the Megalonyx, February 10, 1797," *PTJRS*, 29:291–304; John Stuart to Jefferson, 11 April 1796, *PTJ*, 29:64–65. George Gaylord Simpson, "The Beginnings of Vertebrate Paleontology in North America," *Proceedings of the American Philosophical Society* 80 (1942): 130–188; Martin, *Thomas Jefferson: Scientist*, chapters 4 and 7; Bedini, *Thomas Jefferson and American Vertebrate Paleontology* (Charlottesville: Virginia Division of Mineral Resources, publication 061, Commonwealth of Virginia, 1985), 1; Thomson, *Jefferson's Shadow*, 86–97; Frederic A. Lucas, "Thomas Jefferson: Paleontologist," *Natural History* 26 (1926): 328–330.
90. William Rouse Jillson, *The Extinct Vertebrata of the Pleistocene in Kentucky* (Frankford, Ky: Roberts Printing Co, 1968), 00; Bernard Mayo, "A Peppercorn for Mr. Jefferson," *Virginia Quarterly Review* (1943): 225.
91. Spero, "The Other Presidency," 321.
92. "Jefferson's Notes on the Hessian Fly," *PTJ*, 20:445–449, 456–462; 24:11–14; Jefferson to Charles Thomson, 2 April 1791, *PTJ*, 20:244–245; Jefferson to Thomas Mann Randolph, 1 May 1791, *PTJ*, 20:341–342; Jefferson to Benjamin Barton Smith, 12 May 1791, *PTJ*, 20:395 and 23:430–433; Harry B. Weiss, "Thomas Jefferson and Economic Entomology," *Journal of Economic Entomology* 37, no. 6 (1944): 836–841; Thomson, *Jefferson's Shadow*, 213; Brook Hunter, "The Forgotten Legacy of the Hessian Fly," in *The Economy of Early America: Historical Perspectives & New Directions*, ed. Cathy Matson, (University Park, PA: Penn State Press, 2006), 236–262; Phillip J. Pauly, "Fighting the Hessian Fly: American and British Responses to Insect Invasion," *Environmental History* 7, no. 3 (2002): 486–507.
93. Although *Notes* is commonly described as the only book Jefferson published in his lifetime, he also published the *Manual of Parliamentary Practice* (1801) and the *Proceedings of the Government of the United States, in maintaining the Public Right to the Beach of the Mississippi, Adjacent to New–Orleans* (1812). The phrase "hierarchy of knowledge" comes from George Alan Davy, "Argumentation and Unified Structure in Notes on the State of Virginia." *Eighteenth Century Studies* 26, no.4

(1993), 587–588.

94. Douglas L. Wilson, "The Evolution of Jefferson's Notes on the State of Virginia," *Virginia Magazine of History and Biography* 112 (2004): 98–133; John Ragosta, "Notes on the State of Virginia," *Thomas Jefferson Encyclopedia*, February 22, 2018; Jefferson to the Marquis de Chastellux, 16 January 1784, *PTJ*, 6:466–467; Jefferson to Alexander Donald, 17 September 1787, *PTJ*, 12:132–134; Jefferson to John W. Campbell, 3 September 1809, *PTJRS*, 1:486–488; Jefferson to Alexander von Humboldt, 14 April 1811, *PTJRS* 3:553–555.
95. G. Brown Goode, "The Beginnings of Natural History in America. An Address Delivered at the Sixth Anniversary Meeting of the Biological Society of Washington," 1886, 00. See also Coolie Verner, "Mr. Jefferson Makes a Map," *International Journal of the History of Cartography* 14 (1959): 96–108.
96. Gilbert Chinard, *Thomas Jefferson, the Apostle of Americanism* (Boston: Little, Brown & Co., 1929), 118; Greene, *American Science in the Age of Jefferson*, 188–189, 409; Martin, *Thomas Jefferson: Scientist*, 258; David N. Livingstone, *The Geographical Tradition: Episodes in the History of a Contested Enterprise* (Oxford: Blackwell, 1992), 145; and Austin H. Clark, "Thomas Jefferson and Science," *Washington Academy of Sciences Journal* 33 (1943): 197–198.
97. K. Lehmann Hartleben, "Thomas Jefferson, Archeologist," *American Journal of Archaeology* 47 (1943): 161–163; and Jeffrey L. Hantman and Gary Dunham, "The Enlightened Archaeologist," *Archaeology* 46, no. 3 (1993): 46.
98. Peden, *Notes*, 34–35; Jefferson to Francis Eppes, 11 September 1818, *PTJRS* 13:278; Editorial Note on "Jefferson's Trip to Warm Springs," *PTJRS*, 13:228–229.
99. Oliver, "Thomas Jefferson—Scientist," 461; *Thomas Jefferson's Garden Book*, 172–173; John M. Holmes, *Thomas Jefferson Treats Himself: Herbs, Physicke and Nutrition in Early America* (Fort Valley, Va: Loft Press, 1997); Malone, *Jefferson and His Time, vol. 2, Jefferson and the Rights of Man,* 446.
100. Davy, 582, 584; James L. Golden and Alan L. Golden, *Thomas Jefferson and the Rhetoric of Virtue* (Lanham, Md. : Rowman & Littlefield, 2002), 47–71.
101. For a detailed discussion of Buffon, the esteem he garnered, his thoughts on America, and Jefferson's strategy of refutation, see Henline, "A Study of Notes on the State of Virginia," 233–246 and Martin, *Thomas Jefferson: Scientist,* 148–191.
102. Henline, 245–246 and Peden, *Notes*, 47, 50–52.
103. Peden, *Notes*, 64–65, 276–277. Perhaps because of Jefferson's retort, in later editions of his work, Raynal removed the offending passage. See Cohen, *Science and the Founding Fathers*, 87.
104. Ibid., 160; Jefferson to Benjamin Rush, 23 September 1800, *PTJ*, 32:166–169.
105. Peden, *Notes*, Introductory Comments, xxii–xxiv.
106. Contemporary critical responses included Clement Clarke Moore, *Observations Upon Certain Passages of Mr Jefferson's Notes on Virginia, Which Appears to Have a Tendency to Subvert Religion, and Establish a False Jefferson's Notes on Virginia, Which Appears to Have a Tendency to Subvert Religion, and Establish a False Philosophy* (New York: New York Historical Society, 1804). For a survey of these and other attacks directly or indirectly inspired by the *Notes*, see Martin, *Thomas Jefferson: Scientist*, chapter 9.
107. Jefferson to Charles F. Welles, 3 December 1809, *PTJRS*, 2:51–52; Jefferson to Joseph Delaplaine, 12 April 1817, *PTJRS*, 11:251–252.
108. For a survey of these and other attacks directly or indirectly inspired by the *Notes*, see Martin, *Thomas Jefferson: Scientist*, chapter 9.

109. Peden, *Notes*, 92–108, 139–140.
110. Peden, *Notes*, 137–143 and 286–289; Jefferson to Jared Sparks, 4 February 1824, Library of Congress, *The Thomas Jefferson Papers*, https://www.loc.gov/item/mtjbib024921/; Connor Cruise O'Brien, "Thomas Jefferson: Radical and Racist," *The Atlantic* (October 1996); Stephen Jay Gould, *The Mismeasure of Man* (New York: W.W. Norton & Co., 1996), 64, 422.
111. Constitution of the United States, Article 1, Section 2, Clause 3. The fractional mode of the constitution's three–fifth's clause is explained by concerns about political apportionment as well as perceived racial inferiority. The number was reached as a compromise: the South wanted the enslaved persons to be counted in apportionment of congressional seats but their financial value not to be counted in federal taxation; the North wanted the exact opposite. The compromise applied the three–fifth ratio to both purposes, (and without those extra congressional seats and electoral–college votes based on the enslaved part of the population going to the South, Jefferson would not have won election in 1800). J. Jefferson Looney to author, personal communication, 12 February 2021.
112. "Jefferson's Notes of Proceedings in the Continental Congress, 7 June to 1 August 1776," *PTJ*, 1:130; "Jefferson's Early Career," *PTJRS*, 17:319; and *PTJ*, 2:470–473; *PTJ*, 6:298; *PTJ*, 25:230; Jefferson to Christopher Ellery, 9 May 1803, *PTJ*, 40:337–338; and Jefferson to John Strode, 5 June 1805, Library of Congress, *The Thomas Jefferson Papers*, https://www.loc.gov/item/mtjbib014782/; and William J. Cooper, *Liberty and Slavery: Southern Politics to 1860* (New York: Alfred A. Knopf, 1983), 97.
113. Andrew J. O'Shaughnessy, *The Illimitable Freedom of the Human Mind: Thomas Jefferson's Idea of a University* (Charlottesville: University of Virginia Press, 2021), 183–210.
114. V. Bradley Lewis, The Politics of Pragmatism, 7 February 2013, available at www.americamagazine.org/issue/culture/politics–pragmatism; Jon Meacham, *Thomas Jefferson: The Art of Power* (New York: Random House, 2013), 124, 173 and Jonathan Yardley, "The Complex Thomas Jefferson in his Place and Time," *The Washington Post*, 12 May 2017.
115. Peden, *Notes*, 162–163; Jefferson to Jean Nicolas Démeunier, 26 June 1786, *PTJ*, 10:61–64; Jefferson to Edward Rutledge, 14 July 1787, *PTJ*, 11:587–589; Jefferson to Brissot de Warville, 11 February 1788, *PTJ*, 12:577–578; Jefferson to Edward Coles, 25 August 1814, *PTJRS*, 7:603–605; Jefferson to Thomas Cooper, 10 September 1814, *PTJRS*, 7:649–655; Jefferson to Henri Grégoire, 25 February 1809, Library of Congress, *The Thomas Jefferson Papers*, https://www.loc.gov/item/mtjbib019810/; Jefferson to John Holmes, 22 April 1820, *PTJRS*, 15:550–551; Jefferson to William Short, 8 September 1823, Library of Congress, *The Thomas Jefferson Papers*, https://www.loc.gov/item/mtjbib024751/; Jefferson to Lydia Howard Huntley Sigourney, 18 July 1824, Pierpont Morgan Library; and Jefferson to Edward Everett, 8 April 1826, Library of Congress, *The Thomas Jefferson Papers*, https://www.loc.gov/item/mtjbib025697/. See also Ari Helo and Peter Onuf, "Jefferson, Morality, and the Problem of Slavery," *William and Mary Quarterly* 60, no. 3 (2003): 583–614; Peter Onuf, *The Mind of Thomas Jefferson* (Charlottesville: University of Virginia Press, 2007); Henry Wiencek, *Master of the Mountain: Thomas Jefferson and His Slaves* (New York: Farrar, Straus, and Giroux 2012); Johann N. Neem, "Developing Freedom: Thomas Jefferson, the State, and Human Capability," *Studies in American Political Development*, 2013; Ari Helo, *Thomas*

Jefferson's Ethics and Politics of Human Progress (New York: Cambridge University Press, 2014); and M. Andrew Holochak, *Rethinking Thomas Jefferson's Writings on Slavery and Race* (Newcastle on Tyne: Cambridge Scholars Publishing, 2020).

116. Jefferson to François Jean de Beauvoir, Marquis de Chastellux, 7 June 1785, *PTJ*, 8:184–186. See also Benjamin Banneker to Jefferson, 19 August 1791, *PTJ*, 22:49–54; Jefferson to Banneker, 30 August 1791, *PTJ*, 22:97–98; Jefferson to the Marquis de Condorcet, 30 August 1791, *PTJ*, 22:98–99; Jefferson to Joel Barlow, 8 October 1809, *PTJRS*, 1:588–590, in which Jefferson is dismissive of Banneker's talents; Jefferson's Draft of the Rockfish Gap Report of the University of Virginia Commissioners, 14 August 1818, *PTJRS*, 13:189–208; and Miller, Jefferson and Nature, 66–68.
117. Peden, *Notes*, 143. Eschewing the recent inclination to bash Jefferson, two authors have recently attempted to better contextualize Jefferson's writings on race. See John B. Boles, *Jefferson: Architect of American Liberty* (New York: Basic Books, 2017), 460–469 and Arthur Scherr, "An Honest, Intelligent Man: Thomas Jefferson, the Free Black Patrick Henry, and the Founder's Racist Views in his Last Years," *Virginia Magazine of History and Biography* 127, no. 4 (2019): 300–339.
118. Jefferson to Malesherbes, 11 March 1789, *PTJ*, 7:642. Browne, *Jefferson and the Scientific Trends in His Time*, 462–464; Martin, *Thomas Jefferson: Scientist*, 48–50; Bedini, *Statesman of Science;* and J. G. Crowther, *Francis Bacon: The First Statesman of Science (*London: *The* Creset Press, 1960).
119. Emily Ogden, "He Blinded Me with Science," *Lapham's Quarterly Online* (29 August 2018), https://www.Laphamsquarterly.org/roundtable/he–blinded–me–with–science; Cohen, *Science and the Founding Fathers*, 186–187; Thomson, *Jefferson's Shadow*, 158–159.
120. Charles Thomson to Jefferson, 6 March 1785, *PTJ*, 8:15–17; Jefferson to Thomson, 11 November 1784, *PTJ*, 7:518–519; Jefferson to Rev. James Madison, 11 November 1784, *PTJ*, 7:508; Jefferson to David Rittenhouse, 11 November 1784, *PTJ*, 7:516–517; Jefferson to Francis Hopkinson, 13 January 1785, *PTJ*, 7:602–603; Jefferson to Hugh Williamson, 5 February 1785, *PTJ*, 7:641–643; Jefferson to James Currie, 5 February 1785, *PTJ*, 7:635; Jefferson to Charles Thomson, 21 June 1785, *PTJ*, 8:245–246; and Jefferson to the Rev. William Smith, 21 February 1791, *PTJ*, 19:112–114.
121. Jefferson to Richard Claiborne, 21 February 1795, *PTJ*, 28:273–274; Jeffrey H. Matsuura, "Thomas Jefferson and the Evolution of a Populist Vision of Intellectual Property Rights and Democratic Values." An address given at the symposium *Technology and Democratic Values in the Early Republic* at the University of Virginia, 3 November 2006, available at www.archipelago.org/vol10–34/matsuura.htm.
122. Bedini, *Statesman of Science*, 209–210.
123. Jefferson to Edmund Randolph, 17 March 1793, *PTJ*, 25:398–399, Eli Whitney to Jefferson, 15 October 1793, *PTJ*, 27:240–251; Martin, *Thomas Jefferson: Scientist*, 67–106; Malone, *Jefferson and His Time*, vol. 2, *Jefferson and the Rights of Man*, 281–285. and Silvio A. Bedini, *Thomas Jefferson and his Copying Machines* (Charlottesville: University of Virginia Press, 1984). When the present Patent and Trademark Office celebrated its one-hundredth anniversary, a bust of Jefferson was dedicated recognizing him as one of the fathers of the institution. *Journal of the Patent and Trademark Society* 19 (1937): 3–4, 11, 71–77.
124. Jefferson to Charles Willson Peale, 13 June 1815, *PTJRS*, 8:534–536; Jefferson to George Fleming, 29 December 1815, *PTJRS*, 9:302–304.

125. Jefferson to James Madison, 20 December 1787, *PTJ*, 12:438–243; 31 July 1788, *PTJ*, 13:440–443; 17 October 1788, *PTJ*, 14:16–22; 28 August 1789, *PTJ*, 15:364–369; and 6 September 1789, *PTJ*, 15:392–398.
126. Jefferson to Isaac McPherson, 13 August 1813, *PTJRS* 6:379–386.
127. Jefferson to William Johnson, 4 March 1823, Library of Congress, *The Thomas Jefferson Papers*, https://www.loc.gov/item/mtjbib024584/; Jefferson to Benjamin Waterhouse, 3 March 1818, *PTJRS*, 12:517–519; Matsuura, "Jefferson and the Evolution of a Populist Vision." See also Henry L. Ellsworth, "Patent Act, 1790," *Digest of Patents Issued by the United States, 1790–1839* (Washington D.C.: printed by P. Force, 1840), 3; and Ruth Schwartz Cowan, *A Social History of American Technology* (New York: Oxford University Press, 1997): 121.
128. Jefferson to Benjamin Vaughan, 27 June 1790, *PTJ*, 16:578–580. See also Jefferson to Oliver Evans, 2 May 1807, Library of Congress, *The Thomas Jefferson Papers*, https://www.loc.gov/item/mtjbib017171/.
129. Bedini, *Statesman of Science,* 208–210 and Cowan, *A Social History*, 122.
130. "Jefferson's draft Bill to Promote the Progress of the Useful Arts," 1 December 1791, *PTJ* 22:359–361; E. C. Walterscheid, "Thomas Jefferson and the Patent Act of 1793," *Essays in History* 40 (1998): I–VII; www.stephankinsella.com/2010/06/thomas–jefferson–and–the–patent– act–of–1793/.
131. Walterscheid, "Thomas Jefferson and the Patent Act of 1793," V.
132. Jefferson to Casper Wistar, 20 March 1791, *PTJ*, 19:615–616, Editorial Note on "Experiments in Desalination of Sea Water To Test the Claims of Jacob Isaacks," *PTJ*, 16:608–624; Jefferson's Report on Desalination of Sea Water," 21 November 1791, *PTJ*, 22:318–322; Bedini, *Statesman of Science*, 208–211; and Browne, *Jefferson and Scientific Trends in His Time*, 386.
133. Matsuura, "Jefferson and the Evolution of a Populist Vision." See also Malone, *Jefferson and His Time,* vol. 2, *Jefferson and the Rights of Man*, 284.
134. Jefferson to Isaac McPherson, 13 August 1813, *PTJRS*, 6:379–386.
135. For relevant details, see Jefferson to the Senate and House of Representatives, 18 January 1803, *PTJ*, 39:350–355; Bedini, *Statesman of Science*, 339–372; and Stephen E. Ambrose, *Undaunted Courage: Meriwether Lewis, Thomas Jefferson, and the Opening of the American West* (New York: Touchstone, Simon & Schuster, 1996).
136. Jefferson to George Rogers Clark, 26 November 1782 and 4 December 1783, *PTJ*, 6:204–205, 6:371; Jefferson to John Jay, 14 August 1785, *PTJ*, 8:372–375; Jefferson to Archibald Stuart, 25 January 1786, *PTJ*, 9:217–219; Jefferson to John Ledyard, 27 July 1786, *PTJ*, 10:170–171; Jefferson to Charles Thomson, 20 September 1787, *PTJ*, 12:159–161; Editorial Note on "Jefferson and Michaux's Proposed Western Expedition, January 22, 1793," *PTJ*, 25:75–84; American Philosophical Society's Instructions to André Michaux, [ca. 30 April 1793], *PTJ*, 25:624–626; Jefferson's First Inaugural Address, 4 March 1801, *PTJ*, 33:148–152; and Jefferson to the Senate and House of Representatives, 18 January 1803, *PTJ*, 39:350–355; J. Jefferson Looney, "The Corps of Discovery and Thomas Jefferson: Prehistory and Aftermath," Moulton Lecture, Lewis and Clark Trail Heritage Foundation Conference, 5 August 2020; Bedini, *Statesman of Science*, 339–372; and Peter Marshall and David Manuel, *From Sea to Shining Sea: 1787–1837* (Grand Rapids, Mich., 1985).
137. Jefferson, specifically Jefferson to Meriwether Lewis, 20 June 1803, *PTJ*, 40:176–183.
138. Jefferson to Meriwether Lewis, 20 June 1803, *PTJ*, 40:176–183; Bedini, *Statesman*

of Science, 363; Peter J. Kastor, "The Lewis and Clark Expedition," in *Encyclopedia Virginia, Virginia Foundation for the Humanities* (accessed 20 November 2019), https://www.EncyclopediaVirginia.org/Lewis_and_clark_Expedition_The; Cohen, *Science and the Founding Fathers*, 67–68; and Jeanne E. Abrams, *Revolutionary Medicine: The Founding Fathers and Mothers in Sickness and in Health* (New York: New York University Press, 2013), 207.

139. James Neelly to Thomas Jefferson, 18 October 1809, *PTJRS*, 1:606–608; Gilbert C. Russell to Jefferson, 31 January 1810, *PTJRS*, 2:191–192; Jefferson to Gilbert Russell, 18 April 1810, *PTJRS*, 2:336; Jefferson to Peter S. Du Ponceau, 7 November 1817, *PTJRS*, 12:171–173; Du Ponceau to Jefferson, 5 December 1817, *PTJRS*, 12:235–237; and Editorial Note on Jefferson's Biography of Meriwether Lewis, 18 August 1813, *PTJRS*, 6:417–427. The most complete description is Gary E. Moulton, ed., *The Journals of the Lewis and Clark Expedition*, 13 vols. (Lincoln, NE: University of Nebraska Press, 1983–2001).
140. An act to provide for surveying the coasts of the United States, 10 February 1807, *U.S. Statutes at Large*, 2:413–414; Bedini, *Statesman of Science*, 390–391; and Gaye Wilson, "Jefferson Authorizes the Survey of the Coasts," *Monticello Newsletter*, no. 18, fall 2007.
141. Lawrence H. Cohn, "Contributions of Thomas Jefferson to American Medicine," *The American Journal of Surgery* 138 (1979): 289–292.
142. Robert H. Halsey, *How the President, Thomas Jefferson and Doctor Benjamin Waterhouse Established Vaccination as a Public Health Procedure*, History of Medicine Series (New York: Academy of Medicine, 1936), 5:1–58; John B. Blake, "Benjamin Waterhouse and the Introduction of Vaccination, a Reappraisal," Yale University Department of History of Medicine Monograph, Series 33 (1957), 9–74; Bess Furman, *A Profile of the United States Public Health Service, 1798–1948*, DHEW Publication No. (NIH), 73–369, (Washington, D.C.: United States Government Printing Office, 1974), 23–45; Byrd S. Leavell, "Thomas Jefferson and Smallpox Vaccination," *Transactions of the American Clinical and Climatological Assoc.* 88 (1977): 119–127; and Abrams, *Revolutionary Medicine*, 202–208.
143. Nicolau Barquet and Pere Domingo, "Smallpox: The Triumph over the most Terrible of the Ministers of Death," *Annals of Internal Medicine* 127 (1997): 635–641; Herve Bazin. *The Eradication of Smallpox: Edward Jenner and the First and Only Eradication of a Human Infectious Disease*, trans. Andrew and Glenise Morgan (London and San Diego: Academic Press, 2000); Richard D. Semba, "The Ocular Complications of Smallpox and Smallpox Immunization," *Archives of Ophthalmology* 121 (2003): 715–719.
144. White McKenzie Wallenborn, "Thomas Jefferson and the Medicine of His Day," *Medical Alumni News of the University of Virginia* 11, no. 1 (2002): 4; Phillip Ranlet, "The British, Slaves and Smallpox," *The Journal of Negro History* 84 (1999): 217–26; and Elizabeth A. Fenn, *Pox Americana: The Great Smallpox Epidemic of 1775–82* (New York: Hill and Wang, 2001), 130–133.
145. Genevieve Miller, "Smallpox Inoculation in England and America: A Reappraisal," *William and Mary Quarterly*, third series, 13 (1956): 476–492 and Fenn, *Pox Americana*, 1–43.
146. Anne Eriksen, "Cure or Protection? The meaning of Smallpox inoculation, ca 1750–1775," *Medical History* 57 (2013): 516–536.
147. Cotton Mather, *An Account of the Method and Success of Inoculating the Small–pox, in Boston in New England* (London: J. Peele, 1722), 1–2, 8–11, 14–18, 23–26.

148. Fenner, *Smallpox and Its Eradication*, 257; Otho T. Beall and Richard H. Shyrock, *Cotton Mather: First Significant Figure in American Medicine* (Baltimore: Johns Hopkins University Press, 1954); and Riedel, "Edward Jenner and the History of Smallpox and Vaccination," 21–25.
149. Daniel Bernoulli, *An Attempt at a New Analysis of the Mortality Caused by Smallpox and of the Advantages of Inoculation to Prevent It* (1760).
150. Rosemary Stevens, *American Medicine and the Public Interest* (Berkeley: University of California Press, 1971), 15n and John H. Warner and Janet A. Tighe, *Major Problems in the History of American Medicine and Public Health* (Boston: Houghton Mifflin Co., 2001), 33–34, 48–54.
151. Margot Minardi, "The Boston Inoculation Controversy of 1721–1722: An Incident in the History of Race," *William and Mary Quarterly*, Third Series, 61 (2004): 47–76 and Warner and Tighe, *Major Problems in the History of American Medicine and Public Health*, 30–37.
152. Eriksen, 519–521.
153. Gilmer to John Morgan, 11 May 1766, *PTJ*, 1:18; Jefferson to John Page, 25 May 1766, *PTJ*, 1:18–21; Bedini, *Statesman of Science*, 46.
154. Abrams, *Revolutionary Medicine*, 169–170; Malone, *Jefferson the Virginian*, 100; and Gordon–Reed, *The Hemingses at Monticello*, 215.
155. Jefferson to James Madison, 26 November 1782, *PTJ*, 6:206–207; Todd L. Savitt, *Medicine and Slavery: The Diseases and Health Care of Blacks in Antebellum Virginia* (Urbana, IL: University of Illinois Press, 1981), 294; Bedini, *Statesman of Science*, 310; and Abrams, *Revolutionary Medicine*, 183, 188.
156. Frank L. Dewey, "Thomas Jefferson's Law Practice: The Norfolk Anti–Inoculation Riots," *Virginia Magazine of History and Biography* 91 (1983): 39–53; Halsey, *How the President*, 33–34; Gaye Wilson, "Jefferson: Advocate of Inoculation," *Monticello Newsletter*, no. 15, spring 2004, update available at https://www.monticello.org/site/research–and–collections/innoculation; William W. Hening, *The Statutes at Large: Being a Collection of all the Laws of Virginia* (Richmond, VA, 1809–1823), 8:371–373, 9:371–373. For a contrary interpretation of the Norfolk riots, see Andrew Wehrman, "Thomas Jefferson, Inoculation, and the Norfolk Riots," presented at a symposium on The Spirit of Inquiry in the Age of Jefferson, American Philosophical Society, 7–8 June 2018.
157. Jefferson owned works by Jenner (1749–1823) and by John Coakley Lettsom (1744–1815) detailing their experiments with cowpox. Emily Millicent Sowerby, *Catalogue of the Library of Thomas Jefferson* (Washington, D.C.: Library of Congress, 1952–59), 1:427, 429–432.
158. Robin Weiss and Jose Esparza, "The Prevention and Eradication of Smallpox," *Philosophical Transactions of the Royal Society of London* 370 (2015): 1666; Riedel, "Edward Jenner and the History of Smallpox and Vaccination," 21–22; James F. Hammarsten et al., "Who Discovered Smallpox Vaccination? Edward Jenner or Benjamin Jesty?" *Transactions of the American Clinical and Climatological Association* 90 (1979): 44–55.
159. Jefferson to Benjamin Waterhouse, 25 December 1800, *PTJ*, 32:355.
160. Martin, "Jefferson as a Vaccinator," 28 and Cohn "Contributions of Thomas Jefferson," 288.
161. Halsey, *How the President*, 11–17; Furman, *A Profile of the Public Health Service*, 18, 21–45; Sowerby, *Catalogue*, 1:428–429; Alexandra M. Stern and Howard Markel, "The History of Vaccines and Immunization: Familiar Patterns, New

Challenges," *Health Affairs* 24, no. 3 (2005): 611–621.

162. Jefferson to Benjamin Waterhouse, 25 December 1800; 25 July, 14 and 21 August, 17 September, and 25 December 1801, *PTJ*, 32:355, 34:640–641, 35:91,120–121, and 311–312, 36:203–204; Waterhouse to Jefferson, 1 December 1800, *PTJ*, 32:264–265; 24 July 1801, *PTJ*, 34:629; 2 September 1801, *PTJ*, 35:198–200; and 1 March 1803, *PTJ*, 39:615–616; Jefferson to Dr. John Shore, 12 September 1801, *PTJ*, 35:277–278; Jefferson to James Currie, 30 August 1801, *PTJ*, 35:174; Currie to Jefferson, 23 September 1801, *PTJ*, 35:339–340; Jefferson to Dr. John Vaughn, 5 November 1801, *PTJ*, 35:572–573; Jefferson to Dr. Benjamin Rush, 20 December 1801, *PTJ*, 36:177–178; Jefferson to Martha Jefferson Randolph, 17 January 1802, *PTJ*, 36:387–388; Dr. John Redman Coxe to Jefferson, 23 April 1802, *PTJ*, 37:310–311; Jefferson to Coxe, 30 April 1802, PTJ; 37:364–65, 30 July 1802, *PTJ*, 38:142, and 5 January 1803, *PTJ*, 39:267–268; Halsey, *How the President,* 1–58; Leavell, "Jefferson and Smallpox," 119–27; and Martin, "Jefferson as a Vaccinator," 1–34.
163. John Baron, *The Life of Edward Jenner, with Illustrations and His Doctrines and Selections from His Correspondence* (London: Henry Colburn publisher, 1838), 1:448–449.
164. Jefferson to Dr. John Redman Coxe, 5 November 1801, *PTJ*, 35:572–573 and Halsey, *How the President*, 44–45.
165. Radbill, "Thomas Jefferson and the Doctors," 111.
166. Coxe published some of Jefferson's notes and statistics in 1802 in his *Practical Observations on Vaccination or Inoculation for the Cow–Pock*, sending Jefferson a copy on July 30 of that year. *PTJ*, 38:142. See also Jefferson to Waterhouse, 14 and 21 August 1801, *PTJ*, 35:91 and Jefferson to James Currie, 23 September 1801, *PTJ*, 36:339–340.
167. Jefferson to Dr. John Redman Coxe, 30 April 1802, *PTJ* 37:364–65.
168. Jefferson to Benjamin Waterhouse, 26 June and 25 July 1801, *PTJ*, 34:462 and 640–41; Jefferson to William Wardlaw, 16 July, 1801, *PTJ*, 34:581; Waterhouse to Jefferson, 2 September 1801, *PTJ*, 35:198–200; Jefferson to Martha Jefferson Randolph, 17 January 1802, *PTJ*, 36:387–388; Benjamin Waterhouse, "A Prospect of Exterminating the Small-Pox: Part II (Cambridge: University Press, 1802), 29–31; Furman, *A Profile of the Public Health Service*, 30–31; Courtney R. Hall, "Jefferson on the Medical Theory and Practice of His Day," *Bulletin of the History of Medicine* 31 (1957): 242–243; Andrea Rusnock, "Catching Smallpox: The Early Spread of Smallpox Vaccination," *Bulletin of the History of Medicine* 83 (2009): 26.
169. Waterhouse, "A Prospect of Exterminating the Smallpox: Part II, 34, 37; Martin, "Jefferson as a Vaccinator," 33; Stephen H. Gehlbach, *American Plagues: Lessons from Our Battles with Disease*, updated edition (Lanham, MD: Rowman & Littlefield, 2016), 41–58; and John B. Blake, "Benjamin Waterhouse and the Introduction of Vaccination," *Reviews of Infectious Diseases* 9, no. 5 (1987): 1052.
170. "Jefferson's List of Slave Vaccinations," April–May 1816, *PTJRS*, 9:717–718.
171. Halsey, *How the President,* 18; Robert E. Bartholomew and Benjamin Radford, *The Martians Have Landed: A History of Media–Driven Panic and Hoaxes* (London: McFarland & Co., 2012), 198; Joseph Pierre, "Antivaxxers and the Plague of Science Denial," *Psychology Today*, 8 February 2019; Heidi J. Larson, "The Biggest Pandemic Risk? Viral Misinformation," *Nature* 562 (2018): 309–312; Azhar Hussain, Syed Ali, Madiha Ahmed, and Sheharyar Hussain, "The Antivaccination Movement: A Regression in Modern Medicine," *Cureus* 10, no. 7 (2018): e2919.

Pollsters for the Pew Research Group, Gallup, Kaiser Family Foundation, and Wall Street Journal have reported that 25 to 37 percent of Americans say they will definitely not or probably not get the Covid–19 vaccine. Jeffrey Kluger, "Too Many Americans Still Mistrust the Covid–19 Vaccines. Here's Why," *Time Magazine,* 5 January 2021; and Julie Wernau and Paul Overberg, "Covid–19 Vaccine Hesitancy Present Challenge for Herd–Immunity Push," *Wall Street Journal*, 3 February 2021.

172. Peter J. Hotez, "Vaccine Diplomacy: Historical Perspectives and Future Directions," *PLOS Neglected Tropical Diseases* 8, no. 6 (2014): e2810.
173. The chieftain's identity continues to be debated. Some historians believe it was Little Turtle (c. 1747–1812) of the Miami people, but others say it was Chief Black Hoof (c. 1740–1831) of the Shawnee. Both leaders came to Washington, D.C., as diplomats of Native nations, met with legislative officials in January–February of 1802, and most probably received smallpox vaccinations at the behest of Jefferson, even though one or both had previously undergone inoculation with the live virus. "Editorial Note: Conference with Little Turtle," *PTJ*, 36:274–279; "Address of Black Hoof," 5 February 1802, *PTJ*, 36:517–522; and J. Diane Pearson, "Medical Diplomacy and the American Indian: Thomas Jefferson, the Lewis and Clark Expedition, and the Subsequent Effects on American Health and Public Policy," *Wícazo Sa Review* 19, no. 1 (2004): 106–108. See also Halsey, *How the President*, 54–55; Bedini, *Statesman of Science*, 313–314; Hall, "Jefferson on Medical Theory," 235; Leavell, "Jefferson and Smallpox," 125; and Andrew Cayton, *Frontier Indiana (A History of the Trans–Appalachian Frontier)* (Bloomington, IN: Indiana University Press, 1966).
174. Waterhouse, "A Prospect of Exterminating the Smallpox: Part II," 37–38; Waterhouse to Edward Jenner, 8 April 1802, in Halsey, *How the President*, 54–56; Jefferson to Meriwether Lewis, 20 June 1803, *PTJ*, 40:176–182, quote on 179; Clay Jenkinson, "How Jefferson and Franklin helped End Smallpox in America," *Governing Podcast: The Future in Context*, 20 May 2020; and Savitt, *Medicine and Slavery*, 296.
175. *PTJ*, 2:526–53; *PTJRS*, 12:10–15, 114–27 and 13:173–225.
176. Jefferson to George Washington, 4 January 1786, *PTJ*, 9:150–152; Jefferson to Richard Price, 8 January 1789, *PTJ*, 14:420–424; Jefferson to Charles Yancey, 6 January 1816, *PTJRS*, 9:328–331; Jefferson to Eleuthère I. du Pont de Neumours, 9 September 1817, *PTJRS*, 12:16–17; Jefferson to Marc Antoine Jullien, 23 July 1818, *PTJRS*, 13:153–154; Jefferson to William Charles Jarvis, 28 September 1820, *PTJRS*, 16:287–289; Jefferson to Cornelius Camden Blatchly, 21 October 1822, Library of Congress, *The Thomas Jefferson Papers*, https://www.loc.gov/item/mtjbib024471/.
177. Jefferson to Joseph C. Cabell, 7 February 1826, in Cabell, ed., *Early History of the University of Virginia*, 365–367.
178. Jefferson to Joseph C. Cabell, 14 January 1818, *PTJRS*, 12:357–361.
179. Jefferson to Tadeusz Kosciuszko, 26 February 1810, *PTJRS*, 2:257–261; Jefferson to George Ticknor, 25 November 1817, *PTJRS*, 12:203–205; Jefferson to François D'Ivernois, 6 February 1795, *PTJ*, 28:262–264. See also George Rosen, "Political Order and Human Health in Jeffersonian Thought," *Bulletin of the History of Medicine* 26 (1952): 42–43 and Andrew Burstein, *Jefferson's Secrets: Death and Desire at Monticello* (New York: Basic Books, 2005), 43–44.
180. Jefferson to Joseph Willard, 24 March 1789, *PTJ*, 14:697–699.

181. Jefferson's Bill for Amending the Constitution of the College of William and Mary, [18 June 1779], *PTJ*, 2:535–543; "Jefferson's Early Career," *PTJRS*, 17:328–329; Herbert B. Adams, *Thomas Jefferson and the University of Virginia* (Washington, D.C.: U.S. Bureau of Education, Circular of Information, No. 1, 1888), 41–42.
182. The College of Philadelphia and the King's College of Medicine in New York were founded in 1765 and 1767, respectively. These first two medical schools later became part of the University of Pennsylvania and Columbia University, respectively. The William and Mary School of Medicine was founded in 1779 but closed in 1783, never to reopen. The fourth medical school in America was affiliated with Harvard University and founded in 1783.
183. T. C. Moore and J. A. Shield, "Medical Education at America's First University," *Journal Medical Education* 44 (1969): 241–248. See also Oscar A. Thorup, Jr., "Thomas Jefferson and Academic Medicine," *The Pharos of Alpha Omega Alpha* 40 (1977): 16–22 and Bedini, *Statesman of Science*, 82–84.
184. Stephen Ambrose, *Duty, Honor, Country: A History of West Point* (Baltimore, MD: Johns Hopkins University Press, 1966), 10–11; Robert M. McDonald, *Thomas Jefferson's Military Academy: Founding West Point* (Charlottesville: University of Virginia Press, 2004), xiii, 85, 135; Gordon Brown Goode, "The Beginnings of American Science: The Third Century," 46; Terry S. Reynolds, "The Education of Engineers in America before the Morrill Act of 1862," *History of Education Quarterly* 32, no. 4 (1992): 462, 476; and Joe Albree, David C. Arney, and V. Frederick Rickey, *"A Station Favorable to the Pursuits of Science": Primary Materials in the History of Mathematics at the United States Military Academy* (Providence, RI: American Mathematical Society, 2000).
185. Jefferson to George Washington, 23 February 1795, *PTJ*, 28:275–278.
186. Jefferson to Wilson Cary Nicholas, 23 November 1794, *PTJ*, 28:208–209; Jefferson to John Adams, 6 February 1795, *PTJ*, 28:261–262; Jefferson to François D'Ivernois, 6 February 1795, *PTJ*, 28:262–264.
187. Dorothy H. Twohig et al. eds., *The Papers of George Washington, Presidential Series* (Charlottesville: University of Virginia Press, 1987–2020), 4:543–549.
188. Cohn, "Contributions of Thomas Jefferson," 287 and Martin, *Thomas Jefferson: Scientist*, 60–61.
189. Jefferson to James Madison, 20 December 1787, *PTJ*, 12:438–443; Jefferson to Hutchins G. Burton, Thomas Cooper, and Samuel Brown, 28 September 1821, *PTJRS*, 17:520–522; Martin, *Thomas Jefferson: Scientist*, 60–64; Thomson, *Jefferson's Shadow*, 247.
190. Union of Concerned Scientists (hereafter cited as UCS), Science and Democracy in the United States: A Rich History, 20 August 2012, available at www.ucsusa.org/resources/science–and–democracy–united–states; and Henry S. Pritchett, "Jefferson's Interest in Science," *Alumni Bulletin of the University of Virginia* 6 (1900): 74–75.
191. Jefferson to James Madison, 6 September 1789, *PTJ*, 15:392–398. On constitutional change, see also Jefferson to the Comte de Moustier, 17 May 1788, *PTJ*, 13:173–176; Jefferson to Samuel Kercheval, 12 July 1816, *PTJRS*, 10:222–228; and Jefferson to John Cartwright, 5 June 1824, Library of Congress, *The Thomas Jefferson Papers*, https://www.loc.gov/item/mtjbib025031/.
192. Randolph, *Domestic Life of Thomas Jefferson*, 37.
193. Holton, *Science and Anti–Science*, 109–125 and Barbara Friedberg, "Francis Bacon and the End of Skepticism," *Skeptical Inquirer: The Magazine for Science and Reason*

24, no. 6 (2000): 32–36. See also www.sirbacon.org/friedberg.htm.

194. Holton, *Science and Anti–Science*, 115.
195. Ibid.
196. Francis Bacon, "The New Atlantis," in James Speeding, Robert Leslie Ellis, and Douglas Denon Heath, eds., *The Works of Francis Bacon* (London: Longmans and Co., 1857–1859), 3:156, available at Hathi Trust Digital Library; and A. B. Hill, "The Environment and Disease: Association or Causation?" Proc Royal Society of Med 58 (1965): 295–300. For Monticello, Jefferson ordered portraits of "the three greatest men that have ever lived, without any exception," hanging "Bacon at top Locke next then Newton." Jefferson to John Trumbull, 15 February 1789, *PTJ* 14:561.
197. Jefferson to Benjamin Waterhouse, 3 March 1818, *PTJRS*, 12:517–519.
198. Greene, *American Science in the Age of Jefferson.*

Chapter 2

1. Robley Dunglison (1798–1869) became Jefferson's personal physician in 1825. Recalling the incident in his personal memoranda, Dunglison added that Everette had been annoyed by the quip, which Dunglison regarded as "a harmless jest." He also recorded Jefferson's frequent observation that "It is not to physic that I object so much as physicians." Samuel X. Radbill, ed., "The Autobiographical Ana of Robley Dunglison," *Transactions of the American Philosophical Society* 53 (1963): 26 and John M. Dorsey, *The Jefferson–Dunglison Letters* (Charlottesville: University of Virginia Press, 1960), 105. Charles Everette (d. 1848) practiced medicine in Charlottesville as early as 1798 (*PTJRS*, 3:196).
2. Cynical comments about physicians from medieval times forward are documented in Harry Friedenwald, "The Physician's Aphorisms: A Medieval Hebrew Satire," *Johns Hopkins Hospital Bulletin* 29 (March 1918): 67–71; Richard H. Shryock, "Public Relations of the Medical Profession in Great Britain and the United States: 1600–1870: A Chapter in the Social History of Medicine," *Annals of Medical History* (1930): 308–339; and Shryock, "Empiricism versus Rationalism in American Medicine, 1650–1950," *Proceedings of the American Antiquarian Society* 65 (1965): 106.
3. Jefferson to Dr. Thomas Cooper, 16 January, 25 August, and 7 October 1814, *PTJRS*, 7:124–131, 606–607, 8:12–13; to Peter Carr, 19 August 1785 and 10 August 1787, *PTJ*, 8:405–408, 12:14–19; to Thomas Mann Randolph, 25 November 1785, 27 August 1786, and 6 July 1787, *PTJ*, 9:59–60, 10:305–309, 11:556–559; and to John Adams, 5 July 1814, *PTJRS*, 7:451–455. See also Hall, "Jefferson on Medical Theory," 235–245; Murray, "Thomas Jefferson and Medicine," 146–157; and Abrams, *Revolutionary Medicine*, 170.
4. Jefferson to Caspar Wistar, 21 June 1807. Library of Congress: *The Thomas Jefferson Papers.* This letter, of which excerpts have been frequently quoted, is Jefferson's longest and most detailed criticism of the medical profession.
5. Jefferson to William G. Munford, 18 June 1799, *PTJ*, 31:126–130; to J. D. Crawford, 2 January 1812, *PTJRS*, 4:394–395; to Benjamin Rush, 6 March 1813, *PTJRS*, 5:668–670; to Thomas Cooper, 7 October 1814, PTJRS, 8:12–13; to William Short, 31 October 1819, *PTJRS*, 15:162–166; to Robert Walsh, 21 December 1822, https://www.loc.gov/item/mtjbib024537/; to Robley Dunglison, 26 November 1825, in Dorsey, *Jefferson–Dunglison Letters*, 44–45; and to Joseph

C. Cabell, 7 February 1826, Library of Congress: *The Thomas Jefferson Papers*. In his letter to Dunglison, Jefferson said, "time & experience as well as science are necessary to make a skilful physician, and Nature is preferable to an unskilful one." See also J. S. Spratt, "Thomas Jefferson: The Scholarly Politician and his Influence on Medicine," *Southern Medical Journal* 69 (1976): 660–666.

6. Hellenbrand, *The Unfinished Revolution*, 158; Browne, *Jefferson and Scientific Trends in His Time*, 409–410; and Jefferson to Thomas Mann Randolph, 18 January 1796, *PTJ*, 28:592–593; to Martha Jefferson Randolph, 31 May 1798, *PTJ*, 30:381; and to Gideon Granger, 24 January 1810, *PTJRS*, 2:178–180. In a letter to Benjamin Rush on 6 March 1813 (*PTJRS*, 5:668–670), Jefferson wrote, "observing that there are in the constitution of the animal system some means provided unknown to us which have a tendency to restore order, when disturbed by accident, called by physicians the vis medicatrix naturae, I think it safer to trust to this power, in the unknown cases, than to uncertain conjectures, built on the ever–changing hypothetical systems of medecine."
7. Jefferson to Wistar, 21 June 1807.
8. Thomas Jefferson, *Notes on the State of Virginia*, William Peden, ed. (Chapel Hill: University of North Carolina Press, 1955), 33. See also Jefferson's letters to the Reverend James Madison, 19 July 1788, *PTJ*, 13:379–383, in which Jefferson wrote on false speculations, "It is always better to have no ideas than false ones; to believe nothing, than to believe what is wrong," and to William G. Munford, 18 June 1799, *PTJ*, 31:126–130, in which he says of medicine, "could we divest our self of every thing we suppose we know in it, we should start from a higher ground & with fairer prospects... of disease of doubtful form, physicians have ever had a false knowlege, worse than ignorance."
9. Jefferson to Wistar, 21 June 1807.
10. Ibid.
11. Jefferson to Thomas Cooper, 7 October 1814, *PTJRS*, 8:12–13 and to William G. Munford, 18 June 1799, *PTJ*, 31:126–130. See also Daniel Boorstin, *The Lost World of Thomas Jefferson* (New York: Henry Holt, 1948), 134.
12. Jefferson to Wistar, 21 June 1807.
13. The concept, if not the actual phrase, is traceable to Hippocrates. One translation from his *Epidemics*, Book I, Section XI reads, "As to diseases, make a habit of two things—to help, or at least to do no harm."
14. John Harley Warner, *The Therapeutic Perspective: Medical Practice, Knowledge and Identity in America* (Cambridge, MA: Harvard University Press, 1986) and *Against the Spirit of System: The French Impulse in Nineteenth Century American Medicine* (Princeton, N.J.: Princeton University Press, 1998).
15. The treatment of George Washington during his final illness is also an excellent example of the sort of treatment that Jefferson denounced as unscientific and inhumane.
16. All three physicians were graduates of respectable medical schools: Dr. James Craik (1727–1814) and Dr. Gustavas Richard Brown (1747–1804) from the University of Edinburgh and Dr. Elisha Cullen Dick (1762–1825) from the University of Pennsylvania. Dr. Dick, the youngest, argued that copious bleeding "would only make matters worse" and instead insisted that Washington needed a throat operation (tracheostomy) to clear his airway. The older doctors rejected his pleas in favor of traditional treatments. In later life, Dr. Craik admitted that if the team of physicians had "taken no more blood from him, our good friend might be alive

now." Both Dick and Martha Washington argued against further bleeding, but Craik and Brown prevailed. Abrams, *Revolutionary Medicine*, 75; James T. Flexner, *Washington the Indispensable Man* (Boston: Little, Brown and Co., 1974).

17. Tobias Lear's "Journal Account of the Death of George Washington," 15 December 1799, *PGW, Retirement Series*, 4:542–555; Rudolph Marx, *The Health of the Presidents* (New York: G.P. Putnam, 1960), 24–28; Abrams, *Revolutionary Medicine*, 73–76; and Howard Markel, "Dec. 14, 1799: The Excruciating Final Hours of President George Washington," *PBS NewsHour*, 14 December 2014.
18. Antonio Musa Brasavola (1500–1555), an Italian physician, provided the first scientifically reliable description of a successful tracheostomy in a human case in 1546, saving the life of a patient who was nearly dead from suffocation owing an "abscess in the windpipe." Tracheostomy is one of the oldest, simplest, and most valuable operations in surgical practice. See Peter Szmuk et al., "A Brief History of Tracheostomy and Tracheal Intubation, from the Bronze Age to the Space Age," *Intensive Care Medicine* 34 (2008): 222–228.
19. H. Gaston Hall, "Moliere Satirist of Seventeenth–century French Medicine: Fact and Fantasy," *Proceedings of the Royal Society of Medicine* 70 (1977): 425–431 and Marx, *Health of the Presidents*, 13. Jefferson himself respected surgical procedures more than bleedings and dosing, remarking that, "while Surgery is seated in the temple of the exact sciences, medecine has scarcely entered it's threshold." Jefferson to J. D. Crawford, 2 January 1812, *PTJRS*, 4:394–395.
20. See Randall, *Life of Jefferson*, 1:371, 382; Holmes, *Jefferson Treats Himself*; and Abrams, *Revolutionary Medicine*, 174, 179, and 205.
21. For a salient analysis of Jefferson's reciprocal philosophy of political, social, and health issues, see Rosen, "Political Order and Human Health," 32–44.
22. The phrase has been well known and understood since Roman times. Suggesting that a sound mind is a function of physical health, and vice–versa, it implied that the health of the body must be consciously sought.
23. In 1946, the World Health Organization broadened its definition of health to encompass "physical, mental, and social well–being, and not merely the absence of disease and infirmity." See Faith T. Fitzgerald, "The Tyranny of Health," *New England Journal of Medicine* 33 (1994): 196.
24. See Andrew Burstein, *The Inner Jefferson: Portrait of a grieving optimist* (Charlottesville: University of Virginia Press, 1995), 68–115.
25. By disposition, Jefferson may have meant a healthy equilibrium of opposing tendencies which was similar to the philosophy of the French Idéologues, particularly Pierre–Jean–Georges Cabanis. Louis S. Greenbaum, "Review of *A Review of Cabanis: Enlightenment and Medical Philosophy in the French Revolution*, by Martin S. Staum," *Eighteenth–Century Studies* 16, no. 1 (1983): 337.
26. Jefferson to Martha Jefferson (Randolph), 28 March 1787, 5 May 1787, and 21 May 1787, *PTJ*, 11:250–252, 348–349, 369–370.
27. Jefferson to John Adams, 8 April 1816, *PTJRS*, 9:649–652. The concluding phrase is one of Jefferson's Canons of Conduct that he occasionally passed along as rules for living to young people. See Jefferson to Paul A. Clay, ca. 12 July 1817, *PTJRS*, 11:525–526.
28. Jefferson to John Adams, 8 April 1816, *PTJRS*, 9: 649–652.
29. Jefferson believed that mind-cultivation tactics would allow men at the close of life to "look to it's consummation with the composure of one 'qui summum nec me tuit diem nec optat'" (who neither fears the last day nor prays for it). The quote is

from the Latin poet Martial. See Jefferson to Charles Thomson, 9 January 1816, *PTJRS*, 9:340–342 and to John Adams, 14 March 1820, *PTJRS*, 15:469–470.

30. The University of Virginia stands alone in its claim that one man acted as its architect and general contractor, designed its curriculum and the teaching apparatus to support it, planned and supervised the hiring of its original faculty, and served as the first rector of its governing board.
31. For first–hand accounts of Jefferson's last days, see Dorsey, *Jefferson–Dunglison Letters*, 67–69 and Randall, *Life of Jefferson*, 3:544–549.
32. Jefferson to Vine Utley, 21 March 1819, *PTJRS*, 14:156–158. As Jeanne Abrams has noted, Jefferson promoted healthy eating habits for students in the early years of the University of Virginia, writing, "To strengthen their bodies, Jefferson recommended a daily menu that emphasized fruits and vegetables over meat products." Abrams, *Revolutionary Medicine*, 222 and Jefferson to Peter Laporte, 4 June 1819, *PTJRS*, 14:382–383.
33. Jefferson's biographer, Dumas Malone, states that without exception, "he [Jefferson] did not use tobacco, even though he raised it at Poplar Forest." See Malone, *Jefferson and His Time*, 4:186. On ardent spirits, see Jefferson to Mary Jefferson Eppes, 7 January 1798, *PTJ*, 30:14–16; to Jean Guillaume Hyde de Neuville, 13 December 1818, *PTJRS*, 13:489–490; to Vine Utley, 21 March 1819, *PTJRS*, 14:156–158; and to Samuel Smith, 3 May 1823, MS at the University of Virginia.
34. Margaret Bayard Smith's "Account of a Visit to Monticello, 29 July–2 August 1809," *PTJRS*, 1:386–401. For authoritative studies of Jefferson as a connoisseur of wine, see John R. Hailman, *Thomas Jefferson on Wine* (Jackson: University Press of Mississippi, 2006) and James M. Gabler, *Passions: The Wines and Travels of Thomas Jefferson* (Palm Beach, FL: Bacchus Press Ltd., 2016).
35. Jefferson contrasted "weak wines" with the "ardent wines," taken to mean fortified wines like brandy, port, and sherry. Jefferson to Vine Utley, 21 March 1819, *PTJRS*, 14:156–158.
36. Wallenborn, "Jefferson and Medicine," 8. In this essay, the author does not specify a primary source.
37. Jefferson to Charles Bellini, 30 September 1785, *PTJ*, 8:568–570. Jefferson's favorite granddaughter, Ellen Randolph Coolidge, described the conversation at the many Monticello dinner parties as "completely the feast of reason." See Ann Lucas Birle and Lisa A. Francavilla, eds., *Thomas Jefferson's Granddaughter in Queen Victoria's England: The Travel Diary of Ellen Wayles Coolidge, 1838–1839* (Charlottesville: University of Virginia Press, 2011), p. xx.
38. Jefferson to Thomas Mann Randolph, 6 July 1787, *PTJ*, 11:556–559.
39. Jefferson to Martha Jefferson (Randolph), 28 March 1787, *PTJ*, 11:250–252; to Thomas Mann Randolph, 27 August 1786, *PTJ*, 10:305–309; to Peter Carr, 19 August 1785 and 10 August 1787, *PTJ*, 8:405–408, 12:14–19; to John Garland Jefferson, 11 June 1790, *PTJ*, 16:480–482; to David Howell,15 December 1810, *PTJRS*, 3:257; to William Short, 31 October 1819, *PTJRS*, 15:162–166; and to Benjamin Rush, 16 January and 17 August 1811, *PTJRS*, 3:304–308, 4:87–88. See also Randolph, *Domestic Life of Thomas Jefferson*, 115.
40. Jefferson to John Adams, 21 January 1812 and 15 August 1820, *PTJRS*, 4:428–430, 156–158 and to Vine Utley, 21 March 1819, *PTJRS*, 14:156–158.
41. Randolph, *Domestic Life of Thomas Jefferson*, 338.
42. Jefferson responded to aristocratic sloth in France with frequent admonitions against idleness to his teenage daughter, Martha, and others. See Jefferson to

Martha Jefferson (Randolph), 28 March 1787, 5 May 1787, 21 May 1787, and 26 April 1790, *PTJ*, 11:250–252, 348–349, 369–370, 16:386–387 and to William Short, 31 October 1819, *PTJRS*, 15:162–166. See also Brian Steele, "Thomas Jefferson's Gender Frontier," *Journal of American History* 95, no. 1 (2008): 36.

43. Randolph, *Domestic Life of Thomas Jefferson*, 338; Thomas Jefferson, "Will and Codicil, March 16–17, 1826," *Founders Online*, https://founders.archives.gov/documents/Jefferson/98–01–02–5963; and Hannah Spahn, *Thomas Jefferson's Time and History* (Charlottesville: University of Virginia Press, 2011), 29–42.
44. Isaac Jefferson, one of his enslaved servants, recollected Jefferson having as many as twenty books sprawled across the floor, which he would read in rotation. James A. Bear, Jr., ed., *Jefferson at Monticello* (Charlottesville: University of Virginia Press, 1967), 12.
45. During his lifetime, Jefferson wrote something like 19,000 letters and other published and unpublished works so extensive that the definitive edition of his papers will ultimately extend to well over ninety volumes. J. Jefferson Looney, email to the author, 4 March 2021.
46. At Monticello, Jefferson cultivated at least 16 herbs for their medicinal value. Understanding, moreover, the need to acquire a working knowledge of their use, he obtained many reference volumes, such as William Cullen's *Treatise of the Materia Medica*, Lazarus Riverius's *The Practice of Physick,* James Shipton's *Pharmacopœiæ Londinensis*, Thomas Fuller's *Pharmacopœia Extemporanea,* and Andrew Duncan's expanded edition of William Lewis, *The Edinburgh New Dispensatory.* Holmes, *Jefferson Treats Himself,* 42, 109–111; Sowerby, *Library of Thomas Jefferson*, 1:397–398, 404 (nos. 865, 868, 869, 885).
47. Jefferson to Vine Utley, 21 March 1819, *PTJRS*, 14:156–158 and Daniel Webster, "Notes of Mr. Jefferson's Conversation (1824) at Monticello," in Charles M. Wiltse et al., eds., *The Papers of Daniel Webster, Correspondence* (Hanover, NH: Dartmouth University Press, 1974–1986), 1:370–378. The latter reference says that Jefferson found "retiring" at 9 p.m. "essential to his health & comfort."
48. Ibid. (*PTJRS*, 14:156–158) and Gordon–Reed and Onuf, *Most Blessed of the Patriarchs*, 292.
49. Jefferson to Peter Carr, 19 August 1785, *PTJ*, 8:405–408 and to Thomas Mann Randolph, 9 July 1787, *PTJ*, 11:556–559.
50. Jefferson's library offers evidence of his interest in health maintenance and disease prevention. Relevant books included *Domestic Medicine: or, A Treatise on the Prevention and Cure of Diseases* by William Buchan (9th ed., 1786); *An Epistle to A Friend, On Preserving Health, Promoting Happyness and Prolonging the Life of Man to its Natural Period* by Charles Willson Peale (1803); *The Means of Preserving Health and Preventing Disease* by Shadrach Ricketson (1806); *The Old Man's Guide to Health and Longer Life, with Rules for Diet, Exercise and Physic, for Preserving A good Constitution, and Preventing Disorders in a Bad One* by Sir John Hill (1771); *The Family Companion for Health . . . or . . . Rules which . . . Will . . . Keep Families Free from Diseases and Procure Them a Long Life* by Anonymous (1729); *Observations on The Means of Preserving the Health of Soldiers and Sailors* by Edward Cutbush (1808); and *Psychrolousia: or, The History of Cold Bathing* by Sir John Floyers and Edward Baynard (2d ed., 1706). See Sowerby, *Library of Thomas Jefferson*, 1:406, 413–17 (nos. 891, 907, 908, 912, 914, 918).
51. Abrams, *Revolutionary Medicine*, 1 and Holmes, *Jefferson Treats Himself,* 72.
52. Unlike George Washington and even John Adams, Jefferson's dental health was

quite good throughout his life. Noble E. Cunningham, ed., "The Diary of Frances Few, 1808–1809," *Journal of Southern History* 29, no. 3 (1963): 350; Daniel Webster, "Notes of Mr. Jefferson's Conversation (1824) at Monticello," in Wiltse et al., eds., *The Papers of Daniel Webster, Correspondence*, 1:370–378; and Malvin E. Ring, "The Dental Health of President John Adams," *New York State Dental Journal* 70, no. 7 (2004): 36–37.

53. In the late eighteenth century, Massachusetts was the only state to collect life–expectancy statistics. Of males, only 15 percent reached the age of sixty. Richard B. Morris, *Encyclopedia of American History* (New York: Harper & Row, 1976), 649. See also Randall, *Life of Thomas Jefferson*, 1:133 and Abrams, *Revolutionary Medicine*, 169–198.

54. Jefferson to Benjamin Hawkins, 18 February 1803, *PTJ*, 39:546–549; to Tadeusz Kościuszko, 26 February 1810, *PTJRS*, 2:257–261; to Abigail Adams, 22 August 1813, *PTJRS*, 6:437–438; to Charles Thomson, 9 January 1816, *PTJRS*, 9:340–342; to Benjamin Waterhouse, 3 March 1818, *PTJRS*, 12:517–519; to Vine Utley, 21 March 1819, *PTJRS*, 14:156–158; and to John Adams, 1 June 1822, in Cappon, ed., *Adams–Jefferson Correspondence*, 2:577–579. Jefferson escaped all of the lethal illnesses prevalent during his lifetime: diphtheria, typhoid, yellow fever, smallpox (he was inoculated), and pneumonia. He did complain of gradually increasing rheumatism. But his own evaluation of his health rarely mentions his persistent diarrhea, a serious and enduring impairment with which he struggled beginning in 1801. Jefferson to Benjamin Rush, 28 February 1803, *PTJ*, 39:598–600. Perhaps he considered this problem to be too personal in nature, or a psychological malady connected with the stressful rigors of public life.

55. Abrams, *Revolutionary Medicine*, 173.

56. Spratt, "The Scholarly Politician," 360–366.

57. Malone, *Jefferson and His Time*, 1:426–430, 6:502–503; Holmes, *Jefferson Treats Himself*, 19; Abrams, *Revolutionary Medicine*, Chapters 1–3 on Washington, Franklin, and Adams.

58. J. Worth Estes, "George Washington and the Doctors," *Medical Heritage* (1985): 46 and George Washington to Anthony Whiting, 28 October 1792, in Twohig, ed., *PGW, Presidential Series*, 11:273–278.

59. L. H. Butterfield, et al., eds., *Diary and Autobiography of John Adams* (Cambridge, MA: Belknap Press of Harvard University, 1961–), 1:12–13. The key documents on Adams and tobacco are his letters to Benjamin Waterhouse of 13 and 19 February 1805, *Founders Online,* https://founders.archives.gov/documents/Adams/99–02–02–5069 and https://founders.archives.gov/documents/Adams/99–02–02–5072.

60. Holmes, *Jefferson Treats Himself*, 19. Unlike Jefferson, the Adams family history displayed remarkable longevity. For a comparison of the Adams and Jefferson family histories, see Abrams, *Revolutionary Medicine*, 119–198.

61. Jefferson to Edward Rutledge, 27 December 1796, *PTJ*, 29:231–233 and to James Madison, 9 June 1793, *PTJ*, 26:239–242.

62. Louis S. Greenbaum, "Thomas Jefferson's University of Virginia and the Paris Hospitals on the Eve of the French Revolution," *Medical History* (1992): 306–319. While minister to France, Jefferson worked with and was influenced by several French public–health reformers, including his close friend the Marquis de Condorcet, who proposed the nationalization of health care to replace a charity–based hospital system that linked piety and medical care.

63. Jefferson understood that lack of sanitation and crowded conditions played at least some role in spreading many diseases. Initially he considered yellow fever to be a contagious infection brought to America by passengers on incoming ships, but he later believed it could only be communicated "in a local atmosphere" and "generated near the water side, in close built cities, under warm conditions." He was correct that it was not passed directly from person to person, although an epidemic did require an infected pool of humans as an initiating factor. Only a century later did Walter Reed, a graduate of the University of Virginia Medical School, identify the true culprit, a particular mosquito, *Aedes Aegypti*, as the transmitter of yellow fever. See Jefferson to Thomas Mann Randolph, 2 September 1793, *PTJ*, 27:20–21; to Thomas Pinckney, 27 November 1793, *PTJ*, 27:450–451; to Benjamin Rush, 23 September 1800, *PTJ*, 32:166–169; to John Page, 16 August 1804, *PTJ*, 44:235; and to C. F. C. de Volney, 8 February 1805, *PTJ*, 45:473–77.
64. Thomas Jefferson, "Fifth Annual Message to Congress," *Journal of the Senate*, 9th Cong., 1st sess., 3 December 1805, 4–8.
65. *National Intelligencer*, 11 October 1802.
66. *National Intelligencer*, 1 November 1802.
67. Wilhelmus Bogart Bryan, *History of the National Capital* (New York: MacMillan, 1914), 1:548.
68. John Duffy, *The Sanitarians: A History of American Public Health* (Urbana: University of Illinois Press, 1990), 70–71.
69. Richard Peters, ed., *The Public Statutes at Large of the United States … 1789 to March 3, 1845* (1845–67), 2:806–807.
70. Abrams, *Revolutionary Medicine*, 30.
71. Ibid., 30.
72. Peters, ed., *The Public Statutes at Large of the United States*, 3:677.
73. Richard Williams, *The United States Public Health Service, 1798–1950* (Washington, D.C., 1951), 69–70.
74. William Waller Hening, ed., *The Statutes at Large; being a Collection of all the Laws of Virginia* (Richmond, 1809–23), 10:385–386. Prepayment for medical care of sailors through government was not a new idea. Great Britain had long had a similar law and had collected a tax from its colonies. Williams, *Public Health Service*, 23 and Furman, *A Profile*, 3–4.
75. Hening, *Statutes at Large*, 12:494–495.
76. Williams, *Public Health Service*, 29–31 and Furman, *A Profile*, 16.
77. The Seaman's Act of 1798 required the Department of the Treasury to "provide for the relief and maintenance of ill and disabled seaman" by hiring physicians to staff a series of hospitals to be built in busy seaports. The first government–sponsored marine hospital was constructed in Boston, and by 1818 a total of 26 federally funded facilities were in operation. The government financed the hospitals by a tax of roughly one percent on sailors' monthly wages. Jefferson and his secretary of the treasury, Albert Gallatin, saw to it that these taxes, about 20 cents per month per sailor, were collected and used judiciously.
78. During Jefferson's presidency, an estimated 57,287 seamen received treatment at government–owned marine hospitals. Williams, *Public Health Service*, 40 and William E. Rooney, "Thomas Jefferson and the New Orleans Marine Hospital," *Journal of Southern History* 22, no. 2 (1956): 167–182.
79. John W. Trask, *The United States Marine Hospital, port of Boston: An account of its origin and briefly of its history and of the physicians who have been in charge* (Wash-

ington, D.C.: Federal Security Agency, U.S. Public Health Service, 1940), 56–61.

80. Jefferson to Benjamin Rush, 3 January 1808, Library of Congress, *The Thomas Jefferson Papers*, https://www.loc.gov/item/mtjbib018064/ and Oscar A. Thorup, "Thomas Jefferson and a Few of His Physician Friends," *Transactions of the American Clinical and Climatological Association* 104 (1992): 138–144.
81. Jefferson based his choice of Waterhouse in part on his promotion of vaccination, but he was also the first director of the Boston Marine Hospital with an earned M.D. and extensive European training. Waterhouse to John Adams, 4 June 1821, Massachusetts Historical Society: *The Adams Papers* and Jefferson to Benjamin Rush, 3 January 1808, Library of Congress, *The Thomas Jefferson Papers*, https://www.loc.gov/item/mtjbib018064/.
82. Waterhouse communicated his innovative ideas to Benjamin Lincoln, collector of customs, in a letter dated 9 February 1803. In this letter, he envisaged the hospital serving as a teaching hospital for Harvard medical students, introducing pupils of physic and surgery to the bedside of the sick and to all important chirurgical operations and providing postgraduate education, an "intern service" for better training of military surgeons, and he "set forth the lasting principle that the needs of the patient come first"—that the rules and orders respecting patient care would supersede all others. See *The Benjamin Lincoln Papers* at Massachusetts Historical Society and Furman, *A Profile*, 38–42.
83. C. Everett Koop, "Remarks to the Students and Faculty of the George Washington University School of Medicine," Washington, D.C., 23 April 1986.
84. A lengthy letter from Waterhouse to Jefferson, 21 June 1809, *PTJRS*, 1:295–300, denounces the "infamous intrigue and injustice" of the charges and includes rebuttals by Waterhouse, John Adams, and others. Thorup, "His Physician Friends,"139–141.
85. "Fifth Annual Message to Congress," 4–8.
86. Jefferson to James Madison, 1 and 8 September 1793, *PTJ*, 27:6–8, 61–63; to Thomas Mann Randolph, 2 September 1793, *PTJ*, 27:20–21; to Gouverneur Morris, 11 September 1793, *PTJ*, 27:91; to Martha Jefferson Randolph, 10 November 1793, *PTJ*, 27:345; to Thomas Pinckney, 27 November 1793, *PTJ*, 27:450–451; and to C. F. C. de Volney, 8 February 1805, *PTJ*, 45:473–477. See also Martin Pernick, "Politics, Parties, and Pestilence: Epidemic Yellow Fever in Philadelphia and the Rise of the First Party System," *William and Mary Quarterly*, 3d series, 29 (1997), 559, 568.
87. Resolution of the Board of Visitors of the University of Virginia, 24 April 1826, as cited in Dorsey, *Jefferson–Dunglison Letters*, 47–48.
88. Jefferson to James Buchanan and William Hay, 13 August 1785, *PTJ*, 8:366–368; to David Humphreys, 14 August 1787, *PTJ*, 12:32–33; to Louis Guillaume Otto, 14 January 1787, *PTJ*, 11:42–43; to Thomas Pinckney, 27 November 1793, *PTJ*, 27:450–451; to Joseph Priestley, 18 January 1800, *PTJ*, 31:319–323; to Benjamin Rush, 23 September 1800, *PTJ*, 32:166–169; to John Page, 16 August 1804, *PTJ*, 44:235; to C. F. C. de Volney, 8 February 1805, *PTJ*, 45:473–477; and to the Trustees of the Lottery for East Tennessee College, 6 May 1810, *PTJRS*, 2:365–366. See also John W. Reps, "Thomas Jefferson's Checkerboard Towns," *Journal of the Society of Architectural Historians* 20, no. 3 (1961): 108–114 and Mary Woods, "Thomas Jefferson and the University of Virginia: Planning the Academic Village," *Journal of the Society of Architectural Historians* 44, no. 3 (1985): 266–283.
89. Aaron Antonovsky coined the term salutogenic in his book, *Health, Stress and*

Coping: New Perspectives on Mental and Physical Well–being (San Francisco: Jossey–Bass, 1979). Salutogenesis focuses on factors contributing to the promotion and maintenance of physical and mental well–being, rather than disease.

90. Beginning in the 1790s, Jefferson began adopting a more scientific approach to farming. At Monticello, he practiced "Good husbandry," which meant "abandoning Indian corn and tobacco." He cultivated more diverse crops and raised livestock, with wheat as the leading staple. Although Jefferson's practice "transformed the Monticello landscape and plantation community," it had little effect at his Poplar Forest farm, where he continued to grow tobacco. Moreover, Jefferson reintroduced tobacco growing at Monticello when his financial situation worsened. Jefferson to George Washington, 28 June 1793, *PTJ*, 26:396–398; to Benjamin Vaughan, 27 June 1790, *PTJ*, 16:578–580; "Tobacco Cultivation at Monticello," https://www.monticello.org/slavery/the–plantation/work–on–the–monticello–plantation/crops–produce–and–livestock/tobacco/; and Peden, *Notes*, 166.
91. Jefferson to Martha Jefferson Randolph, 22 December 1783, *PTJ*, 6:416–417 and 9 February 1791, *PTJ*, 19:264; to Nathaniel Burwell, 14 March 1818, *PTJRS*, 12:532–535; Albert Jay Nock, *Jefferson* (New York: Hill and Wang, 1966), 58; Bloch, "Thomas Jefferson 1743 to 1826," 3030–3032; Steele, "Gender Frontier," 17–42.
92. *Datura stramonium* is a plant in the nightshade family and is known by the English name jimsonweed (Jimson weed) or devil's snare. The plant was used in various treatments of traditional medicine and was known for its hallucinogenic and deliriant effects.
93. Jefferson to Dr. Samuel Brown, 14 July 1813, *PTJRS*, 6:292–294.
94. Jefferson's position was contrary to the Hippocratic ban on giving pain relievers to the terminally ill. His preference for the relief of pain may have had its roots in the writings of Sir Francis Bacon, who eloquently defended the use of medication to manage pain in such cases. *The Two bookes of Francis Bacon : of the proficience and advancement of learning, divine and humane* (London: H. Tomes, 1605), 2:42.
95. "Voters in Oregon Allow Doctors to Help the Terminally Ill Die," *New York Times*, 11 November 1994, A28.
96. Examples include letters to William G. Munford, 18 June 1799, *PTJ*, 31:126–30; to Caspar Wistar, 21 June 1807 to John C. Warren, 10 February 1808, *Founders Online,* https://founders.archives.gov/documents/Jefferson/99–01–02–7395; to Robert Walsh, 21 December 1822, https://www.loc.gov/item/mtjbib024537/; and to Joseph C. Cabell, 7 February 1826, Library of Congress, *The Thomas Jefferson Papers*. See also Hall, "Jefferson on Medical Theory," 235–245.
97. Andrew D. Hart, "Thomas Jefferson's Influence on the Foundation of Medical Education at the University of Virginia," *Annals of Medical History* 10 (1938): 47–60. See also Lawrence H. Cohn, "Contributions of Thomas Jefferson to American Medicine," *The American Journal of Surgery* 138 (1979): 286–292.
98. W. B. McDaniel, "A View of 19th Century Medical Historiography in the United States of America," *The Bulletin of the History of Medicine* 33, no. 5 (1959): 415–435.
99. The titles and lengths of the inaugural dissertations, lectures, and essays that were sent to Jefferson before he sold his library to Congress can be found in Sowerby, *Library of Thomas Jefferson*, 193, 399, 419, 423–426, 428–429, 431, 435–436, 439, 440, 442–445, 447, 448, and 494. For two of many later examples, see Jefferson to David Hosack, 3 May 1815, *PTJRS*, 8:467–468, and to Josiah Meigs, 7

April 1816, *PTJRS*, 9:647.

100. If his library is any indication, Jefferson had intimate knowledge of the medical theories and practices of all four of these men. He owned eight books that were authored by the four, two each by Thomas Sydenham and Hermann Boerhaave, three by William Cullen, and one by John Brown, totaling more than 1,700 printed pages. See Sowerby, *Library of Thomas Jefferson*, 399, 402–403, 408, 410–411, and 424 (nos. 871, 881, 895, 897, 900, 902, 903, 937).
101. Daniels, *American Science*, 138.
102. Samuel L. Mitchill, Preface to the American Edition of Erasmus Darwin, *Zoonomia of Laws of Organic Life* (New York, 1796), xxii.
103. The term benighted refers to a contemptible intellectual or moral ignorance. It was used to describe the bloodletting practice in a biography of Benjamin Rush. Robert B. Sullivan, "Rush, Benjamin," *American National Biography* (1999), available online February 2000.
104. David Ramsay, *An Eulogium upon Benjamin Rush, M.D.* (Philadelphia: Bradford & Inskeep, 1813), no. 4, 23 and J. D. Spillane, "Doctors of 1776: I," *British Medical Journal* 1, no. 6025 (1976): 1573–1574.
105. Benjamin Rush, "Lectures on the Practice of Physic" (1796): I, No. 31 and II, No. i, at the Library of The University of Pennsylvania, as cited in Richard H. Shryock, *The Development of Modern Medicine* (Madison: University of Wisconsin Press, 1936), 3 and his *The Medical World of the Eighteenth Century* (Chicago: University of Chicago Press, 1958), 49–55.
106. J. C. Lettsom, *Recollections of Dr. Rush* (London: J. Nichols Sons and Bentley, 1815), 12, 15.
107. For concise summaries of Rush's doctrine and practice, see Richard H. Shryock, *Medicine and Society in America* (Ithaca: Cornell University Press, 1960), 69–72 and his *Medicine in America: Historical Essays* (Baltimore: Johns Hopkins University Press, 1966), 236–238, as well as Corner, *Autobiography of Benjamin Rush*, 361–66 and Appendix 1 for "Rush's Medical Theories."
108. In "A Defence of Blood;Letting as a Remedy for Certain Diseases," in *Medical Inquiries and Observations* (Philadelphia: Thomas Dobson, 1796), 4:181–258, Rush went so far as to suggest (p. 238) that fourth–fifths of the blood in the body could be removed in some cases.
109. Shryock, "Empiricism versus Rationalism," 110.
110. Shryock, *Medicine and Society*, 70.
111. Shryock, "Empiricism versus Rationalism," 110, 112–125 and *Medicine and Society*, 70.
112. The details of this epidemic, including Rush's role, are best described in J. H. Powell, *Bring Out Your Dead: The Great Plague of Yellow Fever in Philadelphia in 1793* (Philadelphia: University of Pennsylvania Press, 1993), updated from the first edition in 1949. See also, Lester S. King, *Transformations in American Medicine: From Benjamin Rush to William Osler* (Baltimore: Johns Hopkins University Press, 1991), 49–60.
113. Benjamin Rush, *An Account of the Bilious remitting Yellow Fever, as It Appeared in the City of Philadelphia in the Year 1793* (Philadelphia: Thomas Dobson, 1794), 271–272, as cited in Robert North, "Benjamin Rush, MD: Assassin or Beloved Healer," *Proceedings (Baylor University Medical Center)* 13, no. 1 (2000): 47 (hereafter, *Account of Yellow Fever, 1793*).
114. Paul E. Kopperman, "'Venerate the Lancet': Benjamin Rush's Yellow Fever Therapy

in Context," *Bulletin of Medical History* 78, no. 3 (2004): 552.

115. Shryock, *Medicine and Society*, 70.
116. Ibid.; Richard Shryock, "The Advent of Modern Medicine in Philadelphia, 1800–1850," *Yale Journal of Biology and Medicine* (1941): 13:715–738; John Harley Warner, *Against the Spirit of System* (Princeton, NJ: Princeton University Press, 1998), 282.
117. Faculty members of the College of Physicians of Philadelphia who opposed Rush's "System" included Benjamin Smith Barton, Alfred Kuhn, and Caspar Wistar; all three incurred Rush's wrath and were never forgiven. "Sure as always, of his opinions, he [Rush] fought them bitterly with spoken words, letters to newspapers and printed pamphlets." George W. Corner, *Two Centuries of Medicine: A History of the School of Medicine, University of Pennsylvania* (Philadelphia: J. B. Lippincott & Co., 1965), 46.
118. Benjamin Rush to Julia Stockton Rush, 25–26 September 1793, in Lyman H. Butterfield, ed., *Letters of Benjamin Rush* (Princeton, N.J.: Princeton University Press, 1951), 2:683–684.
119. *Account of Yellow Fever, 1793*, 92. See also Richard H. Shryock, "The Medical Reputation of Benjamin Rush: Contrasts over Two Centuries," *Bulletin of the History of Medicine* 45, no. 6 (1971): 507–508 and Kopperman, "Venerate the Lancet," 562.
120. Eve Kornfeld, "Crisis in the Capital: The Cultural Significance of Philadelphia's Great Yellow Fever Epidemic," *Pennsylvania History* 51, no. 3 (1984), 197. William Cobbett was the "vituperative publisher of the Porcupine Gazette" who harshly criticized many revolutionary leaders, including Jefferson. See Martin, *Scientist*, 218–219; William Cobbett, *The Rush Light, February 28, 1800* (New York, 1800), 49; and Andrew G. Shuman, Marc Edelman, and Joseph J. Fins, "Bleeding by the Numbers: Rush versus Cobbett" *The Pharos*, (Autumn 2014): 10–14.
121. James T. Flexner, *Doctors on Horseback: Pioneers of American Medicine* (1937; reprinted New York: Fordham University Press, 1992), 57. Dr. William Patterson said of Rush's use of purgatives that "his preparation is of too drastic a nature, is comparable to arsenic, and is a dose for horses; that, as exciting salivation, it is hurtful; that, as adding to the excoriation of the rectum, it contributes to increase inflammation of this part…and that being prescribed indiscriminately, it must do harm to weak habits." William Patterson, *Remarks on Some of the Opinions of Dr. Rush respecting the Yellow Fever which Prevailed in the City of Philadelphia* (Londonderry: G. Douglas, 1795), as cited in Kopperman, "Venerate the Lancet," 545.
122. Benjamin Rush including six hundred of his patented Rush Pills (the "thunderbolts") in furnishing the Lewis and Clark Expedition with medical equipment and supplies. Benjamin Rush to Thomas Jefferson, enclosing Rush's Directions to Meriwether Lewis for Preserving Health, 11 June 1803, *PTJ*, 40:530–531.
123. W. S. W. Ruschenberger, *An Account of the Institution and Progress of the College of Physicians of Philadelphia During a Hundred Years* (Philadelphia: William J. Dornan Publishing, 1887), 59.
124. Cooke published his treatise on Pathology and Therapeutics in 1828. See Elisha Barlett, *The Philosophy of Medical Science* (Philadelphia: Lea & Blanchard, 1844), 233 and Warner, *The Therapeutic Perspective*, 44, 47–52.
125. Thomas D. Mitchell, "Calomel Considered as a Poison," *New Orleans Medical Journal* 5, no. 1 (1844): 28–36.
126. *Richmond Enquirer*, 5 March 1825. See also Shryock, *Development of Modern Medicine*, 253–254.

127. John S. Haller, "Decline of Bloodletting: A Study in 19th–Century Ratiocinations," *Southern Medical Journal* 79, no. 4 (1986): 470.
128. Rush maintained that bleeding "should be repeated" as long as symptoms continue, "till four–fifth of the blood contained in the body is drawn away." Another physician from New York, G. W. Phillips, claimed to have drawn more than 100 barrels of blood during his 47–year career and "had yet to see the first instance in which he had drawn blood to the injury of the patients." Haller, "Decline of Bloodletting," 470; Benjamin Rush, *Sixteen Introductory Lectures, to Courses of Lectures Upon the Institutes and Practice of Medicine* (Philadelphia: Bradford & Inskeep, 1811), 213; Rush to John Coakley Lettsom, 13 May 1804 and to John Syng Dorsey, 23 May 1804, in Butterfield, ed., *Letters of Benjamin Rush*, 2:881–886; Flexner, *Doctors on Horseback*, 109; John B. Blake, "From Buchan to Fishbein: The Literature of Domestic Medicine," in Guenter B. Risse et al., eds., *Medicine Without Doctors* (New York: Science History Publications, 1977), 16.
129. Jefferson to William G. Munford, 18 June 1799, *PTJ*, 31:126–130.
130. Intelligent empiricism, also referred to as scientific empiricism, requires not only the work of the senses but of the mind. Resting on experiment rather than authority, its purpose is to test a hypothesis (i.e., unproved theory) in order to resolve doubts. Successful scientists must doubt until they have collected their own evidence and made their own deductions. They also need to observe accurately and know precisely what to observe. Hellenbrand, *The Unfinished Revolution*, 157–159 and Shryock, "Empiricism versus Rationalism," 99–150.
131. A hallmark of Rush's medical thought was a disdain for nature. He and his disciples disparaged nature as a curative, regarding it as too slow to act. Furthermore, they sometimes neglected to modify their energetic ministration based on the condition of the patient. Bloodletting and purging were used on all categories of patients, including infants, the elderly, and pregnant women. Kopperman, "Venerate the Lancet," 555–559.
132. Jefferson's criticism of Rush and his disciples was in part due to their "complete repudiation of specificity" and affirmation of a wholly unscientific single cause of disease pathology. Shryock, *Medicine and Society*, 75.
133. Jefferson to John Adams, 14 March 1820, *PTJRS*, 15:469–470.
134. Radbill, "Thomas Jefferson and the Doctors," 106–114.
135. Hall, "Jefferson on Medical Theory," 235–245.
136. Jackson, ed., *Lewis and Clark Expedition*, 19.
137. Jefferson to Dr. Edward Jenner, 14 May 1806, Library of Congress, *The Thomas Jefferson Papers*, https://www.loc.gov/resource/mtj1.036_0006_0006/.
138. Jefferson believed that every scientific discovery was potentially valuable. To him, "no discovery is barren. it always serves as a step to something else." Jefferson to Robert Patterson, 17 April 1802, *PTJ*, 37:254.
139. In Jefferson's time, new biological or physiological discoveries rarely resulted in the development and prompt application of effective and safe new techniques, for alleviating pain, preventing disease, shortening illness, or postponing death). Examples include the discovery of the circulation of the blood (1628), of oxygen (1775), and of nitrous oxide (1795). Regarding the disconnect between scientific advance and real medical progress, see David Wootton, *Bad Medicine: Doctors Doing Harm Since Hippocrates* (New York: Oxford University Press, 2006); Thomas S. Kuhn, *The Structure of Scientific Revolutions* (Chicago: University of Chicago Press, 1962); and Ludwik Fleck, *Genesis and Development of Scientific Fact* (Chicago: University of Chicago Press, 1979).

140. Radbill, "Thomas Jefferson and the Doctors," 106–114.
141. Jefferson to Dr. Andrew Kean, 11 November 1818, *PTJRS*, 13:388–390; to Benjamin Rush, 6 March 1813, *PTJRS*, 5:668–670; Jefferson to Dr. Thomas Cooper, 7 October 1814, *PTJRS*, 8: 12–13. In the letter to Rush, Jefferson related the story of Dr. Seymour, a Virginia physician who in Jefferson's youth supposedly tried to employ his medical expertise to cure the ailments of tobacco plants. "He bled some, administered lotions to others, sprinkled powders on a third class, and so on. they only withered & perished the faster." In his letter to Cooper, Jefferson wrote of Rush, "in his theory of bleeding and mercury, I was ever opposed to my friend…whom I greatly loved but who has done much harm in the sincerest persuasion that he was preserving life."
142. Jefferson to William G. Munford, 18 June 17, 99, *PTJ*, 31:126–130.
143. Jefferson to John Crawford, 2 January 1812, *PTJRS*, 4:394–395.
144. Radbill, "Thomas Jefferson and the Doctors," 107 and Savitt, *Medicine and Slavery*, 153–154. However, letters of 28 July 1819 written to their mother by two of Jefferson's grandchildren, Ellen and Cornelia Randolph, describe a case where Dr. William Steptoe bled Burwell Colbert, Jefferson's enslaved butler and personal servant, in his presence after many less intrusive interventions had failed to relieve an intestinal obstruction. Ellen remarked at the time that between herself, Cornelia, and Jefferson, they did not "possess as much medical knowledge as would save a sparrow." Colbert recovered. *PTJRS*, 14:565–567.
145. Savitt, *Medicine and Slavery*, 12.
146. Edwin M. Betts, ed., *Thomas Jefferson's Garden Book* (Philadelphia: American Philosophical Society, 1944), 41, entry for 22 May 1773.
147. Jefferson's Instructions for Poplar Forest Management, December 1811, *PTJRS*, 4:379–382.
148. George Alan Davy, "Argumentation and Unified Structure in Notes on the State of Virginia," *Eighteenth Century Studies* 36, no. 4 (1993): 581–593.
149. Jefferson to James Maury, 16 June 1815, *PTJRS*, 8:542–545.
150. Gilbert Chinard, *Jefferson et les Idéologues* (New York: Arno Press, 1979) reprinted from 1925.
151. Jefferson to Pierre J. G. Cabanis, 13 July 1803, *PTJ*, 41:42–43; Jefferson to Charles Willson Peale, 13 March 1808, in Lillian B. Miller et al., eds., *The Selected Papers of Charles Willson Peale and His Family* (New Haven: Yale University Press, 1983–), 2:1070–1071; to C. F. C. de Volney, 8 February 1805, *PTJ*, 45:473–477; to Peter & Christian Roche, 3 April 1807, in Sowerby, *Library of Thomas Jefferson*, 1:396; to the Marquis de Lafayette, 16 January 1825, in Chinard, ed., *Lafayette and Jefferson*, 427–428.
152. Charles Hunter Van Duzer, *Contributions of the Ideologues to French Revolutionary Thought* (Baltimore: Johns Hopkins University Press, 1935). See also Golden, *Rhetoric of Virtue*, 47–72.
153. Kett, *American Medical Profession*, 151–191.
154. Jefferson to Volney, 17 March 1801, *PTJ*, 33:341–342. The best account of Jefferson's role in publishing Destutt de Tracy's works is in Gilbert Chinard, *Jefferson et les Idéologues*, 97–188 and chapter 14.
155. Martin S. Staum, *Cabanis: Enlightenment and Medical Philosophy in the French Revolution* (Princeton, N.J.: Princeton University Press, 1980).
156. Cabanis, *A Sketch of the Revolutions of Medical Science, and Views relating to its Reform*, translated by Alexander Henderson (London: Bye and Law, 1806). The

original French edition was *Coup d'Oeil sur Les Révolutions et sur la Réforme de la Médicine* (Paris: Crapart, Caille et Ravier, 1804).

157. Cabanis, *An Essay on the Certainty of* Medicine, translated by R. La Roche (Philadelphia: Robert Desilver, 1823), 101, originally printed in French as Du *Degré de Certitude de la Médecine*, (Paris: Crapart, Caille et Ravier, 1803), and his *Sketch of Revolutions of Medical Science* 11–12.
158. Murray, "Thomas Jefferson and Medicine," 150.
159. Rosen, "Political Order and Human Health," 32–41. See also Jefferson to Volney, 8 February 1805, *PTJ*, 45:473–477; to Charles Willson Peale, 13 March 1808, in Miller et al., eds., *Papers of Charles Willson Peale*, 2:1070–1071; and to Thomas Cooper, 10 July 1812, *PTJRS*, 5:223–224, in which Jefferson expresses his unqualified respect for Cabanis, calling his *Rapports du Physique et du Moral de l'homme* "the most profound of all human compositions."
160. In an influential address to the Massachusetts Medical Society, Bigelow argued that disease should often be left to itself as they "cannot, in our present state of knowledge, be eradicated, or abridged." Bigelow, *A Discourse on Self–Limited Diseases* (Boston: Nathan Hale, 1835), 8 and *Nature in Disease* (Boston: Ticknor & Fields, 1854).
161. Bartlett, *An Essay on the Philosophy of Medical Science* (Philadelphia: Lea and Blanchard, 1844), 255.
162. Worthington Hooker, "The present Mental Attitude and Tendencies of the Medical Profession," *New Englander* 10 (1852): 548–568 and Oliver W. Holmes, *Medical Essays* (Boston: Houghton Mifflin Co., 1888), 19.
163. Cabanis to Jefferson, 20 October 1802, *PTJ*, 38:524–525, with which he sent his two-volume work, *Rapports du Physique et du Morale de l'Homme* (Paris: Crapart, Caille et Ravier, 1804). The book, which has been translated as *On The Relation between the Physical and Moral Aspects of Man* by Margaret Duggan Saidi (Baltimore: Johns Hopkins University Press, 1980), is a compilation of a dozen scientific papers that Cabanis wrote in the 1790s on the interrelationship of anatomy, physiology, environment, and the moral faculties of man. See also Jefferson to Cabanis, 13 July 1803, *PTJ*, 41:42–43.
164. Sowerby, *Library of Thomas Jefferson*, Washington, 1952–59, 395–6 (nos. 861, 862).
165. Jefferson to Volney, 8 February 1805. *PTJ*, 45:473–477. For similar praise of Cabanis, see Jefferson to Thomas Cooper, 10 July 1812, *PTJRS*, 5:223–224 and to John Adams, 8 January 1825, in Lester J. Cappon, ed., *The Adams-Jefferson Correspondence: The Complete Correspondence between Thomas Jefferson & Abigail & John Adams* (1959), 2:605–606.
166. Oscar A. Thorup, "Thomas Jefferson and Academic Medicine," *The Pharos* (April 1977): 16–23 and "Thomas Jefferson and Medicine: The Foundations and Development of his Ideas," History of the Health Sciences Lecture Series, University of Virginia, 15 November 1990.
167. Charles E. Rosenberg, *The Care of Strangers: The Rise of America's Hospital System* (New York: Basic Books, 1987), 337. The only two general hospitals in existence in 1800 were the Pennsylvania hospital in Philadelphia, founded in 1751 and the New York hospital (predecessor of the New York-Presbyterian hospital) founded in 1771. The Charity Hospital of New Orleans was opened in 1736, but did not come under American administration until the Louisiana Purchase in 1803.
168. Herein is another similarity with Cabanis, who viewed hospitals as "vicious centers

of abuse and contagion," and who favored keeping medical care in the "natural" and salutary environment of the home. Greenbaum, *A Review of Cabanis,* 337.

169. Jefferson, *Notes on the State of Virginia*, 133–134.
170. Jefferson to Joseph C. Cabell, 16 May 1824, in Cabell, ed., *Early History of the University*, 308–313.
171. This can be seen by comparing Jefferson's *Notes*, Query XIV, to Du Pont's *Idées sur les secours a donner aux pauvres malades dans une grande ville ...* (*Ideas on the Nature, Form and Extent of Assistance to Give the Sick Poor in a large City*), which was written and published in 1786 at the behest of the French Académie des Sciences, and which Du Pont sent to Jefferson on 5 November 1787, *PTJ*, 12:325–326.
172. Louis S. Greenbaum, "Thomas Jefferson, the Paris Hospitals, and the University of Virginia," *Eighteenth-Century Studies* 26, no. 4 (1993): 613.
173. Colin Jones and Michael Sonenscher, "The Social Functions of the Hospital in Eighteenth–Century France: The case of the Hôtel–Dieu of Nîmes," *French Historical Studies* 13, no. 2 (1983): 174.
174. Greenbaum, "Jefferson and the Paris Hospitals," 609 and Wallenborn, "Jefferson and Medicine," 4.
175. Cabanis was named to the Commission for Reforming Hospital care in 1791 on the strength of his *Observations sur les Hospitaux*, published in 1790, in which he described the dreadfully high hospital mortality rates, advocated for smaller hospital units that could cultivate the natural atmosphere of one's own home, and, in connection with this, linked the needs of medical research and teaching to hospital reform.
176. Greenbaum, "Jefferson and the Paris Hospitals," 610.
177. Ibid., 610 and Wallenborn, "Jefferson and Medicine," 5.
178. Greenbaum, "Jefferson and the Paris Hospitals," 611.
179. John D. Thompson and Grace Goldin, *The Hospital: A Social and Architectural History* (New Haven: Yale University Press, 1975), 170–205.
180. Jefferson to Littleton W. Tazewell, 5 January 1805, *PTJ*, 45:303–306.
181. Jefferson associated cities with dissipation and vice, describing New York, "like London," as "a Cloacina [the goddess who presided over the great sewer] of all the depravities of human nature" while in Charlottesville "crime is scarcely heard of, breaches of order rare, and our societies, if not refined, are rational moral and affectionate at least." Jefferson to William Short, 8 September 1823, College of William and Mary, *Thomas Jefferson Papers*, https://digitalarchive.wm.edu/handle/10288/15368.
182. Jefferson to the Trustees of the Lottery for East Tennessee College, May 6, 1810, *PTJRS*, 2:365–366.
183, Richard Guy Wilson, ed., *Thomas Jefferson's Academical Village: The Creation of a Masterpiece* (Charlottesville: University of Virginia Press, 1993), 71.
184. Jefferson to Benjamin Henry Latrobe, 12 June 1817, *PTJRS*, 11:431–432. This letter initiated a correspondence between Jefferson and Latrobe concerning the layout of the University of Virginia. See also Jefferson to Virginia governor Wilson Cary, 2 April 1816, *PTJRS*, 9:623–629, in which Jefferson reiterated his belief that a village design was preferable to a single large building "on account of fire, health, economy, peace & quiet."
185. Greenbaum, "Jefferson and the Paris Hospitals," 623
186. Ibid., 623.
187. Patricia C. Sherwood and Joseph M. Lasala, "Education and Architecture: The

Evolution of the University of Virginia's Academical Village," in Wilson's *Thomas Jefferson's Academical Village*, 9–45; Mary N. Woods, "Thomas Jefferson and the University of Virginia: Planning the Academic Village," *Journal of the Society of Architectural Histories* 44, no. 3 (1985): 266–283; Richard Guy Wilson, "Inspirational Learning. The Architecture of the University of Virginia," *The Journal of Thomas Jefferson's Life and Times* 1, no. 2 (February 2017).

188. Jefferson to William Short, 31 October 1819, *PTJRS*, 15:162–166; Jeanne M. Yarbrough, *American Virtues: Thomas Jefferson on the Character of a Free People* (Lawrence: University Press of Kansas, 1998); Golden, *Rhetoric of Virtue.*

189. Jefferson to George Caines, 21 March1801, *PTJ*, 33:389; to James Breckinridge, 9 April 1822, *PTJRS*, 18:332–334; to Thomas Nelson, 21 February 1781, *PTJ*, 4:677–678; to Peter Carr, 10 August 1787, *PTJ*, 12:14–19; to George Clinton, 31 December 1803, *PTJ*, 42:214–215; to Louis H. Girardin, 27 March 1815, *PTJRS*, 8:384–386.

190. Jefferson's library contained more than 25 books on physiology and medical therapeutics. Sowerby, Chapters IX–XI, 396–455. See also Jefferson to Thomas Cooper, 7 October 1814: "no knolege can be more satisfactory to a man that that of his own frame, it's parts, their functions & actions," *PTJRS*, 8:12–13.

191. Jefferson to John Adams, 28 October 1813, *PTJRS*, 6:562–568.

192. Robley Dunglison, *The Medical Student, or Aids to the Study of Medicine* (Philadelphia, Carey, Lea & Blanchard, 1837): 159–160; Radbill, ed. "Autobiographical Ana," 74; Warner, *The Therapeutic Perspective.*

193. Jefferson to Charles Thomson, 20 September 1787, *PTJ*, 12:159–161; Jefferson to William Johnson, 4 March 1823, Library of Congress, *The Thomas Jefferson Papers*, https://www.loc.gov/item/mtjbib024584/.

194. Jefferson certainly did not avoid all forms of contemporary treatment. He used quinine to help relieve his frequent headaches and laudanum for treating severe diarrhea. And on one occasion, he consented to take mercury for a cutaneous eruption that caused a terrible itch. Jefferson's Notes on Itch Lotion, after 29 May 1818, *PTJRS*, 13:73; Jefferson to Henry Dearborn, 5 July 1819, *PTJRS*, 14:502–504; Dorsey, *Jefferson–Dunglison letters*, 41–42, 50–51, 87; Gaye Wilson, "Medicine," *Thomas Jefferson Encyclopedia*, February 2004.

195. Although Jefferson distrusted most physicians, he extolled the virtues of several who treated him and his family, quite possibly because they mostly shared his aversion to bleeding and excessive doses of purgatives and engaged in more conservative measures that emphasized rest and fresh air augmented by good hydration and nourishing food. In a number of letters, Jefferson expressed his comfort with the practices of Dr. George Gilmer (1743–1795); Dr. Gem, an English physician who treated Jefferson's two daughters, Martha and Maris, while the family was in Paris; Dr. Thomas G. Watkins (1752–1840), who became Jefferson's personal physician in 1819; and Dr. Robley Dunglison (1798–1869), who followed Watkins, and who visited Jefferson no fewer than 35 times during the final eighteen months of his life. See Jefferson to James Madison, 13 and 28 January 1821, *PTJRS*, 16:541–543, 575, and 22 November 1822, *The Papers of James Madison, Retirement Series*, 2:603–604; to Robley Dunglison, 26 November 1825, in Dorsey, *Jefferson–Dunglison Letters*, 44–45; Marx, *Health of the Presidents*, 49; and Abrams, *Revolutionary Medicine*, 190.

Chapter 3

1. *PTJRS*, 16:499–500. The day before he made this justly famous statement, Jefferson similarly promised that the new university would allow the human mind the fullest freedom "to explore and to expose every subject susceptible of its contemplation." Jefferson to Destutt de Tracy, 26 December 1820, *PTJRS*, 16:485–488.
2. For an excellent timeline of the founding of the University of Virginia, see J. Jefferson Looney, "From Academy to College to University: The Prehistory of the University of Virginia," in John A. Ragosta et al., eds., *The Founding of Thomas Jefferson's University* (Charlottesville: University of Virginia Press, 2019), 11–21.
3. Set up for educational purposes with money accrued from state escheats, penalties, and forfeitures. The Literary Fund was to become the main source of financial support for the future University of Virginia. By 1817 it had amassed more than one million dollars. *Richmond Enquirer*, 2 March and 14 December 1816. See also Jefferson to Joseph C. Cabell, 28 November 1820, *PTJRS*, 16:428–430; Joseph C. Cabell to Jefferson, 20 February 1818, *PTJRS*, 12:488–490; and "Jefferson's Estimate of University of Virginia Building Costs," [ca. 28 November 1820], *PTJRS*,16:431–432.
4. Jefferson to Nathaniel Bowditch, 26 October 1818, *PTJRS*, 13:339–341 and Jefferson to Littleton W. Tazewell, 5 January 1805, *PTJ*, 45:303–306.
5. Adams, *Jefferson and UVA*, 148.
6. Virginius Dabney, *Mr. Jefferson's University: A History* (Charlottesville: University of Virginia Press, 1981), 1–2; N.H.R. Dawson, Commissioner of the Bureau of Education, to The Honorable Secretary of the Interior, 9 December 1887, as cited in Adams, *Jefferson and UVA*, 12; Cameron Addis, *Jefferson's Vision for Education, 1760–1845* (New York: Peter Lang, 2003), 155.
7. William F. Norwood, *Medical Education in the United States Before the Civil War* (Philadelphia: University of Pennsylvania Press, 1944), 262–267, 383.
8. "Jefferson's 1779 Bill for the More General Diffusion of Knowledge," *PTJ*, 2:526–535 and his "Draft of the Rockfish Gap Report of the University of Virginia Commissioners," 28 June 1818, *PTJRS*, 13:189–208; Jefferson to John Banister, Jr., 15 October 1785, *PTJ*, 8:635–638; to Elizabeth Trist, 23 November 1816, *PTJRS*, 10:545–546; to Joseph Priestley, 18 January 1800, *PTJ*, 31:319–323; to David Williams, 14 November 1803, *PTJ*, 41:726–728; to William Short, 8 September 1823, *Thomas Jefferson Papers*, Special Collections Research Center, Swem Library, College of William and Mary, https://digitalarchive.wm.edu/handle/10288/15368; to Littleton W. Tazewell, 5 January 1805, *PTJ*, 45:303–306; to Thomas Elder, 25 November 1785, *PTJ*, 9:58–59; to Archibald McCalester, 22 December 1791, *PTJ*, 22:430; to James Breckinridge, 9 April 1822, *PTJRS*, 18:332–333.
9. Jefferson familiarized himself with the American schools of Harvard, Yale, Princeton, William and Mary, the University of Pennsylvania, Baltimore College, Transylvania University, and South Carolina College (later the University of South Carolina); and in Europe, Oxford, and Cambridge in England; Edinburgh University in Scotland; the Swiss college of Geneva; the Paris schools; the Italian schools in Rome, Padua, and Naples; and the German university of Göttingen. The luminaries from whom Jefferson sought counsel and guidance included Joseph Priestley (1733–1804), the discoverer of oxygen; George Ticknor (1791–1871), an eminent linguist from Harvard; Dr. Caspar Wistar (1761–1818), president of the APS from 1815 until his death in 1818; Dr. Samuel Knox (1756–1832), president

of Baltimore College; John Witherspoon (1723–1794), president of the College of New Jersey (later Princeton University); Horace Holley, president of Transylvania University; Dr. Thomas Cooper (1759–1841), a professor and later president of South Carolina College (later the University of South Carolina); Dr. John Augustine Smith (1782–1865), president of the College of William and Mary from 1814 to 1826, the Reverend Timothy Dwight (1752–1817), president of Yale from 1795 to 1817; William Richardson Davie (1756–1820), co–founder of the University of North Carolina; four scholarly Frenchmen—Antoine Louis Claude Destutt de Tracy (1754–1836); Pierre Samuel Du Pont de Nemours (1739–1817); Dr. Alexander–Marie Quesnay de Beaurepaire (1755–1820); and Dr. Pierre Jean Georges Cabanis (1757–1808); two celebrated Swiss men—Marc Auguste Pictet (1752–1825), professor of physics and natural history at the College of Geneva; and the economist and historian François D'Ivernois (1757–1842); and the German naturalist Alexander von Humboldt. Jefferson also consulted many books and essays about European higher education, among the most important of which were Priestley's *Essay on a Course of Liberal Education for Civil and Active Life* (1765) and *Miscellaneous Observations relating to Education* (1778), and Du Pont de Nemours, *National Education in the United States of America*, originally published in 1800, translated from the second French edition of 1812 with an introduction by Bessie Gardner Du Pont (Newark: University of Delaware Press, 1923) (this essay contains many educational ideas that Du Pont and Jefferson shared). See Honeywell, *Educational Work*, 160–173; Adams, *Jefferson and UVA*, 45–52, 72–79; Wagoner, *Jefferson and Education*, 60, 106; Sowerby, *Library of Thomas Jefferson*, 1:505–506 (no. 1112); and John Peter Carey, "Influences on Thomas Jefferson's Theory and Practice of Higher Education," PhD diss., University of Michigan, 1969.

10. Jefferson to Peter Carr, 7 September 1814, *PTJRS*, 7:636–642. This letter has been called "The literary foundation of the University of Virginia" and "the most important document in the early history of the University of Virginia, for it defines Jefferson's educational views as matured after more than thirty years of reflection, from the time when he first draughted a bill for the more general diffusion of knowledge" in 1779. Adams, *Jefferson and UVA*, 61–64. See also Jefferson to Joseph Priestley, 18 January 1800, *PTJ*, 31:319–323; to Thomas Cooper, 14 August 1820, *PTJRS*, 16:187–190; to James Breckinridge, 15 February 1821, *PTJRS*, 16:611–613; and to Edward Livingston, 25 March 1825, Library of Congress: *The Thomas Jefferson Papers*, https://www.loc.gov/item/mtjbib025336/.
11. Roger Geiger, *The History of American Higher Education: Learning and Culture From the Founding to World War II* (Princeton: Princeton University Press, 2015), 179. See also John S. Brubacher and Willis Rudy, *Higher Education in Transition: An American History* (New York: Harper & Brothers, 1958); Lawrence A. Cremin, *American Education: The National Experience, 1783–1876* (New York: Harper & Row, 1980); Richard Hofstadter, *Academic Freedom in the Age of the College* (New Brunswick, N.J.: Aldine Transaction Publishers, 1996); Adams, *Jefferson and UVA*; Hellenbrand, *The Unfinished Revolution*.
12. Jefferson to John Adams, 5 July 1814, *PTJRS*, 7:451–455 and to Thomas Cooper, 14 August 1820, *PTJRS*, 16:187–190.
13. Jefferson to Destutt de Tracy, 26 December 1820, *PTJRS*, 16:485–488 and Robley Dunglison, "College Instruction and Discipline," *American Quarterly Review* 18 (1831): 312–313. In 1993, Joyce Appleby noted that the "true Jefferson legacy is to be hostile to legacies." Appleby, "Jefferson and his Complex Legacy," in Peter S.

Onuf, ed., *Jefferson's Legacies* (Charlottesville: University of Virginia Press, 1993), 2.

14. Honeywell, *Educational Work*, 67–87.
15. Jefferson to Dr. Thomas Cooper, 10 February 1814, *PTJRS*, 7:190–191 and to Joseph C. Cabell, 31 January 1821, *PTJRS*, 16:587–588.
16. During three years in Europe from 1803 to 1806, Cabell studied in or sojourned at Paris, Montpellier, Verdun, Padua, Rome, Naples, Leyden, Cambridge, and Oxford. See Adams, *Jefferson and UVA*, 53–54; and Honeywell, *Educational Work*, 69.
17. Ellen Hickman, "Avoiding 'the appearance of dictating to the Assembly': Thomas Jefferson and the Establishment of the University of Virginia," in Ragosta, et al., eds., *Mr. Jefferson's University*, 95–101; Joseph C. Cabell to Jefferson, 6 March 1822, *PTJRS*, 18:260–265; Clifton Waller Barrett, "The Struggle to Create a University: Founder's Day Address," *Virginia Quarterly Review* 49, no. 4 (1973): 494–506.
18. Bruce, *History of UVA*, 1:3–5.
19. Conveyance of Lands for Central College from John M. Perry and Frances T. Perry to Alexander Garnett, 23 June 1817, *PTJRS*, 11:465–468 and Gene Zechmeister, "Construction of the University, 1817–1826," *Thomas Jefferson Encyclopedia*, https://www.monticello.org/site/research–and–collections/construction–university–1817–1826.
20. Honeywell, *Educational Work*, 67; Adams, *Jefferson and UVA*, 17; William L. Beiswanger, "Jefferson and the Art of Roofing," *Chronicle of Early American Industries Association* 53, no. 1 (2005):18–25; Robert Self, "Thomas Jefferson's Plank–Kilns," *Chronicle of Early American Industries Association* 53, no. 1 (2005): 26–30.
21. "Master List of Subscribers to Central College" [after 7 May 1817], *PTJRS*, 11:328–335 and Honeywell, *Educational Work*, 67.
22. Frederick Daniel, "Virginian Reminiscences of Jefferson," *Harper's Weekly*, 19 November 1904, 48:1766.
23. Honeywell, *Educational Work*, 67; and Ralph Waldo Emerson, *The Essay on Self-Reliance* (New York: The Roycrofters , 1908): 27.
24. Jefferson to Pierre Samuel Du Pont de Nemours, 12 April 1800, *PTJ*, 31:495–496; to Littleton W. Tazewell, 5 January 1805, *PTJ*, 45:303–306; to Joseph Priestley, 18 January 1800, *PTJ*, 31:319–323. In these three letters, Jefferson first revealed his advanced ideas about the character and function of a modern university.
25. Jefferson did not want his university to become another gothic institution, remarking that "Oxford, Cambridge, the Sorbonne &c are now a century or two behind the science of the age." Jefferson to Tazewell, 5 January 1805, PTJ, 45:303–306; to George Ticknor, 25 November 1817, *PTJRS*, 12:203–205; to Charles Yancey, 6 January 1816, *PTJRS*, 9:328–331; to Peter Carr, 7 September 1814, *PTJRS*, 7: 636–642.
26. Jefferson to Destutt de Tracy, 26 December 1820, *PTJRS*,16:485–488.
27. Jefferson to José Corrêa da Serra, 24 October 1820, *PTJRS*, 16:365–379; to Spencer Roane, 9 March 1821, *PTJRS*, 17:31–32; to Edward Livingston, 25 March 1825, Library of Congress: *The Thomas Jefferson Papers*, https://www.loc.gov/item/mtjbib025336/.
28. Jefferson to Wistar, 21 June 1807. This often–quoted letter is Jefferson's longest and most detailed critique of the medical profession. Other relevant letters are Jefferson to William G. Munford, 18 June 1799, *PTJ*, 31:126–130; to John Crawford, 2 January 1812, *PTJRS*, 4:394–395; to William Short, 31 October 1819, *PTJRS*, 15:162–166; to Robley Dunglison, 26 November 1825 in Dorsey,

Jefferson–Dunglison Letters, 44–45.

29. Jefferson to Thomas Cooper, 7 October 1814, *PTJRS*, 8:12–13.
30. Jefferson to Peter Carr, 19 August 1785 and 10 August 1787, *PTJ*, 8:405–408 and 12:14–19; to Thomas Mann Randolph, 25 November 1785, 27 August 1786, and 6 July 1787, *PTJ*, 9:59–60, 10:305–309, and 11:556–559; to John Adams, 5 July 1814, *PTJRS*, 7:451–455.
31. Abrams, *Revolutionary Medicine*, 223.
32. While the only mandated activity was one-and-a-half hours of military drill on Saturday afternoons, in its early years, students at the University of Virginia were expected to exercise regularly and gymnasiums were provided. Minutes of the Board of Visitors of the University of Virginia, October 4–5, 1824, at the University of Virginia.
33. Wagoner, *Jefferson and Education*, 131–132; and *Reports of the Courses of Instruction in the Yale College by a Committee of the Corporation and the Academical Faculty* (New Haven, Yale College, 1828): 15.
34. Minutes of the Board of Visitors of the University of Virginia, October 4–5, 1824, at the University of Virginia.
35. "Enactment of the Board of Visitors of the University of Virginia," July 1831, as cited in Bruce, *History of UVA*, 2:140.
36. Robert S. Gibson, "Medical Education in the Nineteenth Century: Jefferson and Flexner Revisited," in Ragosta, et al., eds., *Mr. Jefferson's University*, 151–189; Norwood, *Medical Education*, 383. See also Dunglison, "College Instruction and Discipline,"283–314; Paul B. Barringer, "A History of the Medical Department of the University of Virginia: Its System of Education, and its Results," An address delivered before the students and alumni, 25 October 1887; Elizabeth A. Rogers, "The Foundation and Early History of the Medical School of the University of Virginia," M.S. Thesis, University of Virginia, 1930; Wyndham B. Blanton, *Medicine in Virginia in the Nineteenth Century* (Richmond: Garrett and Massie, 1933), 19–31; Norwood, *Medical Education*, 262–267; Hart, "Thomas Jefferson's Influence," 47–60; Hall, "Jefferson on Medical Theory," 235–245; William B. Bean, "Mr. Jefferson's Influence on American Medical Education," *Virginia Medical Monthly* 87 (1960): 669–680; Wilhelm Moll, "University of Virginia's 'Firsts' in the History of Medical Education," *Virginia Medical Monthly* 95 (1968):158–161; A. Blinderman, "Thomas Jefferson: Administrator, Practitioner, and Patient," *New York Journal of Medicine* 70, no. 5 (1970): 690–696; Spratt, "The Scholarly Politician," 360–366; Byrd S. Leavell, "Jeffersonian Ideals Endowed the University of Virginia," *Virginia Medical Monthly* 104, no. 2 (1977): 91–96; Thorup, "Thomas Jefferson and Academic Medicine," 16–23; Cohn, "Contributions of Thomas Jefferson," 286–292; Murray, "Jefferson and Medicine," 146–157; and Wallenborn, "Jefferson and Medicine," 3–9.
37. While the rationale underlying this belief is not clearly evident in Jefferson's correspondence, he was painfully aware of major flaws in American education. Unlike many European universities, American colleges were far from richly endowed, and preliminary education was largely neglected there. Honeywell, *Educational Work*, 54–66 and letters from Jefferson to Quesnay de Beaurepaire, 22 December 1787 and 6 January 1788, *PTJ*, 12:452 and 12:499–500; to John Adams, 6 February 1795, *PTJ*, 28:261–262; to François D'Ivernois, 6 February 1795, *PTJ*, 28:262–264; to Marc Auguste Pictet, 5 February 1803, *PTJ*, 39:456–457; to Peter Carr, 7 September 1814, *PTJRS*, 7:636–642.

38. William G. Rothstein, *American Physicians in the Nineteenth Century: From Sects to Science* (Baltimore: Johns Hopkins University Press, 1985), 88; Stevens, *American Medicine and the Public Interest*, 9–33; Kenneth M. Ludmerer, *Learning to Heal: The Development of American Medical Education* (New York: Basic Books, 1985), 14–15, 112; Abraham Flexner, *Medical Education in the United States and Canada* (New York City: The Carnegie Foundation for the Advancement of Teaching, 1910), vii, 7, 8, 12; Thomas Neville Bonner, *Becoming a Physician: Medical Education in Britain, France, Germany, and the United States, 1750–1945* (New York: Oxford University Press, 1995), 175–176; Norwood, *Medical Education*, 384–385; Rothstein, *American Medical Schools*, 29. According to Flexner, one of the necessary first steps in depriving the medical schools of their virtual autonomy came when the parent university began to collect the fees and thenceforth to administer the finances of the department by means of an annual budget, with this first taking place at Harvard in 1871.
39. Barringer, "A History of the Medical Department of the University of Virginia," 6.
40. Minutes of the Board of Visitors of the University of Virginia, October 4–5, 1824, at the University of Virginia.
41. Minutes of the Board of Visitors of the University of Virginia," 5–7 April 1824, at the University of Virginia.
42. Jefferson's letter to the Trustees of the Lottery for East Tennessee College, 6 May 1810, *PTJRS*, 2:365–366, shows that he had developed these ideas long before he began designing the University of Virginia. See also Jefferson to Governor Wilson C. Nicholas, 2 April 1816, *PTJRS*, 9:623–629; to Littleton W. Tazewell, 5 January 1805, *PTJ*, 45:303–306; to William Thornton, 9 May 1817, *PTJRS*, 11:342–343; to George Ticknor, 24 December 1819, *PTJRS*, 15:301–304; to Maria Cosway, 24 October 1822, Library of Congress: *The Thomas Jefferson Papers*, https://www.loc.gov/item/mtjbib024474/; to Tazewell and William C. Rives, 25 November 1825, Library of Congress: *The Thomas Jefferson Papers*, https://www.loc.gov/item/mtjbib025574/.
43. Hellenbrand, *The Unfinished Revolution*, 145; and Jefferson's "Draft of the Rockfish Gap Report [ca. June 28, 1818]," *PTJRS*, 13:189–208.
44. Malone, *Sage of Monticello*, 258.
45. "Minutes of the Board of Visitors of the University of Virginia," 7 October 1822, at the University of Virginia; Harry Clemons, *The University of Virginia Library, 1825–1850, Story of a Jeffersonian Foundation* (Charlottesville: University of Virginia Library, 1954), 6; Bruce, *History of UVA*, 2:36–41, 2:186–190; Jefferson's original catalogue of books to be purchased for the University of Virginia's library, completed on 2 June 1825 and submitted to William Hilliard, the purchasing agent from New York, on 3 June 1825, both at the University of Virginia.
46. Jefferson to Destutt de Tracy, 26 December 1820, *PTJRS*, 16:485–488.
47. For example, the school of medicine of the University of Pennsylvania did not acquire a credible library of its own until 1877. Instead, it relied on the libraries housed in the Pennsylvania Hospital and the College of Physicians of Philadelphia, both of which were far away and rarely visited by medical students. A noteworthy exception was Transylvania University in Kentucky, the medical department of which, founded in 1817, had one of the best libraries in America. Corner, *Two Centuries of Medicine*, 159–160, 257; Flexner, *Medical Education*, 82; Kathleen P. Birchette, "The History of Medical Libraries from 2000 B.C. to 1900 A.D.," *Bulletin of the Medical Library Association* (1973): 302–308; Robert Peter, *History*

of the Medical Department of Transylvania University (Louisville, Ky.: J.P. Morton & Company, 1905), 56; Jefferson to Horace Holley, 5 April 1825, Library of Congress: *The Thomas Jefferson Papers*, https://www.loc.gov/item/mtjbib025355/.

48. Godfrey S. Belleh and Eric v.d. Luft, "Financing North American medical libraries in the nineteenth century," *Bulletin of the Medical Library Association* 89, no. 4 (2001): 388. Whitfield J. Bell, "Private physicians and public collections: Medical libraries in the United States before 1900," in L.G. Stevenson, ed., *A Celebration of Medical History* (Baltimore: Johns Hopkins University Press, 1982).
49. See "Jefferson's Bill to Establish a University" [between 19 November and 14 December 1818], *PTJRS*, 13:401–405, which, with some amendments, became the 'University Act of 25 January 1819" and also the "Rockfish Gap Report" of 4 August 1818, *PTJRS*, 13:179–225, which was mandated by a statute of 21 February 1818.
50. Jefferson's "Bill to Establish a University," 13:401–405. This duty was intended to provide "assurance of fidelity to the Commonwealth" of Virginia and may have derived from Jefferson's 1778–1779 "Bill for the More General Diffusion of Knowledge," which was considered several times by the Virginia General Assembly but not enacted, *PTJ*, 2:526–535.
51. "Minutes of the Board of Visitors of the University of Virginia," 5–7 April 1824, University of Virginia.
52. "Rockfish Gap Report," 217; Ellen Hickman, "Avoiding 'the appearance of dictating to the Assembly': Thomas Jefferson and the Establishment of the University of Virginia," in Ragosta, et al., eds., *Mr. Jefferson's University*, 95–101; Joseph C. Cabell to Jefferson, 24 December 1818, *PTJRS*, 13:514–517; Jefferson to Wistar, 21 June 1807; Jefferson to Cornelius Camden Blatchly, 21 October 1822, , Library of Congress: *The Thomas Jefferson Papers, https://www.loc.gov/item/mtjbib024471/.*
53. During its first 100 years of existence, five attempts were made to "abandon the Medical Department of the University of Virginia and remove it to Richmond." These occurred in 1824, 1834, 1837, 1867, and 1921. For the initial effort in 1824 to move the College of William and Mary to Richmond and to establish a medical school at the relocated site, see Joseph C. Cabell to Jefferson, 5 May 1824 and Jefferson to Cabell, 16 May 1824 in Cabell, ed., *Early History of the University of Virginia*, 305–308, 308–313 and Bruce, *History of UVA*, 1:308–321. A 52–page report published as a supplement to the December 1921 University of Virginia *Alumni News* discusses the history of these five unsuccessful attempts and includes extensive testimony favorable to the University of Virginia from Abraham Flexner, one of the leading authorities of medical education in America, and Dr. William H. Welch of Johns Hopkins University; written opinions from eminent scholars at Harvard, Yale, Stanford, Georgetown, and Washington University and the Universities of California, Chicago, Pennsylvania, Michigan, Iowa, Wisconsin, Kansas, Oregon, and Texas. Woodrow Wilson (former UVA law student and recently retired U.S. President) was moved to write to McLane Tilton, 25 December 1921, that, "I should deplore the removal of the Medical Department of the University of Virginia to Richmond as a very serious detriment to the University and also a deplorable breach in the historical development of education in Virginia."
54. Jefferson to Albert Gallatin, 15 February 1818, *PTJRS*, 12:467–468; Joseph C. Cabell to Jefferson, 24 December 1818, *PTJRS*, 13:514–517.
55. Jefferson to William Short, 8 September 1823, College of William and Mary, *Thomas Jefferson Papers*, https://digitalarchive.wm.edu/handle/10288/15368.

56. The proximity of the University to Monticello also allowed Jefferson to keep an eye on it and enjoy the company of professors and students. For Jefferson's eager anticipation of the company of cultivated professors, see Jefferson to William Short, 31 October 1819, *PTJRS*, 15:162–166.
57. Ludmerer, *Learning to Heal*, 5, 38–4; and Lawrence R. Veysey, *The Emergence of the American University* (Chicago: University of Chicago Press, 1965).
58. Ludmerer, *Learning to Heal*, 25. The failure on two occasions of the University of Pennsylvania to offer a faculty appointment to the prominent physiologist Weir Mitchell illustrates the lack of encouragement offered to 19th–century medical researchers. Bruce Fye, "Weir Mitchell, Philadelphia's Lost Physiologist," *Bulletin of the History of Medicine* 57, no. 2 (1983): 188–202.
59. Jefferson to Thomas Cooper, 25 August 1814, *PTJRS*, 7:606–607. See also Jefferson to Cooper, 16 January 1814, *PTJRS*, 7:124–131.
60. Jefferson to William Short, [29] June 1819 and 31 October 1819, *PTJRS*, 14:488–489 and 15:162–166; Jefferson to Joseph C. Cabell, 3 February 1824 in Cabell, ed., *Early History of the University of Virginia*, 290–292 (there misdated 23 February); Minutes of the Board of Visitors of the University of Virginia, 5–7 April 1824, at the University of Virginia; and Edward Potts Cheyney, *History of the University of Pennsylvania*, 1740–1790 (Philadelpia: University of Pennsylvania Press, 1940), 214–15.
61. Jefferson's expectations of his inaugural professoriate are amply described in his letters to Joseph Priestley, 18 January 1800, *PTJ*, 31:319–323; to Peter Carr, 7 September 1814, *PTJRS*, 7:636–642; to Nathaniel Bowditch, 26 October 1818, *PTJRS*, 13:339–341; to John Adams, 9 July 1819, *PTJRS*, 14:523–525; to William Short, 31 October 1819, *PTJRS*, 15:162–166; to Richard Rush, 26 April 1824, Library of Congress: *The Thomas Jefferson Papers*, https://www.loc.gov/item/mtjbib024998/; to Samuel Parr, 26 April 1824, at the Massachusetts Historical Society.
62. Jefferson to Richard Rush, 26 April 1824, Library of Congress: *The Thomas Jefferson Papers*, https://www.loc.gov/item/mtjbib024998/.
63. Jefferson to Joseph C. Cabell, 3 February 1824, in Cabell, ed., *Early History of the University of Virginia*, 290–292 (there misdated 23 February). See also Bruce, *History of UVA*, 1:336 and Adams, *Jefferson and UVA*, 109–111.
64. Jefferson to Dugald Stewart, 26 April 1824, at the Massachusetts Historical Society. In a letter to Benjamin Rush, 3 January 1808, Library of Congress: *The Thomas Jefferson Papers*, https://www.loc.gov/item/mtjbib018064/, Jefferson said the qualities which make a great man would likewise make a great professor. He listed them as "1. good humor. 2. integrity. 3. industry. 4. science. the preference of the 1st to the 2d quality may not at first be acquiesced in. but certainly we had all rather associate with a good humored light principled man than with an ill tempered rigorist in morality."
65. Jefferson's 1779 "Bill for the More General Diffusion of Knowledge," *PTJ*, 2:526–535.
66. Jefferson to John Adams, 28 October 1813, *PTJRS*, 6:562–568. In this letter, Jefferson states that "there is a natural aristocracy among men. the grounds of this are virtue & talents. . . .there is also an artificial aristocracy founded on wealth and birth, without either virtue or talents; for with these it would belong to the first class."
67. The concept of total devotion to academic life was first expressed in a letter to Joseph Priestley, 18 January 1800, *PTJ*, 31:319–323, when Jefferson wrote, "we

should propose that the professors follow no other calling, so that their whole time may be given to their academical functions." In this same letter, Jefferson announced his interest in recruiting European scholars if necessary. See Bruce, *History of UVA*, 1:334–343 and Malone, *Sage of Monticello*, 397–410.

68. This resolution was first adopted by the Board of Visitors on 7 April 1824 and was modified in March and October 1825 with language that provided some leeway to the medical professors. See "Minutes of the Board of Visitors of the University of Virginia," 5–7 April 1824, 4–5 March 1825, and 3–7 October 1825.
69. The restriction on clinical practice proved to be a significant recruitment barrier. In a letter to Jefferson dated 27 August 1824, Francis Walker Gilmer wrote from London that, "I have had more persons recommended for [the professorship of] anatomy [and medicine] than for any other place; but immediately they find they will not be allowed to practise medicine &c. abroad, they decline proceeding farther. That I fear will prove an insurmountable obstacle to us in this department." Richard Beale Davis, *Correspondence of Thomas Jefferson and Francis Walker Gilmer, 1814–1826* (Columbia: University of South Carolina Press, 1946), 98–100. See also William P. Trent, *English Culture in Virginia: A Study of the Gilmer Letters* (Baltimore: N. Murray, 1889).
70. By American standards, the proposed compensation provisions for the Virginia professors were generous. At most other colleges, nonmedical professors seemed to earn from $600 to $1,200 a year, except at Harvard, South Carolina, and Virginia. In the early nineteenth century, a Harvard professor received an annual salary of $1,500 to $1,700. At South Carolina, Thomas Cooper received $2,500, and at Virginia it was proposed that professors be guaranteed an annual income of $2,500 for five years, the length of the initial contract period. Malone, *Sage of Monticello*, 398; Ludmerer, *Learning to Heal*, 125–126; Frank Stricker, "American Professors in the Progressive Era: Incomes, Aspirations, and Professionalism," *Journal of Interdisciplinary History* 19, no. 2 (1988): 237.
71. Gibson, "Jefferson and Flexner Revisited," 248 and Richard H. Shryock, *Medical Licensing in America, 1650–1965* (Baltimore: Johns Hopkins University Press, 1967), 34.
72. "Minutes of the Board of Visitors of the University of Virginia," 4–5 October 1824. In the early years of Virginia, this contributed to a lower-than-expected student enrollment. Academic sessions at Virginia were also far longer than at many European universities.
73. Davis, *History of Medical Education and Medical Institutions*, 167 and Ludmerer, *Learning to Heal*, 11.
74. The regulations adopted by the Board of Visitors on 7 April and 4 October 1824, respectively, stated that "exercises shall be prescribed to employ the vacant days and hours," and that students were expected to attend military exercises each Saturday for two hours.
75. Jefferson to Robley Dunglison, 26 November 1825, in Dorsey, *Jefferson–Dunglison Letters*, 44–45.
76. Jefferson to Elizabeth Trist, 23 November 1816, *PTJRS*, 10:545–546.
77. "Minutes of the Board of Visitors of the University of Virginia," 5–7 April and 4–5 October 1824.
78. Bruce, *History of UVA*, 2:115. See also Ludmerer, *Learning to Heal*, 12.
79. Jefferson to William G. Munford, 18 June 1799, *PTJ*, 31:126–130; to Caspar Wistar, 21 June 1807; to John Crawford, 2 June 1812, *PTJRS*, 4:394–395; to Ro-

bley Dunglison, 26 November 1825, in Dorsey, *Jefferson–Dunglison Letters*, 44–45.

80. "Rockfish Gap Report," 217. Several letters from Jefferson reveal his belief that "experience alone brings skill," that "all theory must yield to experience," and "a little experience is worth a great deal of reading." Jefferson to William H. Crawford, 14 February 1815, *PTJRS*, 8:258–260; to James Maury, 16 June 1815, *PTJRS*, 8:542–545; to Mary Jefferson Eppes, 26 October 1801, *PTJ*, 35:510–511; to George Fleming, 29 December 1815, *PTJRS*, 9:302–304.
81. Jefferson to John Patten Emmet, 2 May 1826, Library of Congress: *The Thomas Jefferson Papers*, https://www.loc.gov/item/mtjbib025719/.
82. Jefferson to Joseph C. Cabell, 16 May 1824, in Cabell, ed., *Early History of the University of Virginia,* 308–313. Although the medical school of the University of Virginia would come under attack for its "wholly inadequate clinical facilities," this criticism, often self-serving and at times vicious, is unfair, since, in the vast majority of early nineteenth–century American medical schools, instruction was almost entirely didactic. Very few schools offered any meaningful clinical experience. Ludmerer, *Learning to Heal*, 12–13 and Rothstein, *American Medical Schools*, 34.
83. Ralph C. Williams, *The United States Public Health Service, 1798–1950* (Washington, D.C., 1951), 27, 40, 69–70. See also W. E. Rooney, "Thomas Jefferson and the New Orleans Marine Hospital," *The Journal of Southern History* 22, no. 2 (1956): 167–182.
84. C. Edward Koop, "Remarks to the Students and Faculty of the George Washington University School of Medicine," Washington, D.C., 23 April 1986.
85. In Jefferson's time, physiological instruction occupied a dispersed place in the curricula of American medical colleges. No medical school placed a premium on teaching it, and none of the practitioner-teachers who comprised the faculties showed much interest in physiological experimentation or the advancement of principles that impacted clinical practice. Bonner, *Becoming a Physician*, 151–152.
86. Ibid.; John Harley Warner, "Physiology," in Ronald L. Numbers, ed., *The Education of American Physicians* (Berkeley: University of California Press, 1980), 56; *The Catalogue of the Library of the University of Virginia* (Charlottesville: Gilmer, Davis & Company, 1828).
87. C. A. Browne, "Thomas Jefferson's Relation to Chemistry," *Journal of Chemical Education* 20, no. 12 (1943): 574; Jefferson to James Madison, 30 April 1823, *PTJRS*, 3:47–48; Minutes of the Board of Visitors of the University of Virginia," 4–5 October 1824; John G. Waite, et al., *The Chemical Hearth and the First Chemistry Teaching Laboratories and Lecture Rooms at the University of Virginia* (Charlottesville: John G. Waite Associates, Architects, and the University of Virginia, 2017), 7–126 (hereafter referred to as "Waite Report").
88. "Rockfish Gap Report," 217.
89. This series of lectures entitled "The History of the Progress and Theories of Medicine" was one of seven courses that comprised the inaugural medical-school curriculum at the University of Virginia. These lectures, given by Robley Dunglison, were published posthumously in 1872 by his son, Richard Dunglison, M.D. See Robley Dunglison, *History of Medicine from the earliest Ages to Commencement of the Nineteenth Century* (Philadelphia: Lindsay and Blakiston, 1872) and Moll, "University of Virginia's 'Firsts'," 158–161.
90. Jefferson to Robert Skipwith, 3 August 1771, *PTJ*, 1:76–81.
91. Jefferson, *Notes on the State of Virginia*, 148 and preamble to the 1779 "Bill for the More General Diffusion of Knowledge," *PTJ*, 2:526–527.

92. H. Trevor Colbourn, "Thomas Jefferson's Use of the Past," *William and Mary Quarterly*, 3d series, 15, no. 1 (1958): 2 and Genevieve Miller, "Medical History," in Numbers, ed., *The Education of American Physicians*, 290–308.
93. Rothstein, *American Medical Schools*, 55–61.
94. Jefferson to John Adams, 5 July 1814, *PTJRS*, 7:451–455.
95. According to Ludmerer, *Learning to Heal*, 3, 12–13, "Entrance requirements to medical schools were universally low, and in some instances they approached criminal laxity. Most medical students had completed elementary school only, and many were illiterate."
96. Ludmerer, *Learning to Heal*, 3, 10–13: "The Civil War made painfully clear the deficiencies of mid-nineteenth century American medical education. . . . Delusions of an erudite medical profession were shattered by the results of the written examinations of the Military Boards."
97. Ludmerer, *Learning to Heal*, 3.
98. Martin Kaufman, "American Medical Education," in Numbers, ed., *The Education of American Physicians*, 23.
99. Bruce, *History of UVA*, 2:134.
100. "Minutes of the Board of Visitors of the University of Virginia," 4–5 October 1824, at the University of Virginia.
101. "Minutes of the Board of Visitors of the University of Virginia," 4–5 October 1824 and Warner, *Against the Spirit of System*, 24 and 373, n24.
102. Davis, *History of Medical Education and Medical Institutions*, 181–183; Rothstein, *American Physicians in the Nineteenth Century*, 97; Warner, *Against the Spirit of System*, 19.
103. Joseph Kett, "Education," in Merrill D. Peterson, ed., *Thomas Jefferson: A Reference Biography* (New York: Charles Scribner's Sons, 1986), 238.
104. Bruce, *History of UVA*, 2:129 and Dunglison, "College Instruction and Discipline," 310.
105. Dunglison, "College Instruction and Discipline," 312–313.
106. Ibid.
107. Wall, "Students and Student Life at the University," 57.
108. "The University: Its Character and Wants," *Southern Literary Messenger* 22 (April 1856): 241–269 and Barringer, "A History of the Medical Department of the University of Virginia," 9.
109. Dunglison, "College Instruction and Discipline," 309–313; Mary Lovett Smallwood, *An Historical Study of Examinations and Grading Systems in Early American Universities*, PhD diss. (Cambridge: Harvard University Press, 1935); Joseph F. Kett, *Merit: The History of a Founding Ideal from the American Revolution to the Twenty-First Century* (Ithaca: Cornell University Press, 2012), 69–70, 80, 8; Ludmerer, *Learning to Heal*, 3, 12; Davis, *History of Medical Education and Medical Institutions*, 183–188; Bigelow, *Medical Education*, 79; Flexner, *Medical Education*, 7, 10; Norwood, *Medical Education*, 390–391; Warner, *The Therapeutic Perspective*, 172–174.
110. John Shaw Billings, "Literature and Institutions," in Edward H. Clarke, ed., *A Century of American Literature, 1776–1876* (1876), 297.
111. Rothstein, *American Medical Schools*, 33; Eugene C. Massie, "Statutory History of the University of Virginia," *Alumni Bulletin*, 5 (1899): 101–107 and 6 (1899): 10–14; Ludmerer, *Learning to Heal*, 9–28.
112. Norwood, *Medical Education*, 392–393, 422; Robert G. Slawson, "Medical

Training in the United States Prior to the Civil War," *Journal of Evidence–Based Complementary & Alternative Medicine* 17, no. 1 (2012): 18–19; "Catalogue of the Officers and Students of the University of Virginia, Session 1843–44," 23.

113. Stevens, *American Medicine and the Public Interest*, 16n.
114. Ezra Stiles to Jefferson, 14 September 1786, *PTJ*, 10:385–387; Joseph Willard to Jefferson, 24 September 1788, *PTJ*, 13:637–638; Mary Drew Vaughan, *Historical Catalogue of Brown University, 1764–1904* (Providence: Brown University Press, 1905), 525; *General Catalogue of Princeton University, 1746–1906* (Princeton: Princeton University Press, 1908), 402.
115. Bruce, *History of UVA*, 2:135–137. See also Jefferson to John Adams, 28 October 1813, *PTJRS*, 6:562–568.
116. The handful that consistently rejected this practice include the University of Virginia, Massachusetts Institute of Technology, Stanford, Cornell, and Rice. The founder of MIT in 1861, William Barton Rogers (1804–1882), was an alumnus of the University of Virginia who also implemented other Jefferson ideas, including the elective system.
117. Rothstein, *American Medical Schools*, 3; Rothstein, *American Physicians in the Nineteenth Century*, 96.
118. Jefferson to Henry Dearborn, 22 June 1807, Library of Congress: *The Thomas Jefferson Papers*, https://www.loc.gov/item/mtjbib017300/; Jefferson to Peter Carr, 7 September 1814, *PTJRS*, 7:636–642; Jefferson, *Notes on the State of Virginia*, 147–148; Hellenbrand, *The Unfinished Revolution*, 14; Cohn, "Contributions of Thomas Jefferson," 286–292.
119. Martin in *Thomas Jefferson: Scientist*, 60–61.
120. Bean, "Mr. Jefferson's Influence on American Medical Education," 670 and Murray, "Jefferson and Medicine," 151.
121. "Rockfish Gap Report," 221.
122. Jefferson to Destutt de Tracy, 26 December 1820, *PTJRS*, 16:485–488; to Peter Carr, 7 September 1814, *PTJRS*, 7:636–642; to Joseph Priestley, 18 January 1800, *PTJ*, 31:319–323; to John Adams, 15 June 1813, *PTJRS*, 6:193–195.
123. Flexner, *Medical Education*, xv, 19, 154; Rothstein, *American Medical Schools*, 31–32.
124. Jefferson, *Notes on the State of Virginia*, 159 and Jefferson to Peter Carr, 7 September 1814, *PTJRS*, 7: 636–642.
125. Jefferson to James Madison, 20 December 1787, *PTJ*, 12:438–443.
126. Onuf, *Jefferson's Empire*, 119.
127. Jennings L. Wagoner, "Honor and Dishonor at Mr. Jefferson's University: The Antebellum Years," *History of Education Quarterly* 26, no. 2 (1986): 156.
128. The forerunner of the University of Michigan, the University of Michigania, was founded in 1817, 20 years before the territory became a state.
129. Brubacher and Rudy, *Higher Education in Transition*, 140–149.
130. "Rockfish Gap Report," 212–213.
131. Wagoner, "Honor and Dishonor at Mr. Jefferson's University," 164.
132. Jefferson to Thomas Nelson, 21 February 1781, *PTJ*, 4:677–678; to Peter Carr, 10 August 1787, *PTJ*, 12:14–19; to George Clinton, 31 December 1803, *PTJ*, 42:214–215; to Louis H. Girardin, 27 March 1815, *PTJRS*, 8:384–386; to James Breckinridge, 9 April 1822, *PTJRS*, 18:332–333.
133. *A Summary View of the Rights of British America* (Williamsburg: Clementina Rind, 1774) in *PTJ*, 1:121–137, in which Jefferson wrote, "The whole art of government

consists in the art of being honest" (quote on 134); Jefferson to Nathaniel Macon, 12 January 1819, *PTJRS*, 13:571–572. See also Jefferson to Ezra Stiles, 24 December 1786, *PTJ*, 10:629; to Thomas Leiper, 1 January 1814, *PTJRS*, 7:96–99; and to Josephus B. Stuart, 10 May 1817, *PTJRS*, 11:345–347.

134. Yarbrough, *American Virtues*, xix, 27–54.
135. Bean, "Mr. Jefferson's Influence on American Medical Education," 8.
136. Jefferson to Miles King, 26 September 1814, *PTJRS*, 7:704–706 and to John Adams, 14 October 1816, *PTJRS*, 10:458–461.
137. Hellenbrand, *The Unfinished Revolution*, 145.
138. Holowchak, "The Diffusion of Light," 2, 5.
139. Jefferson to Wistar, 21 June 1807.
140. Jefferson to Peter Carr, 19 August 1785, *PTJ*, 8:405–408; "Rockfish Gap Report," 209–224, quote on 219; Radbill, ed., "The Autobiographical Ana of Robley Dunglison," 29–30 (hereafter, "Autobiographical Ana").
141. "Minutes of the University of Virginia Board of Visitors," 4–5 October 1824 and 4–5 March 1825.
142. Radbill, ed., "Autobiographical Ana," 29–30 and Dunglison, "College Instruction and Discipline," 294–298.
143. Paul Starr, *The Social Transformation of American Medicine* (New York: Basic Books, 1982), 9–13, 15; and Hellenbrand, *The Unfinished Revolution*, 90–91.
144. Jefferson to John Adams, 1 August 1816, *PTJRS*, 10:284–286. See also Baker, "Thomas Jefferson on Academic Freedom," 377, 379–381.
145. Jefferson to Benjamin Rush, 23 September 1800, *PTJ*, 32:166–169.
146. Jefferson to Joseph C. Cabell, 1 March 1819, *PTJRS*, 14:79–81; to William Short, 13 April 1820, *PTJRS*, 15:538–541; to Robert Taylor and Chapman Johnson, 16 May 1820, *PTJRS*, 15:602–604; to Thomas Cooper, 14 August 1820, *PTJRS*, 16:187–190. See also Dumas Malone, *The Public Life of Thomas Cooper* (New Haven: Yale University Press, 1926), 245.
147. *PTJ*, 33:148–152.
148. Unfortunately, this philosophy has come under intense partisan scrutiny in recent years. Cardinal John Henry Newman was prescient about the consequences; that by shackling the liberty to investigate and fettering free expression, the ill-formed movement perverts the intellect and misplaces the concerns of the heart, thereby wounding the soul." This last statement, modified slightly, originated from Henry B. Oesman. See editor's note, ii, 2015 reprint of Newman's *The Idea of a University.*
149. Jefferson to Destutt de Tracy, 26 December 1820, *PTJRS*, 16:485–488; and to William Roscoe, 27 December 1820, *PTJRS*, 16:499–500. Several historians have said of these statements, "It is difficult to imagine a more forthright expression" of the academic freedom concept than these familiar words of Jefferson in reference to the University of Virginia." Baker, "Thomas Jefferson on Academic Freedom," 378 and Alan Barth, *The Loyalty of Free Men* (New York: The Viking Press, 1951), 16.
150. Brubacher and Rudy, *Higher Education in Transition*, 296–316; Richard Hofstadter and Walter P. Metzger, *The Development of Academic Freedom in the United States* (New York: Columbia University Press, 1955), 161–177.
151. Jefferson to François D'Ivernois, 6 February 1795, *PTJ*, 28:262–264 and a letter from Francis W. Gilmer to George Long, 21 August 1824, in Thomas Fitzhugh, ed., *Letters of George Long* (Charlottesville: Library of the University of Virginia, 1917), 11–12.

152. Jefferson to Nathaniel Bowditch, 26 October 1818, *PTJRS*, 13:339–341. Although the overriding purpose of tenure was rooted in academic freedom, it may have had another advantage—to make academic medicine a secure career.
153. Jefferson to Joseph C. Cabell, 3 February 1825, in Cabell, ed., *Early History of the University of Virginia,* 339–341.
154. "Minutes of the University of Virginia Board of Visitors," 4–5 March 1825; Jefferson to James Madison, 7 February 1826, *PTJRS*, 3:687–690; Madison to Jefferson, 8 February 1825, *PTJRS*, 3:471–473; Leonard W. Levy, *Jefferson and Civil Liberties: The Darker Side* (Cambridge, Mass.,: The Belknap Press of Harvard University Press, 1963), 151–157.
155. Honeywell, *Educational Work*, 99.
156. Jefferson's dissenting opinion in "Minutes of the Board of Visitors of the University of Virginia," 3–7 April 1826; Bruce, *History of UVA*, 5:8.
157. Jefferson had previously endorsed the principle of rotation in a letter to James Madison, 20 December 1787, *PTJ*, 12:438–443.
158. Jefferson to George Ticknor, 16 July 1823, Library of Congress: *The Thomas Jefferson Papers*, https://www.loc.gov/item/mtjbib024710/ and Long, *Literary Pioneers*, 48.
159. Barth, *The Loyalty of Free Men*, 205 and Roger Geiger, *History of American Higher Education*, 494.
160. Jefferson to Joseph C. Cabell, 24 October 1817, *PTJRS*, 12:133–134; to Cabell, 28 December 1822, in Cabell, ed., *Early History of the University of Virginia,* 260–262; to Joseph Priestley, 18 January 1800, *PTJ*, 31:319–323; to Peter Carr, 7 September 1814, *PTJRS*, 7:636–642.
161. Adams to Jefferson, 26 May 1817, *PTJRS*, 11:382–385.

Chapter 4

1. Sir Astley Cooper, *A Treatise on Dislocations, and on Fractures of the Joints*, 1st American from 3d London edition (Boston: Wells and Lilly, 1825), 98. Jefferson penned a similar statement in a letter to Caspar Wistar, 21 June 1807.
2. Malone, *Sage of Monticello*, 399; "Minutes of University of Virginia Board of Visitors," 29 March 1819, *PTJRS*, 14:176–179; Jefferson to Francis W. Gilmer, 12 October 1824, in Davis, *Correspondence of Jefferson and Gilmer*, 106–109; to Joseph C. Cabell, 5 January 1815, *PTJ*, 8:182–184 and 3 February 1824 in Cabell, ed., *Early History of the University of Virginia*, 290–292 (there misdated 23 February).
3. Jefferson's letter introducing Francis W. Gilmer to Richard Rush, United States minister plenipotentiary to Great Britain, 26 April 1824, Library of Congress: *The Thomas Jefferson Papers*, https://www.loc.gov/item/mtjbib024998/.
4. Jefferson to Hutchins G. Burton, Thomas Cooper, and Samuel Brown, 28 September 1821, *PTJRS*, 17:520–522 and to Robert Greenhow, 29 April 1825, Library of Congress: *The Thomas Jefferson Papers*, https://www.loc.gov/item/mtjbib025385/.
5. Jefferson to Ticknor, 25 October 1818, *PTJRS*, 13:338–339 and Jefferson to Bowditch, 26 October 1818, *PTJRS*, 13:339–341. Jefferson had been so impressed with Cooper's scholarly versatility that at one point he offered him a dual professorship in natural history (chemistry, zoology, botany, mineralogy, and anatomy) and law. Jefferson to Cooper, 1 September 1817, *PTJRS*, 12:3–5.
6. Chad Wellmon, *Organizing Enlightenment: Information Overload and the Invention*

of the Modern Research University (Baltimore: Johns Hopkins University Press, 2016), 221–222.

7. Samuel D. Gross, *Memoir of Robley Dunglison, M.D., LL.D.* (Philadelphia: Collins Printers, 1869), 4 and Dorsey, *Jefferson-Dunglison letters*, 72.
8. Radbill, ed., "Autobiographical Ana," 7.
9. Zachary Cope, "Dr. Charles Thomas Haden (1786-1824), a Friend of Jane Austen," *British Medical Journal* 1, no. 5493 (1966): 974 and Elizabeth P. Cooper, *Miss Austen Regrets: Charles Thomas Haden*. Jane Austen Society of North America, Inc., 2008. A select collection of Haden's writings was published posthumously by Thomas Adcock, along with a biographical sketch, in *Practical Observations on the Management and Diseases of Children* (London: Burgess and Hill, 1827), v–xii.
10. Osmond C. Wu, et al., "The remarkable medical lineage of the Monro family: contributions of Alexander primus, secundus, and tertius," *Journal of Neurosurgery* 116, no. 6 (2012): 1337–1346; Jack B. Morrell, "Practical Chemistry in the University of Edinburgh, 1799–1843," *Ambix* 16, no. 1–2 (1969): 66–80; M. H. Kaufman, "John Barclay (1758–1826) extra–mural teacher of anatomy in Edinburgh: Honorary Fellow of the Royal College of Surgeons of Edinburgh," *Surgeon* 4, no. 2 (2006): 93–100; J. H. Young, "James Hamilton (1767–1839), obstetrician and controversialist," *Medical History* 7, no. 1 (1963): 62–73.
11. Robert J. Graves, *Clinical Lectures on the Practice of Medicine* (London: reprinted from 2d ed. by New Sydenham Society, 1884), 5; and John D. Comrie, *History of Scottish Medicine, 2nd ed.* (Kent, UK: Balliere, Tindall & Cox, 1932), 454.
12. The contents of this notebook kept by Dunglison for his courses in clinical medicine at Edinburgh during the winter and early spring of 1815–1816 are summarized by Jeanne A. Jones and Chalmers L. Gemmill in "The Notebook of Robley Dunglison, Student of Clinical Medicine in Edinburgh, 1815–1816," *Journal of the History of Medicine and Allied Sciences* 22, no. 3 (1967): 261–273. The course given by James Home from early in November 1815 to the middle of January 1816 is the subject of the first volume's 833 pages, the bulk of which details 66 cases examined by Dunglison. The second course was given by Drs. Daniel Rutherford and James Hamilton, the elder, between 31 January and 16 April 1816 and is dealt with more succinctly in the second volume's 70 pages.
13. Ibid., 263–267.
14. Ibid., 262.
15. Dunglison, *The Medical Student*, 164–165.
16. Radbill, "Robley Dunglison, M.D.," 85.
17. Radbill, ed., "Autobiographical Ana," 49.
18. Erwin H. Ackerknecht, *Medicine at the Paris Hospital, 1794–1848* (Baltimore: Johns Hopkins University Press, 1967); Richard Maulitz, "Channel Crossing: The Lure of French Pathology for English Medical Students, 1816–36," *Bulletin of the History of Medicine* 55, no. 4 (1981): 475–496; John Harley Warner, "The Selective Transport of Medical Knowledge: Antebellum American Physicians and Parisian Medical Therapeutics," *Bulletin of the History of Medicine* 59 (1985): 213–231 and *The Therapeutic Perspective*, 24–31, 185–196.
19. For a brief synopsis of Bichat's life, see "Marie François Xavier Bichat (1771–1802)—Tissue Pathologist," *The Journal of the American Medical Association* 203, no. 4 (1968): 291–292.
20. Laennec invented the stethoscope in 1816 and is considered the father of clinical auscultation. See Ariel Roguin, "René Laennec (1781–1826): The Man behind the

Stethoscope," *Clinical Medicine & Research* 4, no. 3 (2006): 230–235.

21. Henry Lonsdale, *The Worthies of Cumberland* (London: George Routledge and Sons, 1867–1875), 6:273.
22. Erwin H. Ackerknecht, "Medical Education in 19th Century France," *Journal of Medical Education* 32, no. 2 (1957): 148–153 and *Medicine at the Paris Hospital*, 31–35.
23. Arnold Chaplin, *Medicine in England during the Reign of George III* (University of California Libraries, 1919), 13. See also Sir D'Arcy Power, *Medicine in the British Isles* (New York: Paul B. Hoebber, 1930), 9.
24. Guildhall Library, 824/1, 22. See also Radbill, ed., "Autobiographical Ana," 7–8.
25. Radbill, ed., "Autobiographical Ana," 194 and A. H. T. Robb-Smith, "Medical Education at Oxford and Cambridge Prior to 1850," in F. N. L. Poynter, ed., *The Evolution of Medical Education in Britain* (London: Pitman Publishing, 1966), 49.
26. John Morgan, *A Discourse Upon the Institution of Medical Schools in America: Delivered at a Public Anniversary Commencement, held in the College of Philadelphia May 30 and 31, 1765* (Philadelphia: William Bradford, 1765).
27. For his views on the state of medicine of his time and the possibilities of future improvement, see Jefferson to William G. Munford, 18 June 1799, *PTJ*, 31:126–130; to Caspar Wistar, 21 June 1807; to John Crawford, 2 January 1812, *PTJRS*, 4:394–395; to Andrew Kean, 11 November 1818, *PTJRS*, 13:388–390; to William Short, 31 October 1819, *PTJRS*, 15:162–166; to Robley Dunglison, 26 November 1825, in Dorsey, *Jefferson-Dunglison letters*, 44–45; and to Joseph C. Cabell, 7 February 1826, in Cabell, ed., *Early History of the University of Virginia*, 365–367.
28. Chalmers L. Gemmill, "The Educational Work of Robley Dunglison, M.D.," *Virginia Medical Monthly* 87 (1960): 1.
29. Birkbeck to Gilmer, 29 August 1824, in William P. Trent, "English Culture in Virginia: A Study of the Gilmer Letters," in Herbert B. Adams, ed., *Johns Hopkins University Studies in Historical and Political Science* (Baltimore: N. Murray, 1898), 97. After he met Dunglison, Gilmer reported to Jefferson on 15 September 1824 that Dunglison was, "a very intelligent & laborious gentleman" and "a writer of considerable eminence on various medical & anatomical subjects. Davis, *Correspondence of Jefferson and Gilmer*, 101–103.
30. Radbill, ed., "Autobiographical Ana," 9.
31. Radbill, ed., "Autobiographical Ana," 4.
32. Dunglison's French accolades included elected memberships in the Linneian Society of Paris, the Royal Society of Arts and Belles Letters of Nancy, the Society of Medicine and Pharmacy of Paris, the Royal Academy of Marseille, and the Academic Society of Medicine of Marseille. See Radbill, ed., "Autobiographical Ana," 194–195.
33. Gross, *Memoir of Robley Dunglison*, 5 and Radbill, ed., "Autobiographical Ana," 10.
34. "Necrology of Robley Dunglison," *American Journal of the Medical Sciences* (1869): 295–297; and Richard J. Dunglison, "Biography of Robley Dunglison," *Western Journal of Medicine* 4 (1869): 495.
35. Dunglison contributed numerous articles to the *London Medical Repository, Monthly Magazine, Medical Intelligencer, London Medical and Physical Journal, British and Foreign Medical Review, Annals of Philosophy, Quarterly Journal of Science and the Arts, London Quarterly Review, Edinburgh Review, Eclectic Review*, and the *Univer-*

sal Review or *Chronicle of the Literature of All Nations*. His first published contribution was an article in the *Monthly Magazine* in 1817 on the "Floating Island in Derwentwater Lake, Cumberland." This was followed by a paper, in the same journal, on the "Wind of a Ball," one on "Anthropoplagi," and one on "Collections of Dietectiea" under the signature of "Philos." For a complete list of his published works, see Radbill, ed., "Autobiographical Ana," 11–18, 196–199 and John Russel Quinan, "Robley Dunglison," *Medical Annals of Baltimore from 1608 to 1880, Including Events, Men and Literature* (Baltimore: Press of Isaac Friedenwald, 1884), 95.

36. Robley Dunglison, "A Communication on Certain Phenomena of Vision Produced by Dilating the Pupil with the Extract of Belladonna," *Annals of Philosophy* 10 (1820): 432.
37. Robley Dunglison, "The Dangers of Quack Medicine," *Monthly Magazine* [of London] 44 (1817), 18–20.
38. The article on malaria attributed to John MacCulloch appeared in volume 72 of the *Edinburgh Review* in 1823. Dunglison's response appeared in the *London Quarterly Review* in October 1823, page 133. See Radbill, ed., "Autobiographical Ana," 15–16; and MacCulloch's lengthy treatise of 1827 entitled *Malaria: An Essay on the Production and Propagation of this Poison, and on the Nature and Localities of the Places by which it is Produced.*
39. Dunglison's views on the cause and treatment of endemic diseases, including malaria, can be found in the *London Quarterly Review*, October 1823; the *Virginia Literary Museum*, July 1829; and several of his major textbooks, such as *Elements of Hygiene and Human Health*, *General Therapeutics*, and *Practice of Medicine,* first published in 1835, 1836, and 1842, respectively.
40. Radbill, ed., "Autobiographical Ana," 13.
41. Ibid., 17.
42. Ibid., 13, 17; Radbill, "Robley Dunglison, M.D.," 76–77. A lengthy anonymous review criticized Dunglison's *Commentaries* "as too partial to purgatives of the drastic kind, particularly scammony, calomel and aloes." See "Critical Analysis of English and Foreign Literature Relative to the Various Branches of Medical Science," *London Medical and Physical Journal* 52 (1824): 493–504.
43. *London Medical Repository* 10 (1 October 1824): 351.
44. The most outspoken critics in the medical elite, all graduates of the University of Pennsylvania, included Nathaniel Chapman (1780–1853); Isaac Hays (1796–1879), who was Chapman's subordinate; and Charles Caldwell (1772–1853). To Dunglison, the claims these men made against him were baseless and malevolent, derogatory and disparaging, and bitterly partisan. See Radbill, ed., "Autobiographical Ana," 75, 84–86, 100–102, and 141–142.
45. Bruce, *History of the UVA*, 1:35, 361–369.
46. Bruce, *History of UVA*, 2:150 and Cameron Addis, *Jefferson's Vision for Education, 1760–1845* (New York: Peter Lange, 2003), 129. For an authoritative work on the subject, see Harry Y. Gamble, *God on Grounds: A History of Religion at Thomas Jefferson's University* (Charlottesville: University of Virginia Press, 2020).
47. Fielding Hudson Garrison, *An Introduction to the History of Medicine: with Medical Chronology, Suggestions for Study and Bibliographic data, Fourth Edition* (Philadelphia: W. B. Saunders, 1929), 500. Another Bostonian, Edward Everett (1794–1865), also criticized the teaching load of the Virginia professors in an anonymous review of the "Rockfish Gap Report" in the *North American Review* 10 [new series,

volume 1] (January 1820): 115–137, which Jefferson commented on in a letter to John Adams, 15 August 1820, *PTJRS*, 16:193–197.

48. Todd L. Savitt, "Jefferson's Vision of Medical Education and his Quest for a Professor of Medicine," *Virginia Medical Quarterly* 122, no. 4 (1995): 245–251 and Francis W. Gilmer to Jefferson, 27 August 1824, in Davis, *Correspondence of Jefferson and Gilmer*, 98–100.
49. Radbill, ed., "Autobiographical Ana," 9.
50. Harriette Leadam, born in 1802, was considered a "very nice looking girl at the time" and was much sought after. When Dunglison was seeking her favor, clergyman Thomas Lee was wooing her. Both suitors arrived on the same day to present their matrimonial request to her father. According to J. Alden Tifft in a personal communication, as cited in Radbill, ed., "Autobiographical Ana," 9, "One was ushered into the drawing room and the other into the consulting room, and Mr. Leadam had to go backwards and forward between them and his daughter to ascertain their respective positions and his daughter's decision. It was a trying day."
51. Bruce, *History of UVA*, 1:357.
52. Radbill, ed., "Autobiographical Ana," 158.
53. University of Virginia: *The Thomas Jefferson Papers.*
54. Shryock, *Medicine and Society* and his *American Medical Research: Past and Present* (New York: Commonwealth Fund, 1947). One of the few exceptions was the University of Pennsylvania, where popular professors drew 300 or more students to their lectures. At $20 per ticket per course, this could yield an annual income of $6,000 from student fees alone. Corner, *Two Centuries of Medicine*, 48, 68.
55. Minutes of the Board of Visitors of the University of Virginia, 5–7 April 1824.
56. Minutes of the Board of Visitors of the University of Virginia, 4–5 March 1825, 3–7 October 1825.
57. After two months of searching throughout Great Britain, Gilmer expressed his frustration to Jefferson on 27 August 1824, writing that, "I have had more persons recommended for [the professorship of] anatomy [and medicine] than for any other place; but immediately they find they will not be allowed to practise medicine &c. abroad [i.e., unfettered private practice], they decline proceeding farther. That I fear will prove an insurmountable obstacle to us in this department." Davis, *Correspondence of Jefferson and Gilmer*, 98–100.
58. Karen Hunger Parshall, "Bonnycastle, Charles (1796–1840)," *Dictionary of Virginia Biography* (Richmond: Library of Virginia, 1998–), 2:77–78 and Bruce, *History of UVA*, 2, 95, 98–99, 126, 145–146. During his career at Virginia, Bonnycastle proved to be an effective teacher who used "updated pedagogy that was borrowed from French mathematicians" and authored a major textbook on *Inductive Geometry*. He also served as chairman of the faculty from 1833 to 1835, and in 1836 he founded the School of Civil Engineering and Applied Science, possibly the first engineering school in the United States to be attached to a comprehensive university.
59. Christopher Stray, "Key, Thomas Hewitt (1799–1875)," *Oxford Dictionary of National Biography* and Bruce, *History of UVA*, 2, 33–36, 144–145. Key was the first member of the original faculty to resign. Evidently finding Charlottesville disagreeable due to its climate, its rebellious students, his unwillingness to discipline them, and his belief that he was overworked and underpaid, Key left to accept a prestigious professorship at the newly founded University of London.
60. Radbill, ed., "Autobiographical Ana," 18–21; Dunglison to Jefferson, 10 February

1825, in Dorsey, *Jefferson–Dunglison Letters*, 11; Bruce, *History of UVA*, 2:9–12. By way of contrast, it took Francis W. Gilmer only 26 days to travel by packet from New York to Holyhead, England. Trent, "English Culture in Virginia," 55.

61. Radbill, ed., "Autobiographical Ana," 21–22.
62. Ibid., 21–23 and Bruce, *History of UVA*, 2:3.
63. Bruce, *History of UVA*, 2:9 and Looney, "From Academy to College to University, 18.
64. The only American-born member of the original faculty was John Tayloe Lomax (1781–1862), professor of law from July 1826 to 1830. Bruce, *History of UVA*, 2:31–34, 102–105, 169.
65. George Long taught Latin, Greek, Hebrew, belles–lettres, rhetoric, ancient history, and geography from 1825 to 1828. Like Thomas Key, he did not complete his five-year term of appointment, resigning to accept the professorship of Greek at University College in London. Later, Long helped found the Royal Geographical Society and the popular *Penny Cyclopedia*. He edited a number of journals, including the *London Journal of Education*. Bruce, *History of UVA*, 1:367–369, 2:33–35, 82–84, 146–151, 263.
66. Blaettermann taught German, Spanish, Italian, and Anglo–Saxon, and he also "was prepared to give lessons in the vernacular of Demark, Sweden, Holland, and Portugal" from 1825 to 1840. His classes were unpopular and not well attended. In 1830, his salary was reduced in order to hire a tutor to assist his students. Blaettermann was a target of student hostility, and other faculty found him to be rude and abrasive. In 1840, the Board of Visitors dismissed Blaettermann after convicting him of twice beating his wife in public. Brent Tarter, "Blaetermann, George Wilhelm (1782–1850)," *Dictionary of Virginia Biography* (Richmond: Library of Virginia, 1998–), 1:533–534 and Bruce, *History of UVA*, 2:38, 90–95, 157–160.
67. Lisa A. Francavilla, "Emmet, John Patten (1796–1842)," *Encyclopedia Virginia*, https://encyclopediavirginia.org/entries/emmet–john–patten–1796–1842/ and Bruce, *History of UVA*, 2:15–17, 100, 107, 188, 299.
68. Tucker served the university as chair of moral philosophy and political economy from March 1825 through the 1845 term, when he retired at the age of seventy. Over the course of his life, his publications totaled about 10,000 pages. Robley Dunglison, "Obituary Notice of Professor George Tucker," *Proceedings of the American Philosophical Society* 9 (1862–1864): 64–70; Sarah Funderburke, "Tucker, George (1775–1861)," *Encyclopedia Virginia*, accessed 12 February 2012, https://encyclopediavirginia.org/entries/tucker–georg–1775–1861; Bruce, *History of UVA*, 2:19–24, 33, 299, 3:188–189.
69. Nathaniel Chapman's lengthy article under the caption of "American Medicine" appeared in the *Philadelphia Journal of Medical and Physical Sciences* 9 (1825): 404–409 and suggested, without specifically mentioning Dunglison, that, "it is probable the American Medical Societies throughout the country will protest against this act of injustice."
70. Trent, "English Culture in Virginia," 307–309; Paul B. Barringer and James M. Garnett, *The University of Virginia: Its History, Influence, Equipment and Characteristics* (New York: Lewis Publishing Company, 1904), 97–98; Radbill, ed., "Autobiographical Ana," 24–26; Irwin Richmond, "Robley Dunglison, M.D.," *Pennsylvania Medicine* 69, no. 11 (1966): 76; "Imported Professors, and Virginia Stump Orators," in the *Central Gazette*, Charlottesville, 25 December 1824; and *The New York Monthly Chronicle of Medicine and Surgery*, Volume 1 (1824–1825),

191. Another newspaper, the *New York American*, was more open–minded, observing of the new faculty that, "they are well known and highly esteemed in England. Their talents and acquirements will doubtless be highly advantageous to the cause of public instruction in the country."

71. Jefferson to John Adams, 8 January 1825 and Adams to Jefferson, 22 January 1825, in Cappon, ed., *Adams–Jefferson Correspondence*, 2:605–607; Jefferson to Joseph Priestley, 18 January 1800, *PTJ*, 31:319–323; University of Virginia Board of Visitors to the Literary Fund Directors, 5 October 1824, University of Virginia.
72. Jefferson to J. Evelyn Denison, 9 November 1825, Library of Congress: *The Thomas Jefferson Papers*, https://www.loc.gov/item/mtjbib025566/.
73. Daniels, *American Science in the Age of Jackson*, 43.
74. Radbill, ed., "Autobiographical Ana," 25, 28. Caldwell's comments appeared in a hostile review of Dunglison's 1842 work entitled *The Practice of Medicine, or A Treatise on Special Pathology and Therapeutics*, which he published in the *Western Journal of Medicine and Surgery* 5 (June 1842): 429–450, quote on 447.
75. *Catalogue of the Offices and Graduates of Yale University in New Haven, Connecticut 1701–1915* (New Haven: Yale University, 1916), 464 and Radbill, ed., "Autobiographical Ana," 25–26.
76. Jefferson to Joseph C. Cabell, 3 February 1824, in Cabell, ed., *Early History of the University of Virginia*, 290–292 (there misdated 23 February). See also Bruce, *History of UVA*, 1:336.

Chapter 5

1. Opening epigram for chapter on Robley Dunglison in Lonsdale, *Worthies of Cumberland*, 6:262–279.
2. Jefferson to Robert Greenhow of New York, 8 March 1825, Library of Congress: *The Thomas Jefferson Papers*, https://www.loc.gov/item/mtjbib025308/.
3. *Professor Dunglison's Valedictory Lecture Delivered to the Medical Class of the University of Virginia, July 9, 1833* (Charlottesville: Watson & Tompkins Printing, 1833), 3, quoted in Radbill, ed., "Autobiographical Ana," 60.
4. Bruce, *History of UVA*, 2:37. Because the library room in the Rotunda was not completed until October 1826, the books and periodicals were initially housed in Pavilion 7.
5. Minutes of the Board of Visitors of the University of Virginia, 7 October 1822, at the University of Virginia; Clemons, *University of Virginia Library*, 6; Bruce, *History of UVA*, 2:36–41, 186–190; Patten, *Jefferson, Cabell and UVA*, Chapter 20 and "A Short Story," 425–427; Cometti, ed., *Jefferson's Ideas on a University Library*; President Jefferson's Catalogue of Books for the University of Virginia Library, 3 June 1825, at the University of Virginia, in Nicholas P. Trist's hand and signed by Jefferson.
6. Bruce, *History of UVA*, 2:36, 39–40; Jefferson to Joseph C. Cabell, 3 February 1825, in Cabell, ed., *Early History of the University of Virginia*, 339–341; Jefferson to James Madison, 8 August 1824, *PTJRS*, 3:355–356; Patten, "A Short Story," 422–425.
7. James Eckman, "Anglo–American Hostility in American Medical Literature of the Nineteenth Century," *Bulletin of the History of Medicine* 9, no. 1 (1941): 31–71.
8. See Flexner, *Medical Education*, 82; Brubacher and Rudy, *Higher Education in Transition*, 185; Birchette, "History of Medical Libraries," 302–308; Belleh and

Luft, "Financing North American medical libraries," 388; and Corner, *Two Centuries of Medicine*, 159–160, 257.
9. Minutes of Faculty Meetings for 14 and 16 February, 15 and 30 March, 15 April, 5 July, 15 August, 14 and 17 October, and 18 December 1826; 10 September 1827; 15 February, 5 July, and 3 and 5 November 1828; 15 April 1829; 7 January and 7 July 1830; 9 July 1831; and 2 November 1832. See also Minutes of Meetings of the Board of Visitors, 14 December 1826, 15 April 1829, and 1 December 1832; letters between Jefferson and Dunglison of 18 and 31 March, 12 and 16 April, and 20 and 21 May 1826, in Dorsey, *Jefferson-Dunglison Letters*, 51–54, 61–62, 63–66; and Cometti, ed., *Jefferson's Ideas on a University Library*, 29, 32, and 34.
10. Clemons, *University of Virginia Library*, 10.
11. Margaret Bayard Smith to her sisters Anna Bayard Boyd and Jane Bayard Kirkpatrick, 2 August 1826, *Margaret Bayard Smith Papers*, Library of Congress. Smith was thus favorably comparing the university's library to the Library of Congress, which at this time still largely consisted of volumes that Jefferson sold to the nation in 1815 and which Smith had herself seen at Monticello in 1809 (*PTJRS*, 1:389–390).
12. Patten, *Jefferson, Cabell and UVA*, 262 and "A Short Story," 425–426.
13. On 30 September 1826, the Proctor reported to the Rector and Board of Visitors that he had paid $35,947.38 for library materials and other teaching apparatus. This figure may not have included the $6,000 allotted to Francis W. Gilmer for the purchase and transportation cost of library books acquired while he was recruiting European professors in 1824. Adding that would boost the total to almost $42,000.
14. The principal sources for the early history of the University of Virginia's first medical library are the catalogue that Dunglison had printed in 1828, *Catalogue of the Library of the University of Virginia Arranged Alphabetically Under Different Heads, with the Number and Size of the Volumes of Each Work, and its Edition Specified* (reproduced in another, more accessible publication: Peden, *1828 Catalogue of the Library of the University of Virginia*, 50–67) and Cometti, ed., *Jefferson's Ideas on a University Library*, 19–49.
15. Dunglison, *The Medical Student*, vii.
16. Cometti, ed., *Jefferson's Ideas on a University Library*, 22–23. Jefferson's original list of medical works included a total of 662 volumes and 329 titles. By comparison, the revised list of 1828 included 710 volumes and 435 titles, not counting 84 volumes and 44 titles under the Chemistry heading.
17. Bruce, *History of UVA*, 2:204.
18. Clemons, *University of Virginia Library*, 14.
19. "University of Virginia Library List of Books Borrowed, 1825–1827," University of Virginia Library, Special Collections.
20. Dorsey, *Jefferson-Dunglison Letters*, 14–16, 18–30 and Jefferson to Robert Greenhow, 29 April 1825, Library of Congress: *The Thomas Jefferson Papers*, https://www.loc.gov/item/mtjbib025385/.
21. Jefferson referred to it as a "Theatre." See *Encyclopedia Virginia*, https://encyclopediavirginia.org/entries.anatomival–thretre/.
22. Dorsey, *Jefferson-Dunglison Letters*, 17–31.
23. Robert Greenhow to Jefferson, 22 March 1825, Library of Congress: *The Thomas Jefferson Papers*, https://www.loc.gov/item/mtjbib025328/.

24. Dunglison to Jefferson, [ca. 21 May 1825], Library of Congress: *The Thomas Jefferson Papers*, https://www.loc.gov/item/mtjbib025412/, available in Dorsey, *Jefferson–Dunglison Letters*, 14–16.
25. Dunglison was a strong proponent of such correlations; specifically, the need to compare pathological findings carefully with the symptoms and signs of disease that preceded death. He lamented the prejudice against examination of bodies after death and encouraged "an exertion of fortitude and philanthropy for its removal." See *Dunglison's Valedictory Lecture*, 5–6, and his Address to the Graduates in Medicine of the University of Maryland, 19 March 1834, 9–10.
26. Report from the Board of Visitors to the President and Directors of the Literary Fund, 3–7 October 1825, University of Virginia. Correspondence between Jefferson and Robert Greenhow of New York dated 8 and 22 March; 14, 23, and 29 April; 22 May; and 16 and 22 June 1825; letters from Jefferson to Granville Sharp Pattison of Baltimore, 12 March 1824 and 12 March 1825; and to Thomas Calloway of London and Rufus King, U.S. ambassador to Great Britain, both dated 28 July 1825. All of these letters are in Library of Congress: *The Thomas Jefferson Papers*. See also Dorsey, *Jefferson-Dunglison Letters*, 17–30.
27. Robert Greenhow to Jefferson, 22 March 1825, Library of Congress: *The Thomas Jefferson Papers*, https://www.loc.gov/item/mtjbib025328/.
28. Dorsey, *Jefferson-Dunglison Letters*, 16, 19.
29. For example, John Collins Warren of Harvard Medical School donated his collection of anatomical and pathological specimens to the college in 1847 (the Warren Anatomical Museum); Thomas Dent Mutter, a surgeon at Jefferson Medical College, presented his collection to the College of Physicians of Philadelphia in 1858, thus founding the Mutter Museum; and in 1820, the Medical College of Maryland (founded in 1807) purchased a large collection from Granville Sharp Pattison. The oldest anatomical museum in North America was housed in Philadelphia's Pennsylvania Hospital. William Pepper, *Descriptive Catalogue of the Pathological Museum of the Pennsylvania Hospital* (Philadelphia: Collins Printers, 1869).
30. Stephen C. Kenny, "The Development of Medical Museums in the Antebellum American South: Slave Bodies in Networks of Anatomical Exchange," *Bulletin of the History of Medicine* 87, no. 1 (2013): 32–62.
31. "Rockfish Gap Report of the University of Virginia Commissioners," 14 August 1818, *PTJRS*, 13:209–224. See also Jefferson to Joseph C. Cabell, 11 January 1825, in Cabell, ed., *Early History of the University of Virginia*, 330–332.
32. Dorsey, *Jefferson-Dunglison Letters*, 16.
33. The medical library of the University of Virginia contained 44 different titles of anatomy books, including works by William Cheselden of Boston, Charles Bell of London, Alexander Monro III and John Lizars of Edinburgh, Xavier Bichat and Jules Cloquet of Paris, and Friedrich Tiedemann of Heidelberg.
34. See Jefferson to James Madison, 30 April 1823, *PTJRS*, 3:47–48 and Radbill, ed., "Autobiographical Ana," 24, n23.
35. Jefferson to Joseph C. Cabell, 11 January and 3 February 1825, in Cabell, ed., *Early History of the University of Virginia*, 330–332, 339–341.
36. Honeywell, *Educational Work of Thomas Jefferson*, 85.
37. Minutes of the Board of Visitors of the University of Virginia, 4–5 March 1825.
38. Puzio, "Anatomical Theatre."
39. Dunglison later recalled that Jefferson agreed on the need for a building dedicated to anatomical purposes, with Jefferson to "choose the position and the architec-

tural arrangement externally, whilst all the interior arrangements should be left to me." See Radbill, ed., "Autobiographical Ana," 23.

40. Corner, *Two Centuries of Medicine*, 50; Puzio, "Anatomical Theatre"; John C. Van Horne et al., eds., *The Correspondence and Miscellaneous Papers of Benjamin Henry Latrobe* (New Haven: Yale University Press, 1984–1988), 2:408–411.
41. Jefferson to Joseph C. Cabell, 4 February 1826, in Cabell, ed., *Early History of the University of Virginia*, 363–364; Jefferson to Arthur S. Brockenbrough, 7 April 1826, Library of Congress: *The Thomas Jefferson Papers*, https://www.loc.gov/item/mtjbib025695/; Dunglison to Jefferson, 21 May 1826, in Dorsey, *Jefferson-Dunglison Letters*, 65–66; Dunglison to Brockenbrough, 8 September 1826. See also Minutes of the University of Virginia Board of Visitors, 10 July 1827.
42. Dunglison, *The Medical Student*, 137, 149.
43. Harvey E. Jordan, *History of the School of Medicine of the University of Virginia* (Charlottesville, 1952), 15; Lauren Massari, Institute for Advanced Technology (IATH) of the University of Virginia, email to the author, 25 September 2017; Minutes of the University of Virginia Board of Visitors, 10 July 1833 and 17 August 1837.
44. Ernie Gates, "Theatre of the Macabre," *Virginia Magazine*, Spring 2017.
45. Blanton, *Medicine in Virginia in the Nineteenth Century*, 69–73; Bruce, *History of UVA*, 2:111–113; Frederick C. Waite, "Grave Robbing in New England," *Bulletin of the Medical Library Association* 33, no. 3 (1945): 279; Savitt, *Medicine and Slavery*, 282, 291–292 and "Use of Blacks for Medical Experimentation and Demonstration in the Old South," *The Journal of Southern History* 48, no. 3 (1982): 332; James O. Breeden, Body Snatchers and Anatomy Professors: Medical Education in Nineteenth-Century Virginia," *Virginia Magazine of History and Biography* 83, no. 3 (1975): 337–338; Robert L. Blakely and Judith M. Harrington, eds., *Bones in the Basement: Postmortem Racism in Nineteenth-Century Medical Training* (Washington, D.C.: Smithsonian Institution Press, 1998); Kenny, "Development of Medical Museums," 50.
46. John B. Blake, "The development of American Anatomy laws," *Journal of Medical Education* 30, no. 8 (1955): 431–439 and Edward C. Halperin, "The Poor, the Black, and the Marginalized as the Source of Cadavers in United States Anatomical Education," *Clinical Anatomy* 20, no. 5 (2007): 490.
47. Breeden, "Body Snatchers," 321, 344; Waite, "Grave Robbing in New England," 272–294; Halperin, "The Poor, the Black, and the Marginalized," 489–495; Raphael Hulkower, "From Sacrilege to Privilege: The Tale of Body Procurement for Anatomical Dissection in the United States," *Einstein Journal of Biology and Medicine* 27, no. 1 (2011): 23–26. See also Sappol, *A Traffic of Dead Bodies* and Daina R. Berry, *The Price for their Pound of Flesh: The Value of the Enslaved, from Womb to Grave, in the Building of a Nation* (Boston: Beacon Press, 2017).
48. For contrasting views, see Todd Savitt, "Use of Blacks for Medical Experimentation," 332; and Kirt von Daacke, "Anatomical Theater," in Maurie D. McInnis and Louis P. Nelson, eds., *Educated in Tyranny: Slavery at Thomas Jefferson's University* (Charlottesville: University of Virginia Press, 2019), 171–198. The latter opinion is also advanced in "President's Commission on Slavery and the University," Report to President Teresa Sullivan, 2018, 44–52.
49. Waite, "Grave Robbing in New England," as cited by Halperin, "The Poor, the Black, and the Marginalized," 493; Hulkower, "From Sacrilege to Privilege," 24; Kenny, "Development of Medical Museums," 55, figure 3.

50. Dunglison's views on medical education were widely disseminated through his published writings, most notably in: College Instruction and Discipline," 283–314 and *The Medical Student, or Aids to the Study of Medicine*, 1837 (323 pages) and 1844 (311 pages). Other sources include *Dunglison's Valedictory Lecture*; *An Introductory Lecture to the Medical Class of the University of Maryland, 31 October 1833* (Baltimore: John D. Toy, Printer); *Address to the Graduates: An Address to the Medical Graduates of the Jefferson Medical College, 11 March 1837* (Philadelphia: Adam Waldie, Printer); *Introductory Lecture to the Course of Institutes of Medicine in Jefferson Medical College* (Philadelphia: William Geddes, Printer, 1839); and other keynote lectures at the Jefferson Medical College, dated 8 November 1843, 25 March 1847, 19 October 1848, 4 March 1854, 8 October 1860, and 10 March 1864.
51. Dunglison, *The Medical Student*, 141.
52. Garrison, *An Introduction to the History of Medicine*, 500; Mayo, "Robley Dunglison: 1798–1869," 709; Radbill, "Dr. Robley Dunglison and Jefferson," 40.
53. Radbill, ed., "Autobiographical Ana," 35.
54. *Dunglison's Valedictory Lecture*, quoted in Radbill, ed., "Autobiographical Ana," 61.
55. Jefferson to Dunglison, 26 November 1825, in Dorsey, *Jefferson-Dunglison Letters*, 47–48; Minutes of the Board of Visitors of the University of Virginia, 3–7 October 1825, 3–7 April 1826, University of Virginia. Around this time, other medical schools were also operating dispensaries or outpatient clinics as a means of providing their students "daily contact with injuries and diseases seen by the general practitioner." Dale C. Smith, "The Emergence of Organized Clinical Instruction in Nineteenth Century Cities of Boston, New York, and Philadelphia," PhD diss., University of Minnesota, 1979, 168.
56. Dorsey, *Jefferson-Dunglison Letters*, 47–48.
57. Dunglison, *The Medical Student*, 46–47.
58. Corner, *Two Centuries of Medicine*, 72–73.
59. Jefferson to William G. Munford, 18 June 1799, *PTJ*, 31:126–130 and to John D. Crawford, 2 January 1812, *PTJRS*, 4:394–395; *Dunglison's Valedictory Lecture*, 8; Dunglison's Introductory Lecture to the Medical Class of the University of Maryland, 31 October 1833, 14–15; Dunglison's 1836 textbook, *General Therapeutics*, 52; *The Medical Student*, 160.
60. Bruce, *History of UVA*, 2:172–173.
61. Dunglison, "College Instruction and Discipline," 310.
62. Dunglison, *The Medical Student*, 143–148.
63. Jefferson made this point very well in the "Rockfish Gap Report," 212–214.
64. *Dunglison's Valedictory Lecture*, 13.
65. The major works that Dunglison published or began during his eight years in Charlottesville were *Syllabus of Lecture on Medical Jurisprudence* (1827); "College Instruction and Discipline" (1831, 31 pages); the first American textbook on *Human Physiology* (1832; 1,058 pages); and *A New Dictionary of Medical Science and Literature* (1833; 1,239 pages) which contained more than 30,000 medical terms with accompanying explanations. Other lesser-known works were essays on *Longevity*, *Infirmities of Men of Genius*, *Gastronomy of the Romans*, and *Popular Superstitions*.
66. Dunglison, *The Medical Student*, 10, 49–54, 104–108.
67. Radbill, "Robley Dunglison, M.D.," 84–93.
68. *Dunglison's Valedictory Lecture*; *Journal of the Chairman* and Meeting Minutes of

the Faculty, http://juel.iath.virginia.edu/resources; Brendan Wolfe, "Slavery at the University of Virginia," *Encyclopedia Virginia*, https://encyclopediavirginia.org/entries/slavery–at–the–university–of–virginia/; "President's Commission on Slavery and the University"; McInnis and Nelson, eds., *Educated in Tyranny*.

69. Gross, *Memoir of Robley Dunglison*, 11, read before the College of Physicians at a Special Meeting held 20 October 1869.
70. Dunglison, "College Instruction and Discipline, " 306–307, 310–313 and *The Medical Student*, 180–182.
71. Minutes of the Board of Visitors of the University of Virginia, 3–7 October 1825, University of Virginia. See also Kett, "Education," 238; Bruce, *History of UVA*, 2:129; and Dunglison, *The Medical Student*, 146, 181.
72. Ludmerer, *Learning to Heal*, 3, 12; Rothstein, *American Medical Schools*, 32; Dunglison, "College Instruction and Discipline, " 310–311.
73. Blanton, *Medicine in Virginia in the Eighteenth Century*, 19 and Smith, *Addresses Commemorative of James L. Cabell, July 1, 1890* (Charlottesville: Chronicle & C. M. Brand, 1890), 19.
74. Dunglison, College Instruction and Discipline, " 312–313; University of Virginia, *Journal of the Chairman*, Minutes of 27 April 1829; Nathan S. Smith, *History of Medical Education and Institutions in the United States* (Chicago: S.C. Griggs & Co., 1851), 185–190.
75. Dunglison, "College Instruction and Discipline," 302–310.
76. Paul B. Barringer, "A History of the Medical Department of the University of Virginia: Its System of Education, and its Results," *North Carolina Medical Journal* 20 (1887): 285.
77. Dunglison, "Valedictory Address Delivered to the Medical Class of the University of Virginia," 1833, 15–17, and *The Medical Student*, 225–226; John Gregory, *Lectures on the Duties and Qualifications of a Physician*—first published in 1772 and republished in 1817 in Philadelphia; Percival, *Medical Ethics; or A Code of Institutes and Precepts, adapted to the Professional Conduct of Physicians and Surgeons* (Manchester: S. Russell, 1803).
78. *Dunglison's Valedictory Lecture*, 12, 14–17 and *The Medical Student*, 8–9.
79. Gert H. Brieger, "Fit to Study Medicine: Notes for a History of Premedical Education in America," *Bulletin of the History of Medicine* 57 (1983): 121 and Daniel Drake, *Practical Essays on Medical Education and the Medical Profession in the United States* (Cincinnati: Roff and Young, 1832), 6.
80. Radbill, ed., "Autobiographical Ana," 48–49, 111–118, 135–136; *Dunglison's Valedictory Lecture*, 6–7; Dunglison, *The Medical Student*, 255–262; Bonner, *Becoming a Physician*, 152.
81. *Dunglison's Valedictory Lecture*, 6–7; Radbill, "Robley Dunglison, M.D.," 84–94; William Bennett Bean, "Jefferson's Influence on American Medical Education," *Virginia Medical Monthly* 87 (1960): 669–680; Grover C. Pitts, "History of Physiology at the University of Virginia," *The Physiologist* 28, no. 5 (1985): 402–403.
82. The 1828 *Catalogue of the Library of the University of Virginia* contained 32 titles and 56 volumes in the physiology section. European scientists wrote 98 percent of the holdings. The only American title included was *A Comparative View of the Sensorial and Nervous Systems of Men and Animals* by Dr. John Collins Warren (1778–1856) of Boston.
83. Corner, *Two Centuries of Medicine*, 73, 75; *Dunglison's Valedictory Lecture*, 7; *The Medical Student*, 48, 111–118, 134, 148, 157–158.

84. Dunglison, *The Medical Student,* 48–49.
85. Moll, "University of Virginia's 'Firsts,'" 158–161 and Radbill, "Robley Dunglison, M.D.," 84–94. For Dunglison's philosophy on teaching history and its value, see *Dunglison's Valedictory Lecture*, 7–13 and *The Medical Student*, 176–180.
86. Dunglison, *The Medical Student,* 17, and Radbill, "Robley Dunglison, M.D.," 93.
87. This emphasis is clearly reflected in the 1828 library catalogue. More than 1,300 of the approximately 8,000 volumes were devoted to historical subjects—ancient, modern, and natural history; histories of mathematics, natural philosophy, botany, chemistry, medicine, zoology, mineralogy, and geology; ecclesiastical history; and histories of mental philosophy, ethics, education, and even the female sex.
88. Eugene F. Cordell, "The Importance of the Study of the History of Medicine," *Medical Library and Historical Journal* 2, no. 4 (1904), 272.
89. Robley Dunglison, *History of Medicine: From the Earliest Ages to the Commencement of the Nineteenth Century*, Richard J. Dunglison, ed. (Philadelphia: Lindsay and Blakiston, 1872), iii–iv and Cordell, "The Importance of the Study of the History of Medicine," 270–272.
90. Dunglison, *History of Medicine*, iv.
91. Hermann F. Kilian, *Die Universitaeten Deutschlands in medicinisch–naturwissenschaftlicher Hinsicht betrachtet* (translated, The Universities of Germany in terms of medicine and science), Heidelberg-Leipzig, 1828 and Guenter B. Risse, "Sprengel, Kurt Polycarp Joachim," https://www.encyclopedia.com/science/dictionaries–thesauruses–pictures–and–press–releases/sprengel–kurt–polycarp–joachim.
92. Dunglison, "College Instruction and Discipline" 307.
93. Dunglison, *History of Medicine*, 117–125.
94. Dunglison, *The Medical Student*, 179 and Cordell, "The Importance of the Study of the History of Medicine," 277.
95. *Dunglison's Valedictory Lecture*, 7–13 and *The Medical Student*, 177–178.
96. Gross, *Memoir of Robley Dunglison*, 294–313.
97. Dunglison, "College Instruction and Discipline, " 283–314; *Dunglison's Valedictory Lecture*, 12; *The Medical Student*; and his many introductory and commencement lectures given to students at the University of Virginia and Jefferson Medical College.
98. Dunglison was quoting a statement made by Dr. Anthony Todd Thomson (1778–1849) in his 1828 *Thoughts on Medical Education: A Plan for Improvement*, addressed to the Council of the University of London, Temple Printing Office. Dunglison, *The Medical Student*, 28–29 and his *Autobiographical Ana*, 155, 197.
99. Dunglison, *The Medical Student*, 29.
100. Ibid., 183–184.
101. Dunglison, *Introductory Lecture to Jefferson Medical College*, 14.
102. Dunglison, *The Medical Student*, 183.
103. Ibid., 163–168, 188.
104. Emmet had previously chaired the natural history department. In 1827, when Charles Bonnycastle assumed that post, Emmet was able to devote himself entirely to the medical department and to the teaching of chemistry, materia medica, and pharmacy.
105. For details on Dunglison's expectations for this course, see *The Medical Student*, 166–167.
106. Barringer, *History, Influence, Equipment and Characteristics*, 24.
107. Chester R. Burns,"Medical Ethics and Jurisprudence," in Numbers, ed., *The Edu-*

cation of American Physicians, 276–289.
108. Radbill, ed., "Autobiographical Ana," 36.
109. Robley Dunglison, *Syllabus of the Lectures on Medical Jurisprudence and on the Treatment of Poisoning and Suspended Animation* (Charlottesville: University of Virginia, 1827).
110. Dunglison, *The Medical Student*, 169–170.
111. P. M. Dunn, "William Potts Dewees (1768–1841) of Pennsylvania: Pioneer of Perinatal Medicine in America," *Archives of Diseases of Children and Fetal Neonatal Education* 75, no. 1 (1996): 69–70; the 1828 *Catalogue of the Library of the University of Virginia* that Dunglison assembled; also Baudelocque's *The Art of Midwifery* (Paris, 1822); Capuron's *Course of Midwifery* (Paris, 1823); Gardien's *Treatise on Midwifery* (Paris, 1824); Maygrier's *Plates on Midwifery, with Descriptions* (Paris, 1825); Blumdell's *Syllabus of Lectures on Midwifery* (London, 1821); Conquest's *On Obstetric Instruments and the Use of Belladonna in Protracted Labor* (London, 1823); Powers's *Treatise on Midwifery* (London, 1823); and Smellie's *Treatise on Midwifery* (Dublin, 1765).
112. Blanton, *Medicine in Virginia in the Eighteenth Century*, 21.
113. Thomas Addis Emmet, Jr., *Memoir of John Patten Emmet, M.D., formerly Professor of Chemistry and Materia Medica in the University of Virginia, with a brief outline of the Emmet family History* (New York: privately printed, 1898), available at the National Library of Medicine, 11–13; Emmet, Jr., "Memoir of Professor John Patten Emmet," *Alumni Bulletin of the University of Virginia* 1, no. 4 (1895): 93–101; Lisa A. Francavilla, "Emmet, John Patten (1796–1842)," *Encyclopedia Virginia*, https://encyclopediavirginia.org/entries/emmet–john–patten–1796–1842/; B. F. D. Runk, "John Patten Emmet," *Magazine of Albemarle County History* 13 (1953): 54–67; Minutes of the Faculty of the University of Virginia, 6 (1842), 38–39. Emmet's papers are at the University of Virginia, Historical Collection Library.
114. Wyndham D. Miles, "William James MacNeven and Early Laboratory Instruction in the United States," *Ambix* 7, no. 3 (1970) and "Waite Report," 19–21; Jefferson to William James MacNeven, 12 January 1822, Gilder Lehrman Collection, https://www.gilderlehrman.org/collection/glc07148.
115. Bruce, *History of UVA*, 2:16.
116. Emmit, Jr., "Memoir of Professor John Patten Emmet," 94.
117. Daniels, *American Science in the Age of Jackson*, 147–148.
118. Emmet, Jr., *Memoir of John Patten Emmet, M.D.*, 25–26.
119. Jefferson to James Madison, 30 April 1823, *PTJRS*, 3:47–48; to Horace Holley, 5 April 1825, University of Virginia; to John Patten Emmet, 16 May 1825 and 2 May 1826, Library of Congress: *The Thomas Jefferson Papers*, http://hdl.loc.gov/loc.mss/mtj.mtjbib025404 and http://hdl.loc.gov/loc.mss/mtj.mtjbib025719; Gilmer to Jefferson, 3 December 1824, in Davis, *Correspondence of Jefferson and Gilmer*; Emmet to Jefferson, 12 May 1825, Library of Congress: *The Thomas Jefferson Papers*, http://hdl.loc.gov/loc.mss/mtj.mtjbib025400 and 27 May 1826, Huntington Library; Minutes of the Board of Visitors of the University of Virginia, 4–5 October 1824, University of Virginia; Bruce, *History of UVA*, 2:14–16; "Waite Report," 12–13, 65, n25. See also Danny Lewis, "The Oldest Chemistry Lab in America?" *Smithsonian Magazine, SmartNews*, 14 October 2015; Susan Svrluga, "America's first chemistry lab discovered accidentally in a building designed by Thomas Jefferson," *Washington Post*, 13 October 2015, II:41; and Brakkton Booker, "Historic Chemistry Lab with Links to Thomas Jefferson Discovered Behind Wall," *NPR*

Radio, 18 October 2015, 4:38 PM ET.

120. "Waite Report," 21–31.
121. Catalogues of the Officers and Students of the University of Virginia and Emmet to Jefferson, 12 May 1825, Library of Congress: *The Thomas Jefferson Papers*, http://hdl.loc.gov/loc.mss/mtj.mtjbib025400.
122. Charles A. Browne, "The History of Chemical Education in America between the Years 1820 and 1870," *Journal of Chemical Education* 9, no. 4 (1932): 712–713 and "Waite Report," 37.
123. Runk, "John Patten Emmet," 63; Tucker, *Memoir of the Life and Character of John Patten Emmet*, 12; "Waite Report," 58.
124. Emmet, Jr., *Memoir of John Patten Emmet, M.D.*, 56–58.
125. Minutes of the Board of Visitors of the University of Virginia, 4–5 October 1824, University of Virginia. Laboratory experiments and demonstrations occurred in the Lower East Oval Room, with lectures in the Lower West Oval Room. See Lewis, "The Oldest Chemistry Lab in America?"
126. "Waite Report," 53; Tucker, *Memoir of the Life and Character of John Patten Emmet*, 22–23; Emmet, Jr., *Memoir of John Patten Emmet, M.D.*, 38–39.
127. Minutes of the Board of Visitors of the University of Virginia, 16, 17, and 19 July 1827, University of Virginia and Gross, *Memoir of Robley Dunglison*, 12. See also Mayo, "Robley Dunglison: 1798–1869," 709 and Dorsey, *Jefferson-Dunglison Letters*, 87.
128. Norwood, *Medical Education*, 269–273.
129. Blanton, *Medicine in Virginia in the Eighteenth Century*, 46.
130. Charles Christian Wertenbaker, "Early Days of the University," *Alumni Bulletin of the University of Virginia* 4, no. 1 (1897): 22.
131. *A Sketch of the History of the University of Virginia, together with A Catalogue of the Professors and Instructors, the Graduates in Law and Medicine since the Foundation of the Institution* (Charlottesville: Chronicle Steam Book and Job Printing House, 1880). See also *Catalogue of the University of Virginia, 1825–1900* and Schele De-Vere's *Semi Centennial Catalogue with Sketches of Student Matriculants, 1835–1875*.
132. John Albert Broadus, *A Memorial of Gessner Harrison, M.D., Professor of Ancient Languages in the University of Virginia* (Charlottesville: Chronicle Steam Printing House, 1874); Brian Neumann, "Harrison, Gessner (1807–1862)," *Encyclopedia Virginia.* https://encyclopediavirginia.org/entries/harrison–gessner–1807–1862.
133. Blanton, *Medicine in Virginia in the Eighteenth Century*, 19–21. See also *Alumni Bulletin of the University of Virginia* 4 (1897): 79 and Bruce, *History of UVA*, 2:109.
134. Kaufman, "American Medical Education," in Numbers, ed., *The Education of American Physicians*, 11.
135. Norwood, *Medical Education*, 267.
136. Kaufman, "American Medical Education," in Numbers, ed., *The Education of American Physicians*, 15–16.
137. Gayle M. Schulman, "Slaves at the University of Virginia," unpublished paper presented to the African-American Genealogy Group of Charlottesville/Albemarle, May 2003; Catherine S. Neale, "Slaves, Freed people, and the University of Virginia," Undergraduate Honors Thesis, Corcoran Department of History, University of Virginia, April 2006; McInnis and Nelson, eds., *Educated in Tyranny*, 2019.
138. Schulman, "Slaves at the University of Virginia," 27, n17; Catherine A. Creighton, "Pavilion X: A Brief History (1820–1895)," http://juel.iath.virginia.edu/resources.

139. Schulman, "Slaves at the University of Virginia," 4; Dunglison to Thomas J. Randolph, University of Virginia Special Collections: *Randolph Family Papers*, Box 2, Folder 10; "Account of Sale of Slaves from Thomas Jefferson's Estate," 1 January 1829, https://www.monticello.org/slaveauction/.
140. Neale, "Slaves, Freedpeople, and the University of Virginia," 78 and Ian Iverson, "The Enslaved Workers of Pavilion X," http://juel.iath.virginia.edu/resources. The professor of modern languages, George Blaettermann, owned 18 enslaved African Americans in 1830. McInnis and Nelson, eds., *Educated in Tyranny*, 74, n10.
141. Schulman, "Slaves at the University of Virginia," 15–16.
142. Radbill, ed., "Autobiographical Ana," 43.
143. Dunglison's consultation and treatment of Jackson occurred in June 1833 while Dunglison was visiting Washington, D.C.
144. Minutes of the Board of Visitors of the University of Virginia, 3–7 April 1826, University of Virginia.
145. Savitt, *Medicine and Slavery*, 189, 283.
146. Bean, "Mr. Jefferson's Influence on American Medical Education," 673. See also Radbill, ed., "Autobiographical Ana," 7–9 and I. Richmond, "Robley Dunglison, M.D.," *Pennsylvania Medicine* 69 (1966): 76–77.
147. Radbill, "Dr. Robley Dunglison and Jefferson," 40–44, 80 and *Dunglison's Valedictory Lecture*, 8–10.
148. This visit occurred on 17 May 1825. During the next two weeks, Dunglison made eight professional visits to the ailing Jefferson. Radbill, ed., "Autobiographical Ana," 26; "Jefferson's Record of Dunglison's Visits," 17 May–20 September 1825, Library of Congress: *The Thomas Jefferson Papers*, https://www.loc.gov/resource/mtj1.055_0106_0108/?sp=1.
149. Robley Dunglison, *A New Dictionary of Medical Science and Literature, Containing a Concise Account of the Various Subjects and Terms with the Synonymes [sic] in Different Languages and Formulae for Various Official and Empirical Preparations* (Boston, 1833), 13.
150. Radbill, ed., "Autobiographical Ana," 26.
151. "Jefferson's Record of Dunglison's Visits."
152. Jefferson to Robley Dunglison, 2 and 4 July, 17 and 26 November 1825, in Dorsey, *Jefferson-Dunglison Letters*, 34–35, 36, 41–43, 44–45.
153. Dunglison to Jefferson, 2 July and 18 November 1825, in Dorsey, *Jefferson-Dunglison Letters*, 35, 43.
154. Wilhelm Moll, "Medical Fee Bills," *Virginia Medical Monthly* 94 (1966): 657–664. See the Fredericksburg *Virginia Herald*, 11 September 1816 and http://blog.hsl.virginia.edu/feebill/ for Charlottesville fee schedules for 1816 and 1848, which allow for conjecture on the amount of money that Dunglison sacrificed by work he did gratis.
155. Bear and Stanton, eds., *Jefferson's Memorandum Books*, 1414, entry for 27 November 1825.
156. William Short to Jefferson, 27 June 1825, Massachusetts Historical Society; Jefferson to Short, 9 August 1825, College of William and Mary, https://digitalarchive.wm.edu/handle/10288/15125.
157. Lee presumably made his offensive comment directly to the family, after which he summarized his visit in a letter that appeared in the *Richmond Enquirer*. Radbill, ed., "Autobiographical Ana," 32, 34.
158. Radbill, ed., "Autobiographical Ana," 32. See also Dunglison to James Madison, 1

July 1826, in Dorsey, *Jefferson-Dunglison Letters*, 66–67.

159. George Tucker, *The Life of Thomas Jefferson, Third President of the United States*, 2 vols. (London: Charles Knight & Co., 1848), 2:552 and Radbill, ed., "Autobiographical Ana," 32.
160. Radbill, ed., "Autobiographical Ana," 32, 34.
161. Thomas Jefferson to James Madison, 17 February 1826, *PTJRS*, 3:355–356.
162. "Memoranda of Dr. Robley Dunglison on the Last Words of Jefferson." Radbill, ed., "Autobiographical Ana," 32–33; "Philadelphia Public Ledger," quoted in *Alumni Bulletin of the University of Virginia* 6 (1894–1900): 79–80. See also Bean, "Mr. Jefferson's Influence on American Medical Education," 672 and Randall, *Life of Jefferson*, 512–519, 547–549, 670–671.
163. On 3 July, Jefferson's abdominal pain was of sufficient concern that Dunglison prescribed laudanum (a tincture of opium with associated alkaloids, including morphine and codeine) and from that point forward, Jefferson was comfortable but stuporous. In a letter to David Hosack, 13 August 1826, Thomas Mann Randolph mentioned that Dunglison had previously recommended daily use of opium for several months leading up to Jefferson's death, *Thomas Jefferson's Monticello*, https://tjrs.monticello.org/letter/463.
164. Radbill, ed., "Autobiographical Ana," 32. See also "Thomas Jefferson Randolph's Account of Thomas Jefferson's Death," *Thomas Jefferson's Monticello*, https://tjrs.monticello.org/letter/1896.
165. Karl C. Wold, *Mr. President, how is your health?* (Milwaukee: Bruce, 1948), 31, 200–211.
166. Russel L. Martin, "Jefferson's Cause of Death," *Thomas Jefferson Encyclopedia*, May 1990; Wold, *Mr. President, how is your health?*, 31; Dorsey, *Jefferson-Dunglison Letters*, 66–67; Marx, *The Health of the Presidents*, 64; James A. Bear, "The Last Few Days in the Life of Thomas Jefferson," *Magazine of Albemarle County History* 32 (1974): 63–79.
167. Radbill, ed., "Autobiographical Ana," 41–42. For the efforts to care for the sick and control the spread of the infection, see Faculty Minutes for 22, 26, 29, and 31 January 1829; 6, 20, 25, and 26 February 1829; and 12 and 14 March 1829, http://juel.iath.virginia.edu/resources; "To the Editors of the Enquirer," *Richmond Enquirer*, 10 March 1829; Bruce, *History of UVA*, 2:243.
168. John V. Ashurst, Justina Truong, and Blair Woodbury, *Salmonella Typni*, 2020, https://www.ncbi.nlm.nih.gov/books/NBK519002/.
169. Dunglison discussed the outbreak in an article on "The Salubrity of The University" published in the *Virginia Literary Museum* on 17 June 1829, and in two of his major textbooks: *Elements of Hygiene* (1835) and *The Practice of Medicine* (1842), 2:544. Radbill, ed., "Autobiographical Ana," 41–42.
170. Bruce, *History of UVA*, 2:244 and Radbill, ed., "Autobiographical Ana," 42.
171. Barringer, Garrett, and Page, eds., *History, Influence, Equipment and Characteristics*, 147.
172. Bruce, *History of UVA*, 2:240–241; Faculty Minutes, 22 January and 6 February 1829, http://juel.iath.virginia.edu/resources; Matt Kelly, "The Past as Prologue: How UVA has Risen to Meet Crises Throughout History," *UVA Today*, 3 April 2020.
173. Faculty Minutes, 22 January 1829.
174. Radbill, ed., "Autobiographical Ana," 42.
175. Faculty Minutes, 12 March 1829, http://juel.iath.virginia.edu/resources and

Bruce, *History of UVA*, 2:244.
176. Faculty Minutes, 26 January, 6 February, and 14 March 1829, http://juel.iath.virginia.edu/resources.
177. Faculty Minutes, 25 February 1829 and *Chairman's Journal*, 26 February, 6 and 15 March 1829, http://juel.iath.virginia.edu/resources.
178. Faculty Minutes, 12 March 1829.
179. Norfolk *Southern Argus*, 3 December 1858, text quoted in full in Radbill, ed., "Autobiographical Ana," 174–175.
180. Dunglison to Madison, 10 and 19 March 1830, requested permission to publish this dedication, Library of Congress: *The James Madison Papers*, https://www.loc.gov/item/mjm020397/ and https://www.loc.gov/resource/mjm.23_0077_0077/.
181. Radbill, ed., "Autobiographical Ana," 48–50, 57, 111, 147–148.
182. Samuel W. Gross and Albert Haller Gross, eds., *Autobiography of Samuel D. Gross, M.D. with Sketches of His Contemporaries* (Philadelphia: G. Barrie, 1887), 329–335.
183. Gross, *Memoir of Robley Dunglison*, 294–313.
184. *Silliman's Journal* 64 (1833): 165.
185. Radbill, ed., "Autobiographical Ana," 49.
186. Ibid., 44–47, 55, 147–148.
187. Gross and Gross, eds., *Autobiography of Samuel D. Gross, M.D.*, 2:330.
188. Cushing, *The Life of Sir William Osler*, 1:238 and Dorsey, *Jefferson-Dunglison Letters*, 85.
189. Gross, *Memoir of Robley Dunglison*, 294–313.
190. Radbill, ed., "Autobiographical Ana," 43.
191. Ibid., 43.
192. Correspondence quoted in Jesse Shire Myer, *Life and Letters of Dr. William Beaumont: Including Hitherto Unpublished Data Concerning the Case of Alexis St. Martin* (St. Louis: C.V. Mosby, 1912) (original publication, updated 1939), 151, 157–168. See also Dunglison's 1832 edition of *Human Physiology* (1832), 476–500, where he discussed gastric physiology.
193. John Duffy, *From Humors to Medical Science* (2nd ed.) (Urbana: University of Illinois Press, 1993), 110; Jerome J. Bylebyl, "William Beaumont, Robley Dunglison, and the Philadelphia Physiologists," *Journal of the History of Medicine and Applied Sciences* 25 (1970): 3–21; Shryock, *Development of Modern Medicine*, 131.
194. Radbill, ed., "Autobiographical Ana," 50–53.
195. Kenneth R. Crispell, "Beaumont and Dunglison: Who was Dunglison?," *Transactions of the American Clinical and Climatological Association* 92 (1981): 194–198; Radbill, ed., "Autobiographical Ana," 52, n15; Myer, *Life and Letters of Dr. William Beaumont*, 216, 219.
196. "Tribute to Dr. John P. Emmett," *Proceedings of the Faculty of The University of Virginia* 6 (1842): 38–39; Chalmers L. Gemmill, "John Patten Emmet, M.D.," in *Pharmacology at the University of Virginia School of Medicine* (Charlottesville: University of Virginia Press, 1966), 27–37; Thomas Addis Emmet, Jr., *Biographical Sketch of Professor John Patten Emmet, M.D.*; Tucker, *Memoir of the Life and Character of John Patten Emmet*.
197. Minutes of the Board of Visitors of the University of Virginia, 5–16 December 1826, University of Virginia; Bruce, *History of UVA*, 2:48–52, 132.
198. Minutes of the Faculty Meetings of the University of Virginia, 1825–1834, https://juel.iath.virginia.edu.

199. Bruce, *History of UVA*, 2:34, 83–84, 148, 157–159; and John S. Patton, "History of Faculty Chairmen of the University of Virginia," *Alumni Bulletin of the University of Virginia* 4, no. 4 (1904): 266.
200. Minutes of the Board of Visitors of the University of Virginia, 10 July 1827, University of Virginia.
201. Dunglison, "College Instruction and Discipline," 289–291.
202. Ibid., 292–293.
203. Bruce, *History of UVA*, 2:258–266; Radbill, ed., "Autobiographical Ana," 29–30; Dunglison, "College Instruction and Discipline," 293–301.
204. *Journal of the Chairman*, minutes of meetings on 2, 3, 5, 6, and 14 October 1825; Minutes of the Board of Visitors of the University of Virginia, 3–7 October 1825, University of Virginia.
205. Wagoner, *Jefferson and Education*, 142–143 and Wagoner, "Honor and Dishonor at Mr. Jefferson's University," 155–180. See also Tucker, *The Life of Thomas Jefferson*, 2:480–481 and Rex Bowman and Carlos Santos, *Rot, Riot, and Rebellion: Mr. Jefferson's Struggle to Save the University that Changed America* (Charlottesville: University of Virginia Press, 2013), 33–41.
206. Dunglison to the Board of Visitors of the University of Virginia, 1 October 1825, with enclosed faculty resolution, in Dorsey, *Jefferson-Dunglison Letters*, 39–41.
207. Jefferson to Henry Tompkinson (a.k.a Samuel Kercheval), 12 July 1816, *PTJRS*, 10:226–227.
208. Wagoner, *Jefferson and Education*, 142–143.
209. Dunglison to the rector and visitors of the University of Virginia, 3 April 1826, University of Virginia, in Dorsey, *Jefferson–Dunglison Letters*, 54–58 and Dunglison, "College Instruction and Discipline," 308.
210. Radbill, ed., "Autobiographical Ana," 39, n84 and Davis, *Correspondence of Jefferson and Gilmer*, 19, n5.
211. Jefferson to the Faculty of the University of Virginia, 7 April 1826, in Dorsey, *Jefferson-Dunglison Letters*, 59–60.
212. Radbill, ed., "Autobiographical Ana," 36 and Dunglison, "College Instruction and Discipline" 308.
213. Harvard University, Annual report of the President (Charles Eliot) and Treasurer of Harvard College (1979–80), 33. See also Charles Eliot, "Public Health Service," *Harvard Alumni Bulletins*, 29 January 1925, 527.
214. Dunglison, *The Medical Student*, 11, 15.
215. Ibid., 17. This quote was extracted from Chitty's *Practical Treatise on Medical Jurisprudence* (Philadelphia: Carey, Lea & Blanchard, 1835), 11.
216. Radbill, ed., "Autobiographical Ana," 36; Dunglison, "College Instruction and Discipline," 308 and *The Medical Student*, 18.
217. Minutes of the Board of Visitors of the University of Virginia, 10 July 1828. Such advertisements were to be issued "under the direction of the Chairman of the Faculty."
218. Meeting Minutes of the Faculty of the University of Virginia, 9 July 1831; Bruce, *History of UVA*, 2:140; Radbill, ed., "Autobiographical Ana," 37.
219. What makes it revolutionary is that for many years thereafter, most schools followed longstanding British tradition and gave this degree out merely as a formality three years after awarding the B.A. J. Jefferson Looney, "The Master's Degree: A Note to Readers," in J. Jefferson Looney and Ruth L. Woodward, eds., *Princetonians, 1791–1794: A Biographical Dictionary* (Princeton, N.J.: Princeton Universi-

ty Press, 1991), 489–490.

220. *A Sketch of the History of the University of Virginia, together with a Catalogue of Professors and Instructors, the Graduates in Law and Medicine, and the Masters and Bachelors of Arts since the Foundation of the Institution* (Washington, D.C.: H. Polkinhorn, 1859), 56–60.
221. Radbill, ed., "Autobiographical Ana," 37 and Bruce, *History of UVA*, 2:172.
222. Letters of inducement from Nathan Ryno Smith, 15 March 1831 and 3 April 1833; Eli Geddings, 26 April 1833; and Nathaniel Potter, 29 April and 8 July 1833 are cited in Radbill, ed., "Autobiographical Ana," 38, 56–60.
223. Dunglison to James Madison, 18 April 1831, Library of Congress: *James Madison Papers*, https://www.loc.gov/item/mjm020924/; Gross, *Memoir of Robley Dunglison*, 6; *Proceedings of the Board of Visitors of the University of Virginia*, 10 July 1833; Radbill, ed., "Autobiographical Ana," 40.
224. Francis W. Gilmer to Thomas Hewett Key, 26 July 1824, in Trent, *English Culture in Virginia*, 75–78.
225. Bruce, *History of UVA*, 2:180–184.
226. Bruce, *History of UVA*, 2:381.
227. Ibid, 381–382.
228. Gross, *Memoir of Robley Dunglison*, 6.
229. Radbill, ed., "Autobiographical Ana," 39, 70; George H. Callcott, *A History of the University of Maryland* (Baltimore: Maryland Historical Society, 1966), 114.
230. Radbill, ed., "Autobiographical Ana," 58, 70.
231. Myer, *Life and Letters of Dr. William Beaumont*, 161, n46.
232. *Dunglison's Valedictory Lecture*, 13.
233. Letter from Robert Y. Conrad to Dr. A. T. Magill, 10 November 1833, quoted in *Alumni Bulletin of the University of Virginia* 4 (1897): 79.

Chapter 6

1. Isaac Newton to Robert Hooke, 5 February 1675 (*Historical Society of Pennsylvania*).
2. Hofstadter, *Academic Freedom in the Age of the College*, 269.
3. Geiger, *History of American Higher Education*, 148; Kaufman, "American Medical Education," in Numbers, ed., *The Education of American Physicians*, 68; Shryock, *Medical Licensing in America*, 27–32; John S. Haller, *American Medicine in Transition, 1840–1910* (Urbana: University of Illinois Press, 1981), 199–203.
4. Sectarian schools promoted alternative modes of healing, often laying claim to some secret formula or gadgetry. Examples include homeopathic, chiropractic (mechano–therapists), botanicomedical, eclectic, and naturopathic schools. Norwood, *Medical Education*, 416–421; Frederick C. Waite, "American Sectarian Medical Colleges before the Civil War," *Bulletin of the History of Medicine* 19, No. 2 (1946): 148–166; Anonymous, "Medical Schools in the United States," *The Journal of the American Medical Association* 51, no. 7 (1908): 575–604; Robert Kenneth Jones, "The Development of Medical Sects," *Journal of Religion and Health* 22, no. 4 (1983): 307–321; John S. Haller, *A Profile in Alternative Medicine* (Kent, OH: Kent State University Press, 1999); *Slawson*, "Medical Training in the United States Prior to the Civil War," 11–27.
5. John Duffy, *The Healers: The Rise of the Medical Establishment* (New York: McGraw-Hill, 1976), 98, 109; Thomas Neville Bonner, *To The Ends of the Earth:*

Women's Search for Education in Medicine (Cambridge: Harvard University Press, 1992).

6. Norwood, *Medical Education*, 380–386; Stephen Smith, *Addresses Commemorative of James L. Cabell* (Charlottesville: Chronicle and C. D. Brand, 1890), 27; Eugene J. F. M. Custers and Olle ten Cate, "The History of Medical Education in Europe and the United States, with Respect to Time and Proficiency," *Academic Medicine* 93, no. 3 (2018 supplement): s49–s54.
7. Rothstein, *American Medical Schools* and Wilhelm Moll, "History of American Medical Education," *British Journal of Medical Education* 2, no. 3 (1968): 173–181.
8. R. H. Fitz, "The Legislative Control of Medical Practice," *Medical Communications of the Massachusetts Medical Society* 16 (1894): 306–307; and Moll, "History of American Medical Education," 173–181.
9. Tuition and added fees in American medical schools were substantially higher than in other college or university departments. When all expenses are aggregated—that is, tuition, matriculation and diploma fees, fees for anatomical dissection and sometimes chemical demonstrations, cost of clinical instruction and living expenses—student costs averaged $300 to $400 for each term; at most schools, only three to four months in length. Costs at UVA were less when the term length of 10+ months is taken into account. Norwood, *Medical Education*, 392–395; Slawson, "Medical Training in the United States Prior to the Civil War," 18–19; Geiger, *History of American Higher Education*, 147; "Catalogue of the Officers and Students of the University of Virginia, Session 1843–44," 23. Kaufman, "American Medical Education," in Numbers, ed., *The Education of American Physicians*, 7–28, 42; James G. Burrow, *Organized Medicine in the Progressive Era: The Move Towards Monopoly* (Baltimore: Johns Hopkins University Press, 1977), 31–32; and J. A. Waddell, "A Study of the Expenditures of Medical Students," *Alumni Bulletin of the University of Virginia* XIV (1921): 160–174.
10. Rothstein, *American Medical Schools*, 52–61; Ludmerer, *Learning to Heal*, 3, 12, 152–155, 219; Davis, *History of Medical Education and Medical Institutions*, 166, 175–176; Edward C. Atwater, "Internal Medicine," in Numbers, ed., *The Education of American Physicians*, 160–163; Bonner, *Becoming a Physician*, 118–119, 132–135; Norwood, *Medical Education*, 398–400; Robert P. Hudson, *Patterns of Medical Education in Nineteenth Century America*, MA Thesis (Baltimore: Johns Hopkins University, 1966).
11. Ludmerer, *Learning to Heal*, 3, 12.
12. Atwater, "Internal Medicine," in Numbers, ed., *The Education of American Physicians*, 160, 164–167; Norwood, *Medical Education*, 368–371; Ludmerer, *Learning to Heal*, 21, 152–155.
13. Shauna Devine, *Learning from the Wounded: The Civil War and the Rise of American Medical Science* (Chapel Hill: University of North Carolina Press, 2014).
14. Ludmerer, *Learning to Heal*, 10–11. See also "Minutes of the Fourteenth Annual Meeting of the American Medical Association," *Transactions of the American Medical Association* 14 (1864): 32 and George Washington Adams, *Doctors in Blue: The Medical History of the Union Army in the Civil War* (Baton Rouge: Louisiana State University Press, 1996), 38–41.
15. For accounts of Dunglison's time in Baltimore and Philadelphia, see Radbill, ed., "Autobiographical Ana," 69–82, 83–185; Eugene F. Cordell, *Historical Sketch of the University of Maryland, School of Medicine (1807–1890)* (Baltimore: Isaac Frie-

denwald, printer, 1891), 76, 124; Callcott, *A History of the University of Maryland*, 67, 116; Larry Pitrof, *University of Maryland School of Medicine: The First Two Centuries, 1807–2007* (Baltimore: Medical Alumni Association of the University of Maryland, 2006), 25–26; Frederick B. Wagner, Jr., *Thomas Jefferson University—Tradition and Heritage* (Philadelphia: Lea & Febiger, 1989); L. M. Rosenfeld, "Physiology at Jefferson Medical College (1842–1982)," *The Physiologist* 27, no. 3 (1984): 113–127; Samuel X. Radbill, "Robley Dunglison: An Eminent Figure in Philadelphia Medicine," *Transactions & Studies of the College of Physicians of Philadelphia* 32, no. 4 (1965): 164–170; Gross, *Memoir of Robley Dunglison*, 3–23.

16. Norwood, *Medical Education*, 382–384 (five classifications of U.S. Medical Schools); 86–93 (Jefferson Medical College); 223–241 (Maryland); and 262–267 (Virginia).
17. Radbill, "Eminent Figure," 166; Radbill, ed., "Autobiographical Ana," 57–58; Gross, *Memoir of Robley Dunglison*, 20; Norwood, *Medical Education*, 240.
18. Cordell, *Historical Sketch*, 15–103; Callcott, *A History of the University of Maryland*, 16–83; Norwood, *Medical Education*, 223–241.
19. Norwood, *Medical Education*, 242–246.
20. Dunglison, *An Introductory Lecture.*
21. Radbill, ed., "Autobiographical Ana," 58.
22. In other lectures and/or publications, Dunglison cited the satirical writings of some of Jefferson's favorites, especially Molière (*L'Amour médecin, Le Malade imaginaire*), Voltaire, and others.
23. These three possibilities derived from Condorcet, and Dunglison may not have taken them all that seriously himself. "Introductory Lecture to the Medical Class of the University of Maryland, 1833," 22–23; and, Dunglison, "Voyage to the Moon," American Quarterly Review, V3, No. 5, 1828, 61–88.
24. *Baltimore Federal Gazette*, 30 May 1833; Radbill,ed., "Autobiographical Ana," 4; Gross, *Memoir of Robley Dunglison*, 10; Callcott, *A History of the University of Maryland*, 116; Pitrof, *University of Maryland School of Medicine*, 25.
25. Norman Moore, "Dunglison, Robley, M.D."; Leslie Stephens and Sidney Lee, eds., *Dictionary of National Biography* (London, 1885–1900), vol. 16; Norwood, *Medical Education*, 397; Gross, *Memoir of Robley Dunglison*, 20; Billings, "Literature and Institutions," in *A Century of American Medicine*, 298–327.
26. Under the title *On the Influence of Atmosphere and Locality; Change of Air and Climate; Seasons; Food, Clothing, etc on Human Health, constituting* Elements of Hygiene (Philadelphia: Carey, Lea & Blanchard, 1835), hereafter cited as Elements of Hygiene.
27. Radbill, ed., "Autobiographical Ana," 72 and Dunglison, *Elements of Hygiene*, iii.
28. *American Journal of the Medical Sciences*, February 1835; *North American Archives of Medical and Surgical Science*, March 1835; *Transylvania Journal of Medicine* 8, no. 4 (1835); *British and Foreign Review* 3, no. 2 (1836).
29. Radbill, ed., "Autobiographical Ana," 74–76, 80, 130, 195.
30. Ibid., 135–136.
31. Ibid., 139.
32. *Philadelphia Medical and Surgical Reporter* 20 (April 1869): 323.
33. Dunglison, *Elements of Hygiene*, iv.
34. Radbill, ed., "Autobiographical Ana," 76 and "Robley Dunglison: American Medical Educator," 91.
35. Norwood, *Medical Education*, 231 and Radbill, ed., "Autobiographical Ana," 103–104.

36. Gross, *Memoir of Robley Dunglison*, 23.
37. Radbill, ed., "Autobiographical Ana," 77–78.
38. Cordell, *Historical Sketch*, 45–46, 83–84.
39. Radbill, ed., "Autobiographical Ana," 70–71.
40. Pitrof, *University of Maryland School of Medicine*, 30.
41. Radbill, ed., "Autobiographical Ana," 71.
42. Ibid., 70, 82–83.
43. Helen Turnbull Waite Coleman, *Banners in the Wilderness: The Early Years of Washington and Jefferson College* (Pittsburgh: University of Pittsburgh Press, 1956), 59–63.
44. "The Proprietary Years of Jefferson Medical College (1824–1895)," in Frederick B. Wagner and J. Woodrow Savacool, eds., *Thomas Jefferson University: A Chronological History and Alumni Directory*, 1992, http://jdc.jefferson.edu/wagner1/14.
45. Norwood, *Medical Education*, 86–93 and "Jefferson Medical College: The Early Struggles," in Wagner and Savacool, eds., *Thomas Jefferson University*, 1989, 1–45, https://jdc.jefferson/wagner2/50.
46. Radbill, ed., "Autobiographical Ana," 84–87 and Radbill, "Eminent Figure," 168.
47. Radbill, "Robley Dunglison: American Medical Educator," 92; Radbill, ed., "Autobiographical Ana," 93.
48. Heber Chase, *The Medical Student's Guide: Being a Compendious View of the Collegiate and Clinical Medical Schools, the Courses of Private Lectures, the Hospitals and Almshouses. . .* (Philadelphia: J. G. Auner, 1842), 17, 63 and Radbill, ed., "Autobiographical Ana," 92.
49. Radbill, ed., "Autobiographical Ana," 92.
50. Catalogues of the Trustees, Professors, and Students of the Jefferson Medical College of Philadelphia (1840–1859); Radbill, ed., "Autobiographical Ana," 93–94; Wagner, *Jefferson Medical College*, 42–107.
51. During the 20–year period covered in the Table, 19 international locations accounted for 57 graduates. These foreign graduates came from Canada (18); Nova Scotia (12); the West Indies (4); England (3); New Brunswick, Cuba, and Barbados (2 each); and St. Thomas, Newfoundland, New South Wales, Switzerland, Hungary, Uruguay, Turkey, Prussia, Montevideo, and Corsica (1 each).
52. John S. Ezell, "A Southern Education for Southrons," *Journal of Southern History* 17 (1951): 303–327; James O. Breeden, "States–Rights Medicine in the Old South," *Bulletin of the New York Academy of Medicine* 52, no. 3 (1976): 348–372; John Harley Warner, "A Southern Medical Reform: The Meaning of the Antebellum Argument for Southern Medical Education," *Bulletin of the History of Medicine* 57, no. 3 (1983): 364–381; Daniel Kilbride, "Southern Medical Students in Philadelphia, 1800–1860: Science and Sociability in the 'Republic of Medicine,'" *Journal of Southern History* 65, no. 4 (1999): 697–732.
53. Breeden, "States–Rights Medicine," 365–366; Harold J. Abrahams, "Secession from Northern Medical Schools," *Transactions and Studies of the College of Physicians of Philadelphia*, 4th ser., 36 (1968–1969): 29–45; John Duffy, "Sectional conflict and medical education in Louisiana," *Journal of Southern History* 23, no. 3 (1957): 298–303; Warner, "Southern Medical Reform," 380; Corner, *Two Centuries of Medicine*, 112–114.
54. Radbill, "Eminent Figure," 165 and Radbill, ed., "Autobiographical Ana," 133.
55. Dunglison, "Valedictory Lecture to the Medical Class of the University of Virginia," 9 July 1833; "Address to the Graduates in Medicine of the University of

Maryland," 19 March 1834; "Address to the Medical Graduates of the Jefferson Medical College," 11 March 1837; "Introductory Lecture to the Course of Institutes of Medicine in Jefferson Medical College," 14 November 1839, 8 November 1843, and 19 October 1848; "Charge to the Graduates of the Jefferson Medical College," 25 March 1847 and 11 March 1854; "Exhortation to the Graduates of the Jefferson Medical College," 10 March 1864.

56. Dunglison, "Valedictory Lecture to the Medical Class of the University of Virginia," 9 July 1833, 15–18; *The Medical Student*, 225–226; "Address to the Graduates in Medicine of the University of Maryland," 19 March 1834, 17; and "Introductory Lecture to the Course of Institutes of Medicine in Jefferson Medical College," 8 November 1843, 8.
57. Bean, "Mr. Jefferson's Influence on American Medical Education," 673; Radbill, ed., "Autobiographical Ana," 7–9; Warner, "Physiology," in Numbers, ed., *The Education of American Physicians*, 56; Richmond, "Robley Dunglison, M.D.," 76–77.
58. *Charge to the Graduates of the Jefferson Medical College, delivered March 25, 1847 by Professor Dunglison* (Philadelphia: John C. Clark, printer), 13.
59. Radbill, ed., "Autobiographical Ana," 108–109, 126–127, 171, 195, 196 and Franklin Peale, *Memorial of the Late Robley Dunglison* (Philadelphia: Collins Printers), 1869.
60. Gross, *Memoir of Robley Dunglison*, 7; Gross and Gross, eds., *Autobiography of Samuel D. Gross, M.D.*, 2:331; Radbill, ed., "Autobiographical Ana," 108–109, 195, 198–199.
61. Mayo, "Robley Dunglison: 1798–1869," 710; Radbill, ed., "Autobiographical Ana," 158–159, 166–167, 185; Gross, *Memoir of Robley Dunglison*, 15.
62. Frank J. Klingberg and Frank W. Klingberg, *The Correspondence Between Henry Stephen Randall and Hugh Blair Grigsby, 1856–1861* (Berkeley: University of California Press, 1952), 35.
63. Cushing, *The Life of Sir William Osler*, 1:238.
64. Gross and Gross, eds., *Autobiography of Samuel D. Gross, M.D.*, 2:329–335 and *Memoir of Robley Dunglison*, 12–13, 22. See also Dorsey, *Jefferson-Dunglison Letters*, 86–87.
65. Allen Johnson and Dumas Malone, eds., *Dictionary of American Biography* (1928–1936, reprint 1968), 5:512–513.
66. Norwood, *Medical Education*, 90; Gross, *Memoir of Robley Dunglison*, 20; Radbill, ed., "Autobiographical Ana," 175.
67. Fortunately, Samuel X. Radbill edited and published Dunglison's "Autobiographical Ana" in the *Transactions of the American Philosophical Society* in 1963, giving new life to a work that he himself never sought to publish.
68. Jones, "The Development of Medical Sects," 313–314.
69. Radbill, ed., "Autobiographical Ana," 121–122 and Gross, *Memoir of Robley Dunglison*, 10.
70. Herbert Clark Hoover, "Presidential Inaugural Address" 4 March 1929 (Gilder Lehrman Collection).
71. Alexander Brown, *The Cabells and Their Kin: A Memorial Volume of History, Biography, and Genealogy* (Richmond: Garrett and Massie, 1939).
72. Blanton in his *Medicine in Virginia in the Eighteenth Century*, 19 and 388–389.
73. Joseph Van Holt Nash and M. Shele deVere, *Students of the University of Virginia: A Semi–Centennial Catalogue, with brief biographical sketches* (Baltimore: C. Harvey & Co., 1878). See also the Matriculation Records of the University of Virginia.

74. Judge William H. Cabell to his brother, Joseph Carrington Cabell, August 1829, University of Virginia: Cabell Family Papers.
75. James L. Cabell to Joseph C. Cabell, Baltimore, 29 January and 13 December 1834, 22 February 1835, University of Virginia: James Lawrence Cabell Papers.
76. James L. Cabell to Joseph C. Cabell, Baltimore, 22 February 1835, University of Virginia: James Lawrence Cabell Papers.
77. Russel M. Jones, "American Doctors in the Parisian Medical World," *Bulletin of the History of Medicine* 47, no. 2 (1973): 177–204 and Russel C. Maulitz, "Channel Crossing: The Lure of French Pathology for English Medical Students, 1816–36," *Bulletin of the History of Medicine* 55, no. 4 (1981): 475–496.
78. James L. Cabell to Joseph C. Cabell, Richmond, 23 and 26 October 1836, University of Virginia: James Lawrence Cabell Papers.
79. James L. Cabell to Joseph C. Cabell, New York, 1 December 1836, and Paris, 28 January and 26 February 1837, University of Virginia: James Lawrence Cabell Papers.
80. Warner, *Against the Spirit of System*, 44–47, 92, 97,101, 254.
81. James L. Cabell to Joseph C. Cabell, Paris, 28 January 1837, University of Virginia: James Lawrence Cabell Papers; Warner, *Against the Spirit of System*, 254; Richard H. Shryock, "Nineteenth Century Medicine: Scientific Aspects," *Journal of World History* 3 (1956): 889.
82. Bruce, *History of UVA*, 3:93.
83. Blanton, *Medicine in Virginia in the Nineteenth Century*, 23, 25–26, 351 and John S. Davis, "History of the Medical Department of the University of Virginia, 1825–1914," *University of Virginia Alumni Bulletin* (July 1914): 6.
84. Minutes of University of Virginia Board of Visitors, 4 July 1840, 4 July 1843, 28 June 1850; Barringer, *History, Influence, Equipment and Characteristics*; Slaughter G. FitzHugh, *Anatomical Laboratory—Dissecting Hall 1833–1928* (manuscript, 1981), 3, University of Virginia: Historical Collections & Services, Claude Moore Health Sciences Library.
85. Joseph Dubose and Curtis Tribble, "James Lawrence Cabell, One of the Most Influential of America's Early Surgeons," *American Surgeon* 81 (2015): 331.
86. Smith, *Addresses Commemorative of James L. Cabell*, 20.
87. Minutes of University of Virginia Board of Visitors, 30 June 1857 and Bruce, *History of UVA*, 3:44–45, 148–150, 4:175.
88. Emily Matson, "John Staige Davis (1824–1885)," *Encyclopedia Virginia*, accessed 13 November 2017, https://www.EncyclopediaVirginia.org/Davis_John_Staige_1824–1885.
89. William A. Christmas and James C. Turner, "Varsity Hall: The Infirmary of the University of Virginia," *Journal of American College Health* 57, no. 3 (2008): 349–351.
90. Gamble, *God on Grounds*, 86.
91. William S. Forbes (a former pupil and patient of Cabell), *Addresses Commemorative of James L. Cabell*, 6; Bruce, *History of UVA*, 3:145–147; Gamble, *God on Grounds*, 76, 82, 86; Harrison, *Memorial Sketch of James L. Cabell, 1889*, 1–5. The parsonage built in the mid-1850s remains intact as 4 Dawson's Row, known now as the Luther P. Jackson House and housing the university's Office of African-American Affairs.
92. J. T. C, "Mr. Rives Address," *Southern Literary Messenger* (9 September 1847): 575 and Dabney, *Mr. Jefferson's University*, 13.

93. Harrison (a former pupil of Cabell, who earned both an MA and M.D. from the University of Virginia), *Addresses Commemorative of James L. Cabell*, delivered at the University of Virginia, 1 July 1890, 9–18.
94. Charlottesville. *Richmond Enquirer*, 30 August 1861, 19 September 1862, 1 and 11 September 1863; Minutes of the General Faculty, 2 October 1860 –5 July 1869, Special Collections of the University of Virginia (S;UVA); Chalmers L. Gemmill, "The Charlottesville General Hospital, 1861–1865," *Magazine of Albemarle County History* 22 (1964): 91–160; Ervin I. Jordan, *Charlottesville and the University of Virginia in the Civil War* (Lynchburg, Va.: H. B. Howard, 1988); Bruce, *History of UVA*, 3:256–340; John H. Moore, "The University of Virginia During the Civil War," *Virginia Cavalcade* 13, no. 3 (Winter 1963–64): 23; H. H. Cunningham, *Doctors in Gray: The Confederate Medical Service* (Baton Rouge: Louisiana State University Press, 1958), 36; Norwood, *Medical Education*, 274–275.
95. *Louis Minor Journal*, October 1861 entries, 99–100; Socrates Maupin, *Journals of the Chairman of the Faculty*, 11 January–6 February 1862.
96. George Llewellyn Christian, *Confederate Memories and Experiences* (Richmond: Clayton Publishing Co., 1915), 25–26.
97. James O. Breeden, "Insights into the Medical Statistics of the Charlottesville General Hospital, 1861–1865," *Magazine of Albemarle County History* 30 (1972): 43–59; Blanton, *Medicine in Virginia in the Nineteenth Century*, 272–315; Gemmill, "The Charlottesville General Hospital," 91–160; Bruce, *History of UVA*, 3:256–340; Jordan, *Charlottesville and UVA*, 45–61; Phillis Wheatley, "Medicine in Virginia during the Civil War," *Encyclopedia Virginia*, accessed 21 April 2020, https://encyclopediavirginia.org/entries/medicine–in–virginia–during–the–civil–war/.
98. Dubose, "James Lawrence Cabell," 332.
99. *Catalogue of the University of Virginia*, 43rd and 44th Sessions and *Richmond Medical Journal*, 19, 14.
100. Jordan, *Charlottesville and UVA*, 55; Margaret Humphreys, *Marrow of Tragedy: The Health Crisis of the American Civil War* (Baltimore: Johns Hopkins University Press, 2013), 229–230.
101. Letter from L. Minor Blackford to his mother written on 26 July 1861, in Gemmill, "The Charlottesville General Hospital," 115 and Edward Warren, *A Doctor's Experiences in Three Continents* (Baltimore: Cushings & Bailey, 1885), 283; and, personal communication, Chimborazo Medical Museum, Richmond National Battlefield Park, October 19, 2022.
102. J. David Hacker, "A Census-Based Account of the Civil War Dead," *Civil War History* 57 (2011): 307–348.
103. Jennifer Davis McDaid, "Oriana Russell Moon Andrews (1834–1883)," *Dictionary of Virginia Biography*, accessed 13 May 2021, http://www.lva.virginia.gov/public/dvb/bio.php?b=Andrews_Oriana_Russell_Moon and Humphreys, *Marrow of Tragedy*, 61.
104. Humphreys, *Marrow of Tragedy*, 293–298, 308.
105. Dubose, "James Lawrence Cabell," 333.
106. James O. Breeden, "Joseph Jones and Confederate Medical History," *Georgia Historical Quarterly* 54, no. 3 (1970): 357–380; Breeden, "Insights," 47; Edward B. Williams, *Rebel Brothers: The Civil War Letters of the Truehearts* (College Station: Texas A&M University Press, 1995), 78; Gemmill, "Charlottesville General Hospital," 115, 117, 121–123.

107. Adams, *Doctors in Blue*, 113.
108. Breeden, "Insights," 49. Jones completed his statistics in the course of an interview with Cabell and Davis, presumably in Virginia, in mid-October 1865.
109. Bruce, *History of UVA*, 3:311.
110. J. L. Cabell, *Richmond Medical Journal* 1 (1866): 43 and Maurice F. Shaw, *Stonewall Jackson's Surgeon: Hunter Holmes McGuire, A Biography* (Lynchburg, Va.: A: H. E. Howard Printing, 1993).
111. Blanton, *Medicine in Virginia in the Nineteenth Century*, 145–146.
112. Robert D. Mainwaring and Curtis C. Tribble, "The cardiac illness of General Robert E. Lee," *Surgery, Gynecology & Obstetrics* 174 (1992): 237–244.
113. W. A. Turner, "The College Fusion Question," To the Editors of the *Richmond Enquirer*, 1867; "Memorial of the Faculty of the University to the Rector and Board of Visitors Touching on the Removal of the Medical Department to Richmond," 2 April 1867, Special Collections Library of the University of Virginia; T. M. L., "Virginia Medical Education," *Richmond Whig*, 5 April 1867; *Richmond Medical Journal* 3 (1867): 392, 487; editorials in the *Lynchburg Daily Virginian*, 9 April 1867 and the *Staunton Valley Virginian*, 24 April 1867; representative letters to Cabell from William Frazier, 30 March 1867, from B. M. Attindon, 28 March 1867, from John Graham, 29 March 1867, from J. A. Cochran, 2 April 1867, from James Beale, 5 April 1867, and from Dr. Houston, 6 April 1867, University of Virginia: James Lawrence Cabell Papers. For earlier efforts, see Cabell, *Early History of the University of Virginia*, 501–517; Bruce, *History of UVA*, 1:308–321, 2:111–116, 3:41–43, 5:192; "Editorial," *Virginia Medical Journal* 9 (1857): 248, 507.
114. "Minutes of the First Annual Meeting," *Transactions of the American Medical Association* 1 (1848): 7.
115. J. L. Cabell, "Report of the Committee on Medical Education," *Transactions of the American Medical Association* 7 (1854): 65.
116. Cabell, "Report," 53–81.
117. Ibid., 72.
118. Act to Regulate the Practice of Medicine and Surgery, 31 January 1884, *Acts and Joint Resolutions Passed by the General Assembly of the State of Virginia during the Session 1883–4* (Richmond: James E. Good Co., 1884), 79.
119. Cabell, "Report," 58–59, 74, 81.
120. "The University: Its Character and Wants," *Southern Literary Messenger* (April 1856): 248–249.
121. Dunglison, *The Medical Student*, 164–165; Davis, *History of Medical Education and Medical Institutions*, 166, 175–176; Hudson, *Patterns of Medical Education*, 108; Gerhart, "Remarks on Clinical Education," *American Journal of Medical Science* 18 (1836): 388.
122. Cabell, "Report," 75.
123. Norwood, *Medical Education*, 422–428; Kaufman, "American Medical Education," in Numbers, ed., *The Education of American Physicians*, 102; James Bordley and A. McGehee Harvey, *Two Centuries of American Medicine, 1776–1976* (Philadelphia: W. B. Saunders, 1976), 20.
124. Lynn E. Miller, "Medical Education Reform Efforts and Failures of U.S. Medical Schools, 1870–1930," *Journal of the History of Medicine and Allied Sciences* 63, no. 3 (2008): 348–387 and Gibson, "Medical Education in the Nineteenth Century," 155–157.
125. J. L. Cabell, *The Testimony of Modern Science to the Unity of Mankind; being a sum-*

mary of the conclusions announced by the highest authorities in the several departments of physiology, zoology, and comparative philology in favor of the Specific Unity and Common Origin of All the Varieties of Man, with an introductory notice by James W. Alexander, D.D. (New York: Robert Carter & Brothers, 1859, updated 1860). The second edition includes a clarifying statement misinterpreted in the inaugural publication. References to Cabell's book are from his second edition, unless otherwise noted.

126. Cabell's lectures early in the 1850s clearly show his thinking, well in advance of the appearance of *On the Origins of Species*. See J. L. Cabell, *Syllabus of the Lectures on Physiology and Histology, including the Outlines of Comparative Anatomy* (Charlottesville: McKinnie & Sons, 1853), 57–60.
127. *Protestant Episcopal Quarterly Review and Church Register*, January 1857. In his book, Cabell refers to this and other critical essays on pages xv, 33, 312, and 334–335, and also provides an equally damning review of Nott and Gliddon's later work, *Indigenous Races of the Earth* (Appendix G, 338–368).
128. Four of the more revealing publications by these men include "The Geographical Distribution of Animals," *Christian Examiner* 48 (March 1850): 181–204; "The Diversity of Origin of the Human Species," *Christian Examiner* 48 (July 1850): 110–145; *Types of Mankind* (Philadelphia: Lippincott, Grambo & Co., 1854); and *Indigenous Races of the Earth* (Philadelphia: J. P. Lippincott, 1857). See also Louis Menand, "Morton, Agassiz, and the Origins of Scientific Racism in the United States," *Journal of Blacks in Higher Education*, no. 34 (Winter 2001–2002): 110–113.
129. Cabell, *Testimony*, xiii, 28.
130. Harrison, *Addresses Commemorative of James L. Cabell*, 13.
131. Harrison, *Memorial Sketch of James L. Cabell*, 1889, 3.
132. Larry Robert Morrison, *The Proslavery Argument in the Early Republic, 1790–1830* (Charlottesville: University of Virginia Press, 1975), 121–122.
133. Darwin's *On the Origins of Species by Means of Natural Selection* was published in 1859, several months after Cabell's Testimony, and *his Descent of Man and Selection in Relation to Sex* appeared in 1871.
134. Cabell, *Testimony*, 35 and Conway Zirkle, "The Early History of the Inheritance of Acquired Characters and of Pangenesis," *Transactions of the American Philosophical Society* 35, no. 2 (1946): 118.
135. This quote comes from Dr. Wilburt Cornell Davison (1892–1972), dean of the School of Medicine of Duke University from 1927 to 1960, on the occasion of the dedication of a new medical building in 1930. Cabell's work so impressed Davison that he named one of the hospital wards after him and had three quotations from *Testimony* framed and hung there. Wilburt Cornell Davison and Wiley D. Forbus, *Fourteen Distinguished Physician and Surgeons: Brief Sketches of Eminent Men for whom Duke Hospital Wards are Named* (Durham: Duke University, 1931), https://duke.box.com/s/h4x0vcqo9sshenv05bi1unedkzyiru3q, Duke University Medical Center Archives: Wilburt Cornell Davison Papers, 1930.
136. Cabell, *Testimony*, 35, 70, 309–310, 314.
137. Josiah Nott, George Gliddon, et al., *Types of Mankind: or Ethnological Researches, based upon the Ancient Monuments, Paintings, Sculptures, and Crania of Races, and upon their Natural, Geographical, Philological, and Biblical History* (Philadelphia: Lippincott, Grambo & Co., 1854). See also James Philemon Holcombe, "Is Slavery Consistent with Natural Law," *Southern Literary Messenger* (1858): 8.
138. Nott and Gliddon, *Types of Mankind*, 255, 269 and Cabell, *Testimony*, 104–108.

139. Gould, *The Mismeasure of Man*, 70. Cabell in his *Testimony*, p, 219, described Humboldt as "the most illustrious of living savans."
140. Edward Lurie, "Louis Agassiz and the Races of Man," *Isis* 45, no. 3 (1954): 227, n3.
141. Cabell, *Syllabus of Lectures on Physiology and Histology, including the Outlines of Comparative Anatomy* (Charlottesville: McKennie and Sons, 1853), 59 and Testimony, 263–267.
142. Dunglison, *Human Physiology*, 467.
143. Alfred L. Brophy, *University, Court, and Slave: Proslavery Academic Thought and Southern Jurisprudence* (New York: Oxford University Press, 2016); Thomas Howard and Alfred Brophy, "Proslavery Thought," in McInnis and Nelson, eds., *Educated in Tyranny*, 141–170; Gwen Dilworth, "The Destinies of the South Must be Entrusted to Our Keeping: 1850s Secessionist and Pro-Slavery Thoughts at the University of Virginia," https://juel.iath.virginia.edu/node/1061.
144. A Citizen of the South [Charles B. Shaw], *Is Slavery a Blessing? A Reply to Prof. Bledsoe's Essay on Liberty and Slavery: With remarks on Slavery as It is* (Boston: Jewett, 1857), 25; Alfred L. Brophy, "The Law of Descent of Thought: Law, History, and Civilization in Antebellum Literary Addresses," *Law and Literature* 20, no. 3 (2008): 343–402; Howard and Brophy, "Proslavery Thought," 146; Clement Eaton, *Freedom of Thought in the Old South* (1940), 206; Bruce, *History of UVA*, 2:357–358, 3:259–261.
145. Brian Neumann, "UVA Unionists: The University of Virginia's Neglected Alumni," *Magazine of Albemarle Charlottesville History* 78 (2020: 73–108; Meggan Cashwell and Elizabeth R. Varon, "The Civil War and Reconstruction," *Legal Knowledge*. Podcast audio, February 20, 2023 (9:15 and 32:05). http://archives.law.virginia.edu/legalknowledgepodcast.
146. Dubsoe, "James Lawrence Cabell," 333.
147. J. L. Cabell, "On Sanitary Conditions in Relation to the Treatment of Surgical Operations and Injuries," *Transactions of the American Surgical Association* 1 (1883): 23–63 and Lindsey Fitzharris, *The Butchering Art: Joseph Lister's Quest to Transform the Grisly World of Victorian Medicine* (New York: Scientific American/Farrar, Straus and Giroux, 2017).
148. Smith, *Addresses Commemorative of James L. Cabell*, 22–24.
149. Cabell was sixty-nine years old when he delivered this speech in 1882, far past his "Fixed Period." In 1905, while giving a farewell to the Johns Hopkins faculty, Dr. William Osler, then the most famous physician in English-speaking countries, put forward his views on aging. He spoke of two fixed periods. The first was the comparative usefulness of men above 40 years of age, being far less than the "15 golden years" between 25 and 40, which are the anabolic or constructive years. Osler's second fixed period applies to men above 60 years of age, a time when professors accomplish almost nothing of value, when their service to a university was no longer required, and when, to facilitate their departure, such men should be chloroformed. William Osler, "The Fixed Period," in Osler, *Aequanimitas and Other Addresses to Medical Students, Nurses and Practitioners of Medicine*, 3rd ed. (Philadelphia: The Blakiston Co., 1932), 373–393; Smith, *Addresses Commemorative of James L. Cabell*, 22. See also Charles S. Bryan, "Osler goes viral: The 'Fixed Period' revisited," *Proceedings of Baylor University Medical Center* 31, no. 4 (2018): 550–553.
150. Smith, *Addresses Commemorative of James L. Cabell*, 22–23 and *In Memoriam: Record of the Death of Professor James Lawrence Cabell.* The Faculty of the University of Virginia Regular Meeting of December 1889, 19. See also Thomas Schlich,

"Asepsis and Bacteriology: A Realignment of Surgery and Laboratory Science," *Medical History* 56, no. 3 (2012): 308–334.

151. Humphreys, *Marrow of Tragedy*, 293, 298.
152. Duffy, *The Sanitarians*, 171; James O. Breeden, "Joseph Jones and Public Health in the New South," *Journal of the Louisiana Historical Association* 32, no. 4 (1991): 365–366; Humphreys, *Marrow of Tragedy*, 300.
153. J. L. Cabell, "Report on Defective Drainage as a Cause of disease within the limits of the State of Virginia," *Transactions of the American Medical Association* 25 (1874): 477–519.
154. Examples include J. L. Cabell, "Report on the Water-Supply as related to Public Health in Virginia," *Transactions of the American Medical Association* 27 (1876): 435–450; "The Etiology of Enteric Fever," *Transactions of the American Medical Association* 28 (1877): 411–459; "The Rise and Progress of International Hygiene," *Public Health Papers and Reports* 7 (1880): 16–31; "On Sanitary Conditions in Relation to the Treatment of Surgical Operations and Injuries," *Transactions of the American Surgical Association* (1883): 23–63; "National Legislation and Attempts at Legislation on Quarantine," *The Sanitarian* (January 1883); "A Review of the Operations of the National Board of Health," *American Public Health Association Reports* 8 (1883): 71–101; *National Board of Health: Remarks Before the Committee on Public Health of the House of Representatives in Support of House Bill 2785, 48th Congress, 1st Session, for the Protection of Public Health* (Washington, D.C.: Gibson Brothers, printer, 1884).
155. Dubose, "James Lawrence Cabell," 333.
156. Humphreys, *Marrow of Tragedy*, 300 and Furman, *Profile of the National Public Health Service*, 128.
157. Stephen Smith's essay in *Addresses Commemorative of James L. Cabell*, 26, 29–38. Unfortunately, this "Act to Prevent the Introduction of Infectious or Contagious Disease into the United States and to establish a National Board of Health" included a sunset clause providing for cessation of federal funding without reauthorization, which proved fatal to the organization. Furman, *Profile of the National Public Health Service*, 151–155; Williams, *The United States Public Health Service*, 77–78; Duffy, *The Sanitarians*, 168, 171.
158. Furman, *Profile of the National Public Health Service*, 177–178 and Smith, *Addresses Commemorative of James L. Cabell*, 34.
159. Dubose, "James Lawrence Cabell," 333.
160. Furman, *Profile of the National Public Health Service*, 65, 105, 157.
161. The graduates of the University of Virginia in the medical corps of the Army made up 13.5 percent of the whole body; in the medical corps of the Navy the figure was 15.5 percent; and in the service of the Marine Hospital system it was nearly 30 percent. Bruce, *History of UVA*, 4:206–211. See also *Alumni Bulletin of the University of Virginia*, 1, no. 2, 28–29; 2, no. 1, 11–13; and 4, no. 2, 34.
162. Norman Howard Jones, *The Scientific Background of the International Sanitary Conferences, 1851–1938* (Geneva, Switzerland: World Health Organization, 1975), 11, 42–45; J. L. Cabell, "The National Board of Health and International Sanitary Conference of Washington," *Transactions of the American Medical Association* 32 (1881): 321–339; letter from Cabell to President Chester A. Author, 4 January 1882, as cited in "Annual Reports of the National Board of Health, 1879–1885," binder 882, 23–24; Cabell, "A Review of the Operations of the National Board of Health," *American Public Health Association Reports* 8 (1883), 71–101. These latter

citations illustrate Cabell's tenacity in pursuing international health cooperation.

162. James A. Jacobs, "James Lawrence Cabell," in John T. Kneebone et al., eds., *Dictionary of Virginia Biography*, 2:484–486; and *Virginia Medical Monthly* 16 (1889): 492.

163. Harrison, *Memorial Sketch of James L. Cabell*, 1889, 1.

164. "Address of William S. Forbes, M.D., Professor of Anatomy at Jefferson Medical College," in Harrison, *Addresses Commemorative of James L. Cabell*, 7.

165. Harrison, *Addresses Commemorative of James L. Cabell*, 10.

Bibliography

Primary Sources

Adams, John. *Diary and Autobiography of John Adams*, edited by L. H. Butterfield. Cambridge: Belknap Press of Harvard University, 1961.

——. "An Essay on Man's Lust for Power by John Adams, August 29, 1763." In *The Papers of John Adams* vol. 1, edited by Robert J. Taylor. Cambridge: Harvard University Press, 1977.

——. *The Pas of John Adams*, edited by Robert J. Taylor, Mary-Jo Kline, and Gregg L. Lint. Cambridge: The Belknap Press of Harvard University Press, 1977.

Adams, John and Abigail, and Thomas Jefferson. *The Adams-Jefferson Correspondence: The Complete Correspondence Between Thomas Jefferson & Abigail & John Adams*, edited by Lester J. Cappon. Chapel Hill: The Omohundro Institute of Early American History and Culture and The University of North Carolina Press, 1959.

Bartlett, Elisha. *An Essay of the Philosophy of Medical Science*. Philadelphia: Lea & Blanchard, 1844.

Bigelow, Henry J. *Medical Education in America: Annual Address read before the Massachusetts Medical Society, June 7, 1871*. Cambridge, Mass.: Welch, Bigelow and Company, 1871.

Bigelow, Jacob. *Discourse on Self-Limited Disease, A Lecture Delivered before the Massachusetts Medical Society, May 27, 1835*. Boston, Nathan Hale, 1835.

——. *Nature in Disease, illustrated in various Discourses and Essays. To which are added Miscellaneous Wittings, chiefly on Medical Subjects*. Boston: Ticknor & Fields, 1854.

Billings, John S. "Ideals of Medical Education: The Address in Medicine." Reprinted in *The New Englander* and *Yale University Review* (August 1891).

——. "Literature and Institutions." In *A Century of American Literature, 1776–1876*, edited by Edward H. Clarke, New York: Burt Franklin, 1876.

Boylston, Zabdiel. *An Historical Account of the Small-Pox Inoculated in New England, upon All Sorts of Persons, Whites, Blacks, and All Ages and Constitutions*. London: S. Chandler at Cross-Keys, 1726.

Cabanis, Pierre-Jean-Georges. *An Essay on the Certainty of Medicine*. Translated by

R. La Roche. Philadelphia: Robert Desilver, 1828.

——. *On the Relation between the Physical and Moral Aspects of Man.* Translated by Margaret Duggan Saidi. Baltimore: Johns Hopkins University Press, 1980.

——. *Sketch of the Revolutions of Medical Science and Views Relating to its Reform.* Translated by Alexander Henderson. London: Bye and Law, 1806.

Cabell, James L. *Lecture Introductory to the Course on Anatomy and Surgery in the University of Virginia.* Charlottesville: James Alexander, printer, 1838.

——. *Syllabus of the Lectures on Physiology and Histology; including the Outlines of Comparative Anatomy.* Charlottesville: McKennie & Son, 1853.

——. "Report of the Committee on Medical Education." *Transactions of the American Medical Association* 7 (1854): 53–81.

——. *The Testimony of Modern Science to the Unity of Mankind; being a Summary of the Conclusions announced by the Highest Authorities in Several Departments of Physiology, Zoology, and Comparative Anatomy in Favor of the Specific Unity and Common Origin of all the Varieties of Man.* New York: Robert Carter & Brothers, 1859 and 1860.

——. *An Account of the Hot Springs, Bath County, Virginia, and Analysis of the Waters.* Richmond: Clemmitt & Jones, 1873.

——. "Report on Defective Drainage as a Cause of Disease within the Limits of the State of Virginia." *Transactions of the American Medical Association* 25 (1874): 477–519.

——. "Report on the Water-Supply as Related to Public Health in Virginia." *Transactions of the American Medical Asso*ciation 27 (1876): 435450.

——. "Etiology of Enteric Fever." *Transactions of the American Medical Association* 28 (1877): 411–459.

——. "Address in State Medicine and Public Hygiene." *Transactions of the American Medical Association* 29 (1878): 551–583.

——. "Brief Notice of the Rise and Progress of International Hygiene." *American Public Health Association Papers* 7 (1881): 16–31.

——. "The National Board of Health and the International Sanitary Conference of Washington." *Transactions of the American Medical Association* 32 (1881): 321–339.

——. "On Sanitary Conditions in the Treatment of Surgical Operations and Injuries." *Transactions of the American Surgical Association* 1 (1883): 23–63.

——. "A Review of the Operations of the National Board of Health." *American Public Health Association Reports* 8 (1883): 71–101.

Cabell, Nathaniel Francis, ed. *Early History of the University of Virginia as Contained in the Letters of Thomas Jefferson and Joseph C. Cabell.* Richmond, Va.: J. W. Randolph, 1856. Available at Hathi Trust.

Cappon, Lester J., ed. *The Adams-Jefferson Letters.* New York: Simon & Schuster, 1971.

Crawford, John D. *A Lecture, Introductory To a Course of Lectures On the Cause, Seat, and Cure of Diseases.* Baltimore: Edward J. Coale, 1811.

Davis, Richard Beale, ed. *Correspondence of Thomas Jefferson and Francis Walker Gilmer, 1814–1826.* Columbia: University of South Carolina Press, 1946.

Dorsey, John M. *The Jefferson-Dunglison Letters.* Charlottesville: University of Virginia Press, 1960.

Dunglison, Robley. *Papers.* College of Physicians of Philadelphia.

——. *Commentaries on Diseases of the Stomach and Bowels of Children.* London: G. B. Whittaker, 1824.

——. *Syllabus of the Lectures on Medical Jurisprudence*. Charlottesville: Clement & McKinnie, printer, 1827.

——. "Voyage to the Moon." *American Quarterly Review* 3, no. 5 (1828): 61–88.

——. "The Salubrity of the University." *Virginia Literary Museum*, 17 June 1829.

——. "College Instruction and Discipline." *American Quarterly Review* 9 (1831): 283–314.

——. *Human Physiology*. Philadelphia: Carey, Lea & Blanchard, 1833.

——. *A New Dictionary of Medical Science and Literature*. Boston: Charles Bowen, 1833.

——. *A Valedictory Lecture Delivered to the Medical Class of the University of Virginia*. Charlottesville: Watson & Tompkins, 1833.

——. *An Introductory Lecture Delivered to the Medical Class of the University of Maryland*. Baltimore: John D. Toy, printer, 1833.

——. *An Address Delivered to the Graduates in Medicine of the University of Maryland*. Baltimore: William Woody, printer, 1834.

——. *On the Influence of Atmosphere, Locality; Change of Air; Seasons; Food; Clothing, Bathing; Exercise; Sleep; Corporeal and Intellectual Pursuits, &c. &c on Human Health; constituting Elements of Hygiene*. Philadelphia: Carey, Lea & Blanchard, 1835.

——. *General Therapeutics or Principles of Medical Practice*. Philadelphia: Carey, Lea & Blanchard, 1836.

——. *The Medical Student; or Aids to the Study of Medicine*. Philadelphia: Carey, Lea & Blanchard, 1837 and 1844.

——. *Address to the Medical Graduates of the Jefferson Medical College of Philadelphia*. Philadelphia: Adam Waldie, printer, 1837.

——. *An Appeal to the People of Pennsylvania: On the Subject of an Asylum for the Insane Poor of the Commonwealth*. Philadelphia: Committee on an Asylum for the Insane Poor of Pennsylvania, 1838. A second appeal was published in 1840.

——. *Introductory Lecture to the Course of Institutes of Medicine in Jefferson Medical College*. Philadelphia: William F. Geddes, printer, 1839.

——. "Liability of Vaccine Virus to Deterioration." *Proceedings of the American Philosophical Society* 1 (January 4, 1839): 68.

——. *New Remedies: The Method of Preparing and Administering Them; their Effects on the Healthy and Diseased Economy*. Philadelphia, 1839.

——. *On Certain Medical Delusions: An Introductory Lecture in the Course of Lectures on Institutes of Medicine in Jefferson Medical College in Philadelphia*. Philadelphia, 1842.

——. *The Practice of Medicine, or A Treatise on Special Pathology and Therapeutics*. Philadelphia, 1842.

——. *An Introductory Lecture to the Course of Institutes of Medicine in Jefferson Medical College*. Philadelphia: Merrihew & Thompson, printer, 1843.

——. *Charge to the Graduates of Jefferson Medical College*. Philadelphia: John C. Clark, printer, 1847.

——. "Obituary Notice of Professor George Tucker" (read at the 3 October 1862 meeting of the American Philosophical Society). *Proceedings of the American Philosophical Society* 9, no. 68 (1862): 64–70.

——. "Obituary Notice of George W. Bethune, DD." (read at the 3 October 1862 meeting of the American Philosophical Society). *Proceedings of the American Philosophical Society* 9, no. 68 (1862):70–85.

——. *Exhortation to the Graduates of the Jefferson Medical College of Philadelphia.* Philadelphia: Collins, printer, 1864.

——. *History of Medicine from the Earliest Ages to the Commencement of the Nineteenth Century by Robley Dunglison*, edited by Richard J. Dunglison. Philadelphia: Lindsay and Blakiston, 1872.

Dunglison, Richard J. "Biography of Robley Dunglison," *Western Journal of Medicine* 4 (1869): 493–497.

Eliot, Charles W. "Annual Report of the President and Treasurer of Harvard College," Cambridge, Harvard University (1879–80).

Ellsworth, Henry L. *A Digest of Patents, Issued by the United States, from 1790 to January 1, 1839.* Washington, D.C.: P. Force, printer, 1840.

Emmet Family Papers. University of Virginia, Special Collection Library.

Franklin, Benjamin. *Papers of Benjamin Franklin.* Edited by Barbara Oberg, Claude-Anne Lopez, Ellen R. Cohn, Leonard W. Labaree, Whitfield J. Bell, and William B. Wilcox. 43 vols. to date. New Haven and London: Yale University Press, 1959–.

Franklin, Benjamin and William Heberden. *Some Account of the Success of Inoculation for the Smallpox in England and America.* London: William Strahan, 1759.

Graves, Robert J. *Clinical Lectures on the Practice of Medicine.* London: reprinted from 2d ed. by New Sydenham Society, 1884.

Gregory, John. *Lectures on the Duties and Qualifications of a Physician.* London: W. Strahan & T. Cadell, 1772.

Gross, Samuel W., and Albert Haller Gross, eds., *Autobiography of Samuel D. Gross, M.D., emeritus professor of surgery in the Jefferson medical college of Philadelphia: with sketches of his contemporaries.* 2 vols. Philadelphia: G. Barrie, 1887.

Hench, Philip S. *Walter Reed Yellow Fever Collection.* University of Virginia. Historical Collections, Claude Moore Health Sciences Library.

Hening, William W. *The Statutes at Large: Being a Collection of all the Laws of Virginia,* VIII and IX. Richmond: George Cochran, printer, 1822.

Jackson, Donald, ed. *Letters of the Lewis and Clark Expedition with Related Documents: 1783–1854.* 2 vols. Urbana: University of Illinois Press, 1978.

Jefferson, Thomas. *Coolidge Collection of Thomas Jefferson's Manuscripts.* Boston: Massachusetts Historical Society, 1957.

——. "Fifth Annual Message to Congress, December 3, 1805." Yale Law School, Avalon Project. https://analon.yale.edu/19th_.jeffmes5.asp.

——. *Jefferson's Memorandum Books: Accounts with Legal Records and Miscellany, 1767–1826.* 2 vols. Edited by James A. Bear, Jr. and Lucia C. Stanton. Princeton: Princeton University Press, 1997.

——. *Notes on the State of Virginia*, edited by William Peden. New York: W. W. Norton & Co., 1954.

——. *The Papers of Thomas Jefferson.* Early Access Digital Archive, Thomas Jefferson Foundation and Founders Online. https://founders.archive.gov/documents/Jefferson.

——. *The Papers of Thomas Jefferson.* 43 vols. Edited by Julian P. Boyd (vols. 1–20), Charles T. Cullen (vols. 2223), John Catanzariti (vols. 24-28), Barbara B. Oberg (vols. 29–41), and James P. McClure (vols. 42–43). Princeton, N.J.: Princeton University Press, 1950–.

——. *The Papers of Thomas Jefferson: Retirement Series*. 17 vols. Edited by J. Jefferson Looney. Princeton: Princeton University Press, 2005–2021.

——. *A Summary of the Rights of British America*. Williamsburg: Clementina Rind, 1774.

——. *Thomas Jefferson's Farm Book*, edited by Edwin Morris Betts. Princeton: Princeton University Press, 1953.

——. *Thomas Jefferson's Garden Book, 1766–1824*, edited by Edwin Morris Betts. Philadelphia: American Philosophical Society, 1944.

——. *Thomas Jefferson Papers*. Library of Congress, Manuscript Division, Washington, D.C. https://www.loc.gov. and https://hdl.loc.gov/loc.mss.

——. *The Works of Thomas Jefferson*. 2 vols. Edited by Paul Leicester Ford. New York: Putnam, 1904–1905.

——. *Thomas Jefferson's Writings: Autobiography, Notes on the State of Virginia, Public and Private Papers, Addresses, Messages and Relies*, edited by Merrill D. Peterson. New York: Library of America, 1984.

——. "Will and Codicil." 16–17 March 1826. Founders Online. https://founders.Archives.gov/documents/Jefferson/98-01-02-5963.

——. *The Writings of Thomas Jefferson*. 20 vols. Edited by Andrew A. Lipscomb and Albert E. Bergh. Washington, D.C.: Thomas Jefferson Memorial Foundation, 1903-1907

Jefferson, Thomas and Du Pont de Nemours. *The Correspondence of Jefferson and Du Pont de Nemours*, edited by Gilbert Chinard. Baltimore: Johns Hopkins University Press, 1931, reprint 1979. Available at HathiTrust.

Jefferson, Thomas, James Wilkinson, George Turner, Caspar Wistar, Adam Seybert, C. W. Peale, and John Williams. "Circular Letter." *Transactions of the American Philosophical Society* 4 (1799): xxxvii.

Jefferson Trust. "Jefferson's University . . . the early life (JUEL)." Resources of original primary documents: journals of the chairman of the faculty, minutes of faculty meetings, university enactments, board of visitor's meeting minutes, and university catalogues. https://juel.iath.virginia.edu.

Jenner, Edward. *An Inquiry into the Causes and Effects of the Variolae Vaccinae, a Disease Discovered in Some Parts of the Western Counties of England, Particularly Gloucestershire and Known by the Name of Cow Pox*. London: Sampson Low Co., 1798.

Jurin, James, and John Osborne. "A letter to the learned Dr. Caleb Cotesworth, F. R. S. of the College of Physicians, London, and Physician to St. Thomas's Hospital; containing a statistical comparison between the danger of the natural smallpox, and of that given by inoculation." *Philosophical Transactions of the Royal Society of London* 32, no. 374 (1723).

Juvenal. *Juvenal and Persius: With an English Translation by G. G. Ramsay*. London: William Heinemann; G. P. Putnam's Sons, 1918.

Kaminski, John K. *The Quotable Jefferson*. Princeton: Princeton University Press, 2006.

Kirkpatrick, James. *An Essay on Inoculation Occasioned by Smallpox Being Brought into South Carolina in the Year 1738*. London: J. Huggonsohn, 1743.

Koch, Adrienne, and William Peden, eds. *The Life and Selected Writings of Thomas Jefferson*. New York: The Modern Library, 1944.

——. *The Life and Selected Writings of Thomas Jefferson*. New York: Random House, 1993.

Koop, C. Everett. *The C. Everett Coop Papers*. https://profiles.nlm.nih.gov/spotlight/qq.

——. "Remarks to the Students and Faculty of the George Washington University

School of Medicine." Washington, D.C., 23 April 1986.

Lafayette, Marquis de, and Thomas Jefferson. *The Letters of Lafayette and Jefferson,* edited by Gilbert Chinard. Baltimore: Johns Hopkins University Press, 1929, reprint 1979.

Latrobe, Benjamin Henry. *The Correspondence and Miscellaneous Papers of Benjamin Henry Latrobe, 1984–1988*, edited by John C. Van Horne, et al. New Haven: Yale University Press, 1984-1988.

Lettsom, John Coakley. *Recollections of Dr. Rush.* London: J. Nichols Sons and Bentley, 1815.

Lewis, Meriwether, and William Clark. *The Journals of the Lewis and Clark Expedition.* 13 vols. Edited by Gary E. Moulton. Lincoln, Nebr.: University of Nebraska Press, 2002.

Library of Congress, Thomas Jefferson, and Emily Millicent Sowerby. *Catalogue of the Library of Thomas Jefferson.* Washington, D.C.: The Library of Congress, 1952–59. Available from *HeinOnline.*

Lincoln, Benjamin. *The Benjamin Lincoln Papers.* Boston: Massachusetts Historical Society.

Long, George. *Letters of George Long,* edited by Thomas Fitzhugh. Charlottesville: Library of the University of Virginia, 1917.

Madison, James. *James Madison Papers.* Washington, D.C.: Library of Congress.

——. *The Papers of James Madison, Retirement Series, edited by* David Mattern et al. Charlottesville: University of Virginia Press, 2009-.

Mather, Cotton. *An Account of the Methods and Success of Inoculating the Small-pox in Boston in New England.* London: J. Peele, 1722.

Maury, James. "A Dissertation on Education in the Form of a Letter from James Maury to Robert Jackson, July 17, 1762, edited and with an Introduction by Helen D. Bullock," *The Magazine of the Albemarle County History* 2 (1942).

Moore, Clement Clarke. *Observations upon certain passages in Mr. Jefferson's Notes on Virginia, which appears to have a tendency to subvert religion, and establish a false philosophy.* New York: New York Historical Society, Gilder Lehrman Collection, 1804.

Morgan, John. *A Discourse Upon the Institution of Medical Schools in America: Delivered at a Public Anniversary Commencement, held in the College of Philadelphia May 30 and 31, 1765.* Philadelphia: William Bradford, 1765.

Peden, William, ed. *1828 Catalogue of the Library of the University of Virginia.* Charlottesville: Alderman Library, University of Virginia, 1945.

Peters, Richard, ed. *The Public Statutes at Large of the United States . . . 1789 to March 3, 1845.* Boston: Charles S. Little and James Brown, 1845–67.

Radbill, Samuel X., ed. "The Autobiographical Ana of Robley Dunglison, M.D." *Transactions of the American Philosophical Society* 53 (1963).

Ramsay, David. *An Eulogium upon Benjamin Rush, M.D., Professor of the Institutes and Practice of Medicine and of Clinical Practice in the University of Pennsylvania.* Philadelphia: Bradford & Inskeep, 1813.

Randolph, Sarah N. *The Domestic Life of Thomas Jefferson: Compiled from Family Letters and Reminiscences by His Great-Granddaughter. New York:* Harper & Brothers Co., 1871.

Randolph Family Papers. Charlottesville: University of Virginia Special Collections, Alderman Library.

Reports of the Courses of Instruction in the Yale College by a Committee of the Corporation and the Academical Faculty (New Haven, Yale College, 1828).

Rush, Benjamin. *The Autobiography of Benjamin Rush: His "Travels Through Life" Together with His Commonplace Book for 1789–1813*, edited by George W. Corner. Princeton: Princeton University Press, 1948.

——. *In Defense of Bloodletting, as a Remedy for Certain Diseases.* Philadelphia: Dobson, 1796.

——. *Lectures on the Practice of Physicians 1796.* 1, no. 31; 2, no. 1. Philadelphia: Library of the University of Pennsylvania.

——. *The Letters of Benjamin Rush*, edited by L. H. Butterfield. Princeton: Princeton University Press, 1951.

——. *Sixteen Introductory Lectures, to Courses of Lectures Upon the Institutes and Practice of Medicine.* Philadelphia: Bradford & Inskeep, 1811.

Sundry Documents on the Subject of a System of Public Education for the State of Virginia. Richmond, Va.: Ritchie, Trueheart & Duval, 1817. [Literary Fund.]

Tennent, John. *Every Man His Own Doctor.* Philadelphia: printed and sold by Benjamin Franklin, 1751.

Trent, William P. "English Culture in Virginia: A Study of the Gilmer Letter." In *Johns Hopkins University Studies in Historical and Political Science*, edited by Herbert B. Adams. Baltimore: N. Murray, 1889.

Thomas Jefferson's Scrapbooks: Poems of Nation, Family, and Romantic Love Collected by America's Third President, edited by Jonathan Gross. Chapel Hill: University of North Carolina Press, 2006.

University of Virginia. *Enactments by the Rector and Visitors of the University of Virginia, for Constituting, Governing & Conducting That Institution.* Charlottesville: C. P. M'Kennie, 1825.

University of Virginia (Corporate Author). *A Sketch of the History of the University of Virginia together with a catalogue of professors and instructors, the graduates in law and medicine, and the masters and bachelors of arts, since the foundation of the institution.* Washington, D.C.: H. Polkinhorn, 1859.

University of Virginia Library List of Books Borrowed, 1825–1827. Charlottesville: University of Virginia Library, Special Collections.

Washington, George. *The Papers of George Washington, Presidential Series.* 21 vols. Edited by David R. Hoth, Dorothy Twohig, William M. Ferraro, Carol S. Ebel, Edward G. Lengel, Philander D. Chase, Christine Sternberg Patrick, Adrina Garbooshian-Huggins, Theodore Crackel, and William W. Abbot. Charlottesville: University of Virginia Press, 1987–2020.

——. *The Writings of George Washington.* 14 vols. Edited by Worthington Chauncey Ford. New York: G. P. Putnam's Sons, 1889–1893.

Waterhouse, Benjamin. *A Prospect of Exterminating the Smallpox: Part II, Being a Continuation of a Narrative of Facts Concerning the Progress of the New Inoculation in America; Together with Practical Observations on the Local appearance, Symptoms, and Mode of Treating the Variola Vaccina, or Kine Pock.* Cambridge: Cambridge University Press, 1802.

Wayland, Francis. "Report to the Corporation of Brown University, on Changes in the System of Collegiate Education." In *American Higher Education: A Documentary History*, edited by Richard Hofstader and Wilson Smith. Chicago: University of Chicago Press, 1961.

Webster, Daniel. *The Papers of Daniel Webster, 1798–1852.* 15 vols. Edited by Harold D. Moser and Charles M. Wiltse. Hanover, N.H.: Dartmouth University Press,

1974–1989.
——. *The Private Correspondence of Daniel Webster*, edited by Fletcher Webster. Boston: Little, Brown and Co., 1857.
Welch, William H. *Papers and Addresses.* Baltimore: Johns Hopkins University Press, 1930.

Secondary Sources: Books on Science

Albree, Joseph, David C. Arney, and V. Frederick Rickey. *Station Favorable to the Pursuits of Science: Primary Materials in the History of Mathematics at the United States Military Academy*. (History of Mathematics 18). Providence, R.I.: American Mathematics Society, 2000.
Bacon, Francis. *The Works of Francis Bacon,* vol 3. Edited by James Speeding, Robert Leslie Ellis, and Douglas Denon Heath. London, Longmans and Co., 1857–1859.
Bedini, Silvio A. *Jefferson and Science*. Thomas Jefferson Foundation and University of North Carolina Press, 2002.
——. *Thomas Jefferson and his Copying Machines*, Charlottesville: University Press of Virginia, 1984.
——. *Thomas Jefferson and American Vertebrate Paleontology*. Charlottesville: Virginia Division of Mineral Resources publication 061, Commonwealth of Virginia, 1985.
——. *Thomas Jefferson: Statesman of Science*. New York: Macmillan Publishing Co., 1990.
Benson, C. Randolph. *Thomas Jefferson as Social Scientist*. Cranberry, N.J.: Fairleigh Dickinson University Press, 1971.
Breeden, James O. *Joseph Jones, M.D.: Scientist of the Old South*. Lexington, Ky.: University Press of Kentucky, 1975.
Browne, Charles A. *Thomas Jefferson and the Scientific Trends of His Time*. Waltham, Mass.: The Chronica Botanical Co., 1944.
Cannon, Walter B. *The Way of an Investigator: A Scientist's Experiences in Medical Research*. New York: Norton, 1945.
Chaplin, Joyce. *The First Scientific American: Benjamin Franklin and the Pursuit of Genius.* New York: Basic Books, 2006.
Clagett, Martin. *Scientific Jefferson Revealed.* Charlottesville: University of Virginia Press, 2009.
Cohen, I. Bernard. *Science and the Founding Fathers: Science in the Political Thought of Jefferson, Franklin, Adams and Madison*. New York: W.W. Norton & Co., 1995.
Daniels, George H. *American Science in the Age of Jackson*. New York: Columbia University Press, 1968.
Dorr, Gregory Michael. *Segregation Science: Eugenics & Society in Virginia*. Charlottesville: University of Virginia Press, 2008.
Greene, John C. *American Science in the Age of Jefferson.* Ames, Iowa: Iowa State University Press, 1984.
Holton, Gerald. *Science and Anti-Science*. Cambridge, Mass.: Harvard University Press, 1993. 1984.
Jillson, William Rouse. *The Extinct Vertebrata of the Pleistocene in Kentucky*. Frankford, Ky.: Roberts Printing Co, 1968.
Johnson, Steven. *The Ghost Map: The Story of London's Most Terrifying Epidemic and How*

It Changed Science, Cities, and the Modern World. New York: Riverside Books, 2006.

Kraemer, Sylvia. *Science and Technology Policy in the United States: Open Systems in Action.* New Brunswick, N.J.: Rutgers University Press, 2006.

Lederer, Susan E. *Subjected to Science: Human Experimentation in America before the Second World War.* Baltimore: Johns Hopkins University Press, 1995.

Livingstone, David N. *The Geographical Tradition: Episodes in the History of a Contested Enterprise.* Oxford: Blackwell, 1992.

Marshall, Peter, and David Manuel. *From Sea to Shining Sea: 1787–1837.* Grand Rapids, Mich.: Fleming H. Revell Co., 1985.

Martin, Edwin T. *Thomas Jefferson: Scientist.* New York: Henry Schuman, 1952.

Miller, Charles A. *Jefferson and Nature: An Interpretation.* Baltimore: Johns Hopkins University Press, 1988.

Numbers, Ronald L., and Todd L. Savitt, eds. *Science and Medicine in the Old South.* Baton Rouge, La.: Louisiana State University Press, 1989.

Thomson, Keith. *Jefferson's Shadow: The Story of His Science.* New Haven: Yale University Press, 2012.

———. *A Passion for Nature: Thomas Jefferson and Natural History.* Thomas Jefferson Foundation and Chapel Hill: University of North Carolina Press, 2008.

Woodward, Augustus B. *A System of Universal Science.* Philadelphia, Pa.: published by Edward Earle, Harrison Hall, and Moses Thomas, 1816.

Secondary Sources: Books of Medical Practice, Education, and Literature

Abrams, Jeanne E. *Revolutionary Medicine: The Founding Fathers and Mothers in Sickness and in Health.* New York: New York University Press, 2013.

Ackerknecht, Erwin H. *Medicine at the Paris Hospital, 1794–1848.* Baltimore: Johns Hopkins University Press, 1967.

Adams, George Washington. *Doctors in Blue: The Medical History of the Union Army in the Civil War.* Baton Rouge, La.: Louisiana State University Press, 1996.

Antonovsky, Aaron. *Health, Stress, and Coping: New Perspectives on Mental and Physical Well-being.* San Francisco: Jossey-Bass, 1979.

Baron, John. *The Life of Edward Jenner, with Illustrations and His Doctrines and Selections from His Correspondence,* vol. 1. London: Henry Colburn publisher, 1827.

Bartholomew, Robert E., and Benjamin Radford. *The Martians Have Landed: A History of Media-Driven Panic and Hoaxes.* London: McFarland & Co., 2012.

Bazin, Herve. *The Eradication of Smallpox: Edward Jenner and the First and Only Eradication of a Human Infectious Disease.* Translated by Andrew and Glenise Morgan. London and San Diego, Calif.: Academic Press, 2000.

Beall, Otho T., and Richard H. Shyrock. *Cotton Mather: First Significant Figure in American Medicine.* Baltimore: Johns Hopkins University Press, 1954.

Berry, Daina Ramey. *The Price for Their Pound of Flesh.* Boston: Beacon Press, 2017.

Binger, Carl. *Revolutionary Doctor: Benjamin Rush, 1746–1813,* New York: W. W. Norton, 1966.

Blanton, Wyndham B. *Medicine in Virginia in the Eighteenth Century.* Richmond, Va.: Garrett and Massie, 1931.

———. *Medicine in Virginia in the Nineteenth Century.* Richmond, Va.: Garrett and Massie, 1933.

Bonner, Thomas Neville. *Becoming a Physician: Medical Education in Britain, France, Germany, and the United States, 1750–1945*. New York: Oxford University Press, 1995.

——. *To the Ends of the Earth: Women's Search for Education in Medicine*. Cambridge, Mass.: Harvard University Press, 1992.

——. *Iconoclast: Abraham Flexner and a Life in Learning*. Baltimore: Johns Hopkins University Press, 2002.

Bordley, James, and A. McGehee Harvey. *Two Centuries of American Medicine, 1776–1976*. Philadelphia: W. B. Saunders, 1976.

Brieger, Gert H., ed. *Medical America in the Nineteenth Century: Reading from the Literature*. Baltimore: Johns Hopkins University Press, 1972.

Brodsky, Alyn. *Benjamin Rush: Patriot and Physician*, New York, Truman Tally Books, 2004

Buchan, William. *Domestic Medicine: A Treatise on the Prevention and Cure of Disease, by Regimen and Simple Medicine*. Originally published in 1772. Available through Hathi Trust Digital Library.

Burr, Ann R. *S. Weir Mitchell: His Life and Letters*. New York, Duffield, 1929.

Burrow, James G. *Organized Medicine in the Progressive Era: The Move Towards Monopoly*. Baltimore: Johns Hopkins University Press, 1977.

Cash, Phillip. *Dr. Benjamin Waterhouse: A Life in Medicine and Public Service*. Sagamore Beach, Mass.: Boston Medical Library and Scientific Publications, 2006.

Chaplin, Arnold. *Medicine in England During the Reign of George III: The Fitzpatrick Lectures Delivered at the Royal College of Physicians, 1917–18*. London: Henry Kimpton, 1919.

Chase, Heber. *The Medical Student's Guide: Being a Compendious View of the Collegiate and Clinical Medical Schools, the Courses of Private Lectures, the Hospitals*. Philadelphia, Pa.: J. G. Auner, 1842.

Chitty, Joseph. *Practical Treatise on Medical Jurisprudence*. Philadelphia, Pa.: Carey, Lea & Blanchard, 1835.

Christian, George Llewellyn. *Confederate Memories and Experience*. Virginia Historical Society, Richmond, Va.: Clayton Publishing Co., 1915.

Clarke, Edward H., Henry J. Bigelow, Samuel D. Gross, Theodore G. Thomas, and John S. Billings. *A Century of American Medicine, 1776–1867*. Philadelphia, Pa.: Lea, 1876.

Comrie, John Dixon. *History of Scottish Medicine to 1860*, 2nd edition. London: Bailliere, Tindall & Cox, 1932.

Cooper, Sir Astley Paston. *A Treatise on Dislocations and Fractures of the Joints*. Philadelphia, Pa.: Blanchard and Lea, 1851.

Cordell, Eugene Fauntleroy. *Historical Sketch of the University of Maryland School of Medicine*. Baltimore: I. Friedenwald Press, 1891.

Corner, George W. *Two Centuries of Medicine: A History of the School of Medicine*. University of Pennsylvania. Philadelphia, Pa.: J. B. Lippincott Co., 1965.

Coxe, John Redman. *Practical Observations on Vaccination or Inoculation for the Cow-Pock*. Philadelphia, Pa.: James Humphreys, 1802.

Cunningham, H. H. *Doctors in Gray: The Confederate Medical Service*. Baton Rouge, La.: State University Press, 1958.

Cushing, Harvey. *The Life of William Osler*, Vol. 1. Oxford, England: The Clarendon Press, 1925.

Davis, Nathan S. *Medical Education and Institutions in the United States from the First*

Settlement of the British Colonies to the Year 1850. Chicago: Griggs, 1851.

Devine, Shauna. *Learning from the Wounded: The Civil War and the Rise of American Medical Science*. Chapel Hill, N.C., University of North Carolina Press, 2014.

Drake, Daniel. *Practical Essays on Medical Education and Medical Profession in the United States*. Cincinnati, Ohio: Roff and Young, 1832.

Duffy, John. *The Sanitarians: A History of American Public Health*. Urbana, Ill.: University of Illinois Press, 1990.

——. *From Humors to Medical Science: A History of American Medicine*. Urbana, IL: University of Illinois Press, 1993.

——. *The Healers: The Rise of the Medical Establishment*. New York: McGraw-Hill, 1976.

Emmet, Thomas Addis. *A Memoir of John Patten Emmet, M.D.: formerly Professor of Chemistry and Materia Medica in the University of Virginia, with a Brief Outline of the Emmet Family History*. New York: Privately published, 1898. Available at the National Library of Medicine, Bethesda, Md.

Estes, J. Worth, and Billy G. Smith, eds., *A Melancholy Scene of Devastation: The Public Response to the 1793 Philadelphia Yellow Fever Epidemic*, Canton, Mass.: Science History Publications/USA for the College of Physicians of Philadelphia and the Library Company of Philadelphia, 1997.

Fenn, Elizabeth A. *Pox Americana: The Great Smallpox Epidemic of 1775–82*. New York: Hill and Wang, 2001.

Fenner, Frank, Donald A. Henderson, Isao Arita, Zhenek Jezek, and Ivan Danilovich Ladnyi. *Smallpox and Its Eradication*. History of International Public Health, No. 6. Geneva: World Health Organization, 1988.

Fitzharris, Lindsey. *The Butchering Art: Joseph Lister's Quest to Transform the Grisly World of Victorian Medicine*. New York: Scientific American/Farrar, Straus and Giroux, 2017.

Fleming, Donald. *William H. Welch and the Rise of Modern Medicine*. Boston: Little Brown, 1954.

Flexner, Abraham. *Medical Education in the United States and Canada*. Carnegie Foundation for the Advancement of Teaching, Bulletin No. 4, 1910. Available through Hathi Trust Digital Library.

——. *Medical Education in Europe*. New York: Carnegie Foundation for the Advancement of Teaching, Bulletin No. 6, 1912.

——. *Medical Education: A Comparative Study*. New York: Macmillan Co., 1925.

Flexner, James T. *Doctors on Horseback: Pioneers of American Medicine*. New York: Fordham University Press, 1992 (originally published 1937).

Flexner, Simon, and James Flexner. *William Henry Welch and the Heroic Age of American Medicine*. New York: Viking Press, 1941.

Fried, Stephen. *Rush: Revolution, Madness, and Benjamin Rush, The Visionary Doctor who became a Founding Father*, New York, Broadway Books, 2018.

Friedrich, Johann. *Elements of Physiology*. Translated by Charles Caldwell. 2 vols. Philadelphia, Pa.: Thomas Dobson, 1795.

Furman, Bess. *A Profile of the United States Public Health Service, 1798–1948*. U.S. Department of Health, Education, and Welfare, DHEW Publication No. (NIH) 73-369, Washington, D.C.: U. S. Government Printing Office, 1974.

Garrison, Fielding Hudson. *An Introduction to the History of Medicine: With Medical Chronology, Suggestions for Study and Bibliographic Data*, Fourth Edition. Philadelphia, Pa.: W. B. Saunders, 1929.

Gehlbach, Stephen H. *American Plagues: Lessons from Our Battles with Disease*, updated edition. Lanham, Md.: Rowman & Littlefield, 2016.

Gemmill, Chalmers L., and Mary Jeanne Jones. *Pharmacology at the University of Virginia*. Charlottesville: University of Virginia Printing, 1966.

Haden, Charles. *Practical Observations on the Management and Diseases of Children.* London: Burgess and Hill, 1827.

Haller, John S. *American Medicine in Transition, 1840–1910*. Urbana, Ill.: University of Illinois Press, 1981.

——. *A Profile in Alternative Medicine*. Kent, Ohio: Kent State University Press, 1999.

Halsey, Robert H. *How the President, Thomas Jefferson and Doctor Benjamin Waterhouse Established Vaccination as a Public Health Procedure*, History of Medicine Series, vol. 5. New York: Academy of Medicine, 1936.

Harrington, Thomas F. *The Harvard Medical School: A History and Documentary. 1782–1905*. New York and Chicago: Lewis Publishing Co., 1905.

Hogarth, Rana A. *Medicalizing Blackness: Making Racial Differences in the Atlantic World.* Chapel Hill, N.C.: University of North Carolina Press, 2018.

Holmes, John S. *Thomas Jefferson Treats Himself: Herbs, Physicke and Nutrition in Early America*. Fort Valley, Va.: Loft Press, 1997.

Holmes, Oliver W. *Medical Essays, 1842–1882*, 5 eds. Boston: Houghton, Mifflin & Co., 1888.

Humphreys, Margaret. *Marrow of Tragedy: The Health Crisis of the American Civil War.* Baltimore: Johns Hopkins University Press, 2013.

——. *Yellow Fever and the South*. New Brunswick, N.J.: Rutgers University Press, 1992.

Kastor, John A. *Governance of Teaching Hospitals: Turmoil at Penn and Hopkins*. Baltimore: Johns Hopkins University Press, 2004.

Kett, Joseph F. *The Formation of the American Medical Profession 1780–1860*. New Haven: Yale University Press, 1968.

King, Lester S. *Transformations in American Medicine: From Benjamin Rush to William Osler*. Baltimore: Johns Hopkins University Press, 1991.

Kohn, Livia, and Stephen Jackewicz. *Health and Long-Life, The Chinese Way*. Three Pines Press, 2005.

Ludmerer, Kenneth M. *Learning to Heal: The Development of American Medical Education*. New York: Basic Books, Inc., 1985.

——. *Let Me Heal: The Opportunity to Preserve Excellence in American Medicine*. New York: Oxford University Press, 2015.

——. *Time to Heal: American Medical Education from the Turn of the Century to the Era of Managed Care*. New York: Oxford University Press, 1999.

Makary, Marty. *Unaccountable: What Hospitals Won't Tell You and How Transparency Can Revolutionize Health Care*. New York: Bloomsbury Press, 2012.

Marx, Richard. *The Health of the Presidents,* New York: Van Rees Press, 1960.

Myer, Jesse Shire. *Life and Letters of Dr. William Beaumont: Including Hitherto Unpublished Data Concerning the Case of Alexis St. Martin*. St. Louis, Mo.: C. V. Mosby, original publication 1912, updated 1939.

Nicholson, C. Brid. *Documents of the Lewis and Clark Expedition*, Santa Barbara, Calif., ABC-CLIO, LLC, 2019.

Norwood, William F. *Medical Education in the United States Before the Civil War*. Philadelphia, Pa.: University of Pennsylvania Press, 1944.

Numbers, Ronald L., ed. *The Education of American Physicians*. Berkeley, Calif.: University of California Press, 1980.

Ogden, Emily. *Credulity: A Cultural History of U.S. Mesmerism*. Chicago: University of Chicago Press, 2018.

Oshinsky, David M. *Bellevue: Three Centuries of Medicine and Mayhem at America's Most Storied Hospital*. New York: Doubleday, 2016.

Osler, William. *The Evolution of Modern Medicine: A Series of Lectures Delivered at Yale University on the Silliman Foundation in April 1913*. New Haven: Yale University Press, 1922.

——. *The Fixed Period in Aequanimitas and Other Addresses to Medical Students, Nurses and Practitioners of Medicine,* 3rd ed. Philadelphia, Pa.: the Blakiston Co., 1932.

Peale, Charles Wilson. *An Epistle to a Friend on Preserving Health, Promoting Happiness and Prolonging the Life of Man to its Natural Period.* Philadelphia, Pa.: Jane Aitkin, printer, 1803. Available through U.S. National Library of Congress Digital Collections.

Percival, Thomas. *Medical Ethics; or a Code of Institutes and Precepts, adapted to the Professional Conduct of Physicians and Surgeons*. London: Cambridge University Press, 1803.

Pernick Martin S. *A Calculus of Suffering*. New York: Columbia University Press, 1985.

Peter, Robert. *The History of the Medical Department of Transylvania University*. Louisville, Ky.: J. P. Morton & Co., 1905.

Pitrof, Larry. *University of Maryland School of Medicine: The First Two Centuries, 1807-2007*. Baltimore: Medical Alumni Association of the University of Maryland, 2006.

Powell, J. H. *Bring Out Your Dead: The Great Plague of Yellow Fever in Philadelphia in 1793*. Philadelphia, Pa.: University of Pennsylvania Press, first published in 1949, updated 1993.

Power, Sir D'Arcy. *Medicine in the British Isles*. New York: Paul B. Hoeber, Inc., 1930.

Poynter, Frederick Noel Lawrence. *The Evolution of Medical Education in Britain*. London: Pitman Publisher, 1966.

Quinan, John Russel. "Robley Dunglison," In *Medical Annals of Baltimore from 1608 to 1880, Including Events, Men and Literature*, Baltimore, Press of Isaac Friedenwald, (1884).

Ravitch, Mark M. *A Century of Surgery: The History of the American Surgical Association*. 2 vols. Philadelphia, Pa.: J. B. Lippincott, 1981.

Richerand, Anthelme. *Elements of Physiology*. Translated by Robert Kerrison. Philadelphia: Hopkins and Earle, 1808.

Risse, Guenter B., Ronald L. Numbers, and Judith Walzer Leavitt. *Medicine Without Doctors: Home Health Care in American History*. New York: Science History Publications, 1977.

Rosenberg, Charles E. *The Care of Strangers: The Rise of American's Hospital System*. New York: Basic Books, 1987.

——. *Explaining Epidemics and Other Studies in the History of Medicine*. New York: Cambridge University Press, 1992.

Rothstein, William G. *American Physicians in the 19th Century: From Sects to Science*. Baltimore: Johns Hopkins University Press, 1985.

——. *American Medical Schools and the Practice of Medicine: A History*. New York: Oxford University Press, 1987.

Ruschenberger, W. S. W. *An Account of the Institution and Progress of the College of Physicians of Philadelphia During a Hundred Years*. Philadelphia: William J. Dornan Publishing, 1887.

Sappol, Michael. *A Traffic of Dead Bodies: Anatomy and Embolden Social Identity in Nineteenth-Century America*. Princeton: Princeton University Press, 2002.

Savitt, Todd L. *Medicine and Slavery: The Diseases and Health Care of Blacks in Antebellum Virginia*. Urbana, Ill.:University of Illinois Press, 1981.

——. *Race and Medicine in Nineteenth- and Early Twentieth-Century America*. Kent,Ohio: Kent State University Press, 2007.

Shaw, Maurice F. *Stonewall Jackson's Surgeon: Hunter Holmes McGuire, a Biography*. Lynchburg, Va.: H. E. Howard Printing, 1993.

Shryock, Richard Harrison. *American Medical Research: Past and Present*, reprint edition. New York: Arno Press, 1980.

——. *The Development of Modern Medicine: An Interpretation of the Social and Scientific Factors Involved*. Madison: University of Wisconsin Press, 1979.

——. *Medical Licensing in America, 1650–1965*. Baltimore: Johns Hopkins University Press, 1967.

——. *The Medical World of the Eighteenth Century*. Chicago: University of Chicago Press, 1958.

——. *Medicine and Society in America: 1660–1860*. Ithaca, N.Y.: Cornell University Press, 1960.

——. *Medicine in America: Historical Essays*. Baltimore: " Johns Hopkins University Press, 1966.

Sigerist, Henry E. *The Great Doctors: A Biographical History of Medicine*. New York: Dover Publications, 1971, an unabridged republication of the English translation originally published by W. W. Norton & Co., 1933.

Somers, Herman M., and Anne R. Somers. *Doctors, Patients, & Health Insurance: The Organization and Financing of Medical Care*. Washington, D.C.: The Brookings Institution, 1961.

Starr, Paul. *The Social Transformation of American Medicine*. New York: Basic Books, 1982.

Staum, Martin S. *Cabanis: Enlightenment and Medical Philosophy in the French Revolution*. Princeton: Princeton University Press, 1980.

Stevens, Rosemary. *American Medicine and the Public Interest*. Berkeley, Calif.: University of California Press, 1971.

Stevenson, Lloyd G., ed. *A Celebration of Medical History.* Baltimore: Johns Hopkins University Press, 1982.

Stowe, Steven M. *Doctoring in the South: Southern Physicians and Everyday Medicine in the Mid-Nineteenth Century*. Chapel Hill: University of North Carolina Press, 2004.

Thompson, John D., and Grace Goldin. *The Hospital: A Social and Architectural History*. New Haven: Yale University Press. 1975.

Von Haller, Albrecht. *First Lines of Physiology*. First American edition. Translated from 3rd Latin edition. New York: Obadish Penniman & Co., 1803.

Wagner, Frederick B., ed. *Thomas Jefferson University: Tradition and Heritage*. Philadelphia, Pa.: Jefferson Digital Commons 1989. http://jdc.jefferson.edu/wagner2/50

Waite, Frederick C. *The First Medical College in Vermont: Castleton, 1818–1862*. Montpelier Vermont Historical Society 67 (1949).

Warner, John Harley. *Against the Spirit of System: The French Impulse in Nineteenth Century American Medicine*. Princeton: Princeton University Press, 1998.

——. *The Therapeutic Perspective: Medical Practice, Knowledge and Identity in America*. Cambridge, Mass.: Harvard University Press, 1986.

Warner, John Harley, and Janet A. Tighe. *Major Problems in the History of American Medicine and Public Health*. Boston: Houghton Mifflin Co., 2001.
Warren, Edward. *A Doctor's Experience in Three Continents*. Baltimore: Cushings & Bailey, 1885.
Williams, Richard. *The United States Public Health Service, 1798–1950*. Washington, D.C.: 1951.
Willrich, Michael. *Pox: An American History*. New York: Penguin Press, 2011.
Wooten, David. *Bad Medicine: Doctors Doing Harm Since Hippocrates*. Oxford, England: Oxford University Press, 2006.

Secondary Sources: Books on Higher Education

Adams, Herbert B. *Thomas Jefferson and the University of Virginia*. Washington, D.C.: Government Printing Office for the Bureau of Education, 1888.
Addis, Cameron. *Jefferson's Vision for Education*. New York: Peter Lang, 2003.
Ambrose, Stephen. *Duty, Honor, Country: A History of West Point*. Baltimore: Johns Hopkins University Press, 1966.
Axtell, James. *Wisdom's Workshop: The Rise of the Modern University*. Princeton: Princeton University Press, 2016.
Barringer, Paul B., and James M. Garrett and Rosewell Page, eds. *The University of Virginia: Its History, Influence, Equipment and Characteristics*. New York: Lewis Publishing Co., 1904.
Barth, Alan. *The Loyalty of Free Men*. New York: Viking Press, Inc., 1951.
Bowman, Rex, and Carlos Santos. *Rot, Riot, and Rebellion: Mr. Jefferson's Struggle to Save the University that Changed America*. Charlottesville: University of Virginia Press, 2013.
Bronson, Walter C. *History of Brown University, 1764–1914*. Providence R.I.: University Press, 1914.
Brophy, Alfred L. *University, Court, and Slave: Proslavery Academic Thought and Southern Jurisprudence*. New York: Oxford University Press, 2016.
Bruce, Phillip A. *History of the University of Virginia: 1819–1919*. New York: MacMillan, 1920.
Brubacher, John S., and Willis Rudy. *Higher Education in Transition: An American History*. New York: Harper and Brothers, 1958.
Callcott, George H. *A History of the University of Maryland*. Baltimore: Historical Society, 1966.
Cheyney, Edward Potts. *History of the University of Pennsylvania, 1740–1790*. Philadelphia: University of Pennsylvania Press, 1940.
Clemons, Harry. *The University of Virginia Library, 1825–1850, Story of a Jeffersonian Foundation*. Charlottesville: University of Virginia Library, 1954.
Cometti, Elizabeth, ed. *Jefferson's Ideas on a University Library: Letters from the Founder of the University of Virginia to a Boston Bookseller*. Charlottesville: Tracy W. McGregor Library, University of Virginia, 1950.
Cremin, Lawrence A. *American Education, the National Experience*. New York: Harper and Row, 1988.
Dabney, Virginius. *Mr. Jefferson's University*. Charlottesville: University Press of Virginia, 1981.
Dyer, Thomas G. *The University of Georgia: A Bicentennial History*. Athens: The University of Georgia Press, 1985.

Gamble, Harry Y. *God on Grounds: A History of Religion at Thomas Jefferson's University*. Charlottesville: University of Virginia Press, 2020.

Geiger, Roger. *The History of American Higher Education: Learning and Culture from the Founding to World War II*. Princeton: Princeton University Press, 2015.

Hellenbrand, Harold. *The Unfinished Revolution: Education and Politics in the Thoughts of Thomas Jefferson*. Newark, Del.: University of Delaware Press, 1990.

Hofstradter, Richard, and Walter P. Metzger. *The Development of Academic Freedom in the United States*. New York: Columbia University Press, 1955.

——. *Academic Freedom in the Age of the College*. New Brunswick, N.J.: Aldine Transaction Publishers, 1996.

——. *American Higher Education: A Documentary History*. Chicago: University of Chicago Press, 1961.

Honeywell, Roy J. *The Educational Work of Thomas Jefferson*. Cambridge: Harvard University Press, 1931.

Knight, Edgar W., ed. *A Documentary History of Education in the South Before 1860*. 5 vols. Chapel Hill: University of North Carolina Press, 1945-1953.

Koch, Adrienne. *The Philosophy of Thomas Jefferson*. New York: Columbia University Press, 1943.

Lee, Gordon C. *Thomas Jefferson on Education*. New York: Bureau of Publications, Teachers College, Columbia University, 1961.

Levy, Leonard W. *Jefferson and Civil Liberties: The Darker Side*. Cambridge: Belknap Press of Harvard University, 1963.

Looney, J. Jefferson. *From Academy to College to University: The Prehistory of the University of Virginia*, In The Founding of Thomas Jefferson's University, edited by John A. Ragosta et al, Charlottesville, 2019

Malone, Dumas D. *Mr. Jefferson's University: A History*. Charlottesville: University Press of Virginia, 1981.

McDonald, Robert M. *Thomas Jefferson's Military Academy: Founding West Point*. Charlottesville: University of Virginia Press, 2004.

McInnis, Maurie D., and Louis P. Nelson. *Educated in Tyranny: Slavery at Thomas Jefferson's University*. Charlottesville: University of Virginia Press, 2019.

Morpurgo, Jack E. *The Majesties Royal Colleges: The College of William and Mary in the Seventeenth and Eighteenth Century*. Washington D.C.: Hennage Creative Printers, 1976.

Nash, Joseph Van Holt, and Shele deVere M., eds. *Students of the University of Virginia: a Semi-Centennial Catalogue, with Brief Biographical Sketches*. Baltimore: C. Harvey & Co., 1878.

Neff, Joseph. *Sketch of a Plan and Method of Education Founded on an Analysis of Human Faculties and Natural Reason Suitable for the Offspring of a Free People, and for all Rational Beings*. Philadelphia, Pa.: unknown publisher, 1808.

de Nemmours, Pierre Samuel du Pont. *National Education in The United States of America*. Translated by B. G. Du Pont. Newark, Del.: University's Gordon-Reed, Annette, and Peter S. Onuf. *Most Blessed of the Patriarchs: Thomas Jefferson and the Empire of the Imagination*. New York: Liveright Publishing Corp., 2017.

Gross, Samuel D. *Memoir of Robley Dunglison*. Philadelphia: Collins Printers, 1869.

Hailman, John R. *Thomas Jefferson on Wine*. Jackson: University Press of Mississippi, 2006.

Hays, Kevin J. *The Road to Monticello: The Life and Mind of Thomas Jefferson*. New York: Oxford University Press, 2008.

——. *Jefferson in His Own Time: A Biographical Chronical of His Life, Drawn from Recollections, Interviews, and Memoirs by Family, Friends, and Associates*. Iowa City, Iowa: University of Iowa Press, 2012.

Helo, Ari. *Thomas Jefferson's Ethics and Politics of Human Progress*. New York: Cambridge University Press, 2014.

Holochak, M. Andrew. *Rethinking Thomas Jefferson's Writings on Slavery and Race*. Newcastle on Tyne: Cambridge Scholars Publishing, 2020.

Johnston, William Dawson. *History of the Library of Congress: 1800–1864,* vol 1. Washington, D.C.: Government Printing Office, 1904.

Kerber, Linda. *Federalists in Dissent: Imagery and Ideology in Jeffersonian America*. Ithaca, N.Y.: Cornel University Press, 1970.

Kern, Susan. *The Jeffersons at Shadwell*. New Haven: Yale University Press, 2010.

Kett, Joseph F. *Merit: The History of a Founding Ideal from the American Revolution to the Twenty-First Century*. Ithaca, N.Y.: Cornell University Press, 2012.

Kimball, Marie. *Jefferson, the Road to Glory, 1743–1776*. N.Y.: Coward-McCann, 1943.

Kirkland, Richard Bevier. *George Wythe: Lawyer, Revolutionary and Judge*. New York: Garland, 1986.

Klingberg, Frank J., and Frank W. Klingberg, eds. *The Correspondence Between Henry Stephen Randall and Hugh Blair Grigsby, 1856-1861*. Berkeley: University of California Press, 1952.

Lehmann, Karl. *Thomas Jefferson, American Humanist*. New York: The Macmillan Co., 1947.

Long, William. *Literary Pioneers: Early American Explorers of European Culture*. Cambridge, Mass.: Harvard University Press, 1934.

Malone, Dumas. *Jefferson and His Time,* 6 volumes. (Boston: Little Brown and Co., 1948–1981).

——. *The Public Life of Thomas Cooper, 1783–1839*. New Haven: Yale University Press, 1926.

McCullough, David. *John Adams*. New York: Simon and Schuster, 2001.

McLachlan, James. *Princetonians, 1748–1768: A Biographical Dictionary*. Princeton: Princeton University Press, 1976.

Meacham, Jon. *In the Hands of the People*. New York: Random House, 2020.

——. *Thomas Jefferson: The Art of Power*. New York: Random House, 2013.

Morrison, Larry Robert. *The Proslavery Argument in the Early Republic, 1790–1830*. Charlottesville: University of Virginia Press, 1975.

Mott, Frank Luther. *American Journalism, A History of Newspapers in the United States through 250 Years, 1690 to 1940*. New York: MacMillan, 1941.

Oast, Jennifer. *Institutional Slavery: Slaveholding Churches, Schools, Colleges, and Businesses in Virginia, 1680–1860*. New York: Cambridge University Press, 2016.

Onuf, Peter S. *Jefferson's Empire*. Charlottesville: University Press of Virginia, 2000.

——. *The Mind of Thomas Jefferson*. Charlottesville: University of Virginia Press, 2007.

Padover, Saul. *The Complete Jefferson*. New York: Tudor Publishing Company, 1943.

Parton, James. *Life of Thomas Jefferson*. Boston: J. R. Osgood, 1874.

Peterson, Merrill D. *Thomas Jefferson and the New Nation: A Biography*. New York: Oxford University Press, 1970.

Randall, Henry S. *Life of Thomas Jefferson,* 3 vols. New York: Derby & Jackson, 1858.

Randall, Willard Stein. *Thomas Jefferson: A Life*. New York: Henry Holt and Co., 1993.

Roberts, Cokie. *Founding Mothers: The Women Who Raised Our Nation*. New York: William Morrow, 2004.

La Rochefoucauld-Liancourt, Francois. *Travels Through the United States of North America*. London: R. Phillips, 1800.
Schachner, Nathan. *Thomas Jefferson: A Biography*. New York: Thomas Yoseloff, 1957.
Schlesinger, Arthur M., Jr. *A Thousand Days: John F. Kennedy in the White House*. Boston: Houghton Mifflin, Co. and the Riverside Press, 1965.
Smith, James Morton. *Republic of Letters: The Correspondence between Thomas Jefferson and James Madison*. New York: W. W. Norton, 1995.
Smith, Richard Norton Patriarch. *George Washington and the New American Nation*. Boston: Houghton Mifflin Co., 1993.
Sowerby, E. Millicent. *Catalogue of the Library of Thomas Jefferson*. Washington, D.C.: Library of Congress, 1952–1959.
Spahn, Hannah. *Thomas Jefferson's Time and History*. Charlottesville: University of Virginia Press, 2011.
Stanton, Lucia C. *Those Who Labor for My Happiness: Slavery at Thomas Jefferson's Monticello*. Charlottesville: University of Virginia Press, 2012.
Steele, Brian Douglass. *Thomas Jefferson and American Nationhood*. New York: Cambridge University Press, 2012.
Tucker, George. *Life of Thomas Jefferson*. Philadelphia: Carey, Lea and Blanchard, 1837.
——. *Memoir of the Life and Character of John Patten Emmet, Professor of Chemistry and Materia Medica in the University of Virginia*. Philadelphia: C. Sherman, 1845.
——. *The Valley of Shenandoah: or Memoirs of the Graysons*, 3 vols. New York: C. Wiley, 1824–25.
Tyler, Lyon G. *Williamsburg, The Old Colonial Capital*. Richmond, Va.: Whittet & Shepffersow Publishing, 1907.
Uglow, Jenny. *The Lunar Men*. London: Farber and Farber, 2002.
Van Doren, Carl. *Benjamin Franklin*. New York: Viking Press, 1938.
Van Duzen, Charles Hunter. *Contributions of the Ideologues to French Revolutionary Thought*. Baltimore: Johns Hopkins University Press, 1935.
Weymouth, Lally, ed. *Thomas Jefferson: The Man, His World, His Influence*. London: Weiderfield and Nicholson, 1973.
Wiencek, Henry. *Master of the Mountain: Thomas Jefferson and His Slaves*. New York: Farrar, Straus, and Giroux, 2012.
Wilson, Douglas L. *Jefferson's Books*. Charlottesville, Va.: Thomas Jefferson Memorial Foundation, 1996.
Wold, Karl C. *Mr. President – How is Your Health?* St. Louis, MO: Bruce Publishing Co, 1948.
Wood, Gordon S. *The Creation of the American Republic: 1776–1787*. Chapel Hill: University of North Carolina Press, 1969.
Yarbrough, Jeanne M. *American Virtues: Thomas Jefferson on the Character of a Free People*. Lawrence, KS: University Press of Kansas, 1998.

Secondary Sources: Essays, Chapters, Magazines, Journals, Newspapers, and Video Recordings

Ackerknecht, Erwin H. "Medical Education in 19th Century France," *Journal of Medical Education* 32, no. 2 (1957):148–153.
Ambuske, James P., and Randall Flaherty. "Reading Law in the Early Republic: Legal Education in the Age of Jefferson," in *The Founding of Mr. Jefferson's University*, Charlottesville: University of Virginia Press, 2019: 224–257.

Anonymous. "Critical Analysis of English and Foreign Literature Relative to the Various Branches of Medical Science." *The London Medical and Physical Journal* 52 (1824): 402–432.

Anonymous. "Medical Schools in the United States." *Journal of the American Medical Association* LI, no. 7, 1908: 607–609.

Anonymous. "Marie Francois Xavier Bichat (1771-1802)—Tissue Pathologist." *Journal of the American Medical Association* 203, no. 4 (1968): 129–130.

Appleby, Joyce. *Jefferson and his Complex Legacy,* In Jefferson's Legacies, edited by Peter S. Onuf, Charlottesville: University of Virginia Press, 1993: 1–16.

Atwater, Edward C. "Internal Medicine." In *The Education of the American Physician*, edited by Ronald L. Numbers. Berkeley: University of California Press, 1980: 143–174.

Baker, Gordon E. "Thomas Jefferson on Academic Freedom," *Bulletin of the American Association of University Professors* 39, no. 3 (1953): 377–387.

Barnett, Clifton Waller. "The Struggle to Create a University: Founder's Day Address," *Virginia Quarterly Review* 49, no. 4 (1973): 494–506.

Barquet, Nicolau, and Pere Domingo. "Smallpox: The Triumph over the Most Terrible of the Ministers of Death." *Annals of Internal Medicine* 127 (1997): 635–642.

Barringer, Paul B. "A History of the Medical Department of the University of Virginia: Its System of Education, and Its Results." An address delivered before the students and alumni, October 25, 1887, *North Carolina Medical Journal* 20 (1888): 278–286.

Bean, William Bennett. "Mr. Jefferson's Influence on American Medical Education." *Virginia Medical Monthly* 87 (1960): 669–680.

Bear, James A. "The Last Few Days in the Life of Thomas Jefferson." *The Magazine of Albemarle County History* 32 (1974): 63–79.

Bedini, Silvio. "Godfather of American Invention." In *Smithsonian Book of Invention*, edited by Alexis Doster III, Joe Goodwin, and Jame M. Ross. Washington, D.C,: Smithsonian Exposition Books, 1978: 82–83.

Beiswanger, William L. "Jefferson and the Art of Roofing," *Chronicle of Early American Industries Association* 53, no. 1 (2005): 18–25.

Bell, Whitfield J. "Private Physicians and Public Collections: Medical Libraries in the United States before 1900." In *A Celebration of Medical History*, edited by L. G. Stevenson. Baltimore: Johns Hopkins Press, 1982: 85–102.

Belleh, Godfrey S., and Eric V. D. Luft. "Financing North American Medical Libraries in the Nineteenth Century, *Bulletin of the Medical Library Association* 89, no. 4 (2001): 386–394.

Birchette, Kathleen P. "The History of Medical Libraries from 2000 B.C. to 1900 A.D." *Bulletin of the Medical Library Association* 61, no. 3 (1973): 302–308.

Blake, Aaron. "Here's How Many Americans Are Actually Anti-vaxxers," *Washington Post*, February 9, 2015.

Blake, John Ballard. "Benjamin Waterhouse and the Introduction of Vaccination, a Reappraisal," Yale University Department of History of Medicine Monograph, Series 33 (1957): 9–74.

——. "Benjamin Waterhouse and the Introduction of Vaccination." *Reviews of Infectious Diseases* 9, no. 5 (1987): 1044–1052.

——. "From Buchan to Fishbein: The Literature of Domestic Medicine." In *Medicine Without Doctors*, edited by Guenter B. Risse, Ronald L. Numbers, and Judith Walzer Leavitt. New York: Science History Publications, 1977: 11–30.

——. "The Development of American Anatomy Laws." *Journal of Medical Education* 30 (1955): 431–439.

Blinderman, Abraham. "Thomas Jefferson: Administrator, Practitioner, and Patient." *New York Journal of Medicine* 70, no. 5 (1970): 690–696.

Bloch, H. "Thomas Jefferson 1743 to 1826: Thoughts on Medicine, Child Care and Welfare." *New York State Journal of Medicine* 72, no. 24 (1972): 3030–3032.

Bonner, Thomas Neville. "Abraham Flexner as Critic of British and Continental Medical Education." *Medical History* 33 (1989): 472–479.

——. "Abraham Flexner and the Historians," *Journal of the History of Medicine and Allied Health Sciences* 45, no. 1 (1990): 3–10.

Booker, Brakkon. *Historic Chemistry Lab with Links to Thomas Jefferson Discovered Behind the Rotunda Wall.* NPR Radio, 4:38 PM ET, October 18, 2015.

Breeden, James O. "Body Snatchers and Anatomy Professors: Medical Education in Nineteenth-Century Virginia." *The Virginia Magazine of History and Biography* 83, no. 3 (1975): 321–345.

——. "Insights into the Medical Statistics of the Charlottesville General Hospital," *Magazine of the Albemarle History* 30 (1972): 43–60.

——. "Joseph Jones and Confederate Medical History." *Georgia Historical Quarterly* 54, no. 3 (1970): 357–380.

——. "Joseph Jones and Public Health in the New South." *Journal of the Louisiana Historical Association* 32, no. 4 (1991): 341–370.

——. "States-Rights Medicine in the Old South." *Bulletin of the New York Academy of Medicine* 52, no. 3 (1976): 348–372.

Brieger, Gert H. "Fit to Study Medicine: Notes for a History of Premedical Education in America." *Bulletin of the History of Medicine* 57 (1983): 1–20.

Brinton, John H. "The Faculty of 1841: A Lecture Delivered before the Alumni Association of the Jefferson Medical College," Philadelphia: Collins, Printer, 1880: 3–14.

Brophy, Alfred L. "The Law of Descent of Thought: Law, History, and Civilization in Antebellum." *Literary Addresses, Law and Literature* 20, no. 3 (2008): 343–402.

Browne, Charles A. "The History of Chemical Education in America between the Years 1820 and 1870." *Chemical Education in America* 9, no. 4 (1932): 696–729.

——. "Thomas Jefferson and Agricultural Chemistry." *The Scientific Monthly* 60, no. 1 (1945): 55–62.

——. "Thomas Jefferson's Relation to Chemistry." *Journal of Chemical Education* 20, no. 12 (1943): 574–576.

Bryan, Charles S. "Osler Goes Viral: The 'Fixed Period' Revisited." *Proceedings Baylor University Medical Center* 31, no. 4 (2018): 550–553.

Burns, Chester R. "Medical Ethics and Jurisprudence." In *The Education of American Physicians*, edited by Ronald L. Numbers. Berkeley: University of California Press, 1980: 273–289.

Bylebyl, Jerome J. "William Beaumont, Robley Dunglison, and the Philadelphia Physiologists." *Journal of History of Medicine and Applied Sciences* 25 (1970): 3–21.

Carpenter, James. "Thomas Jefferson and the Ideology of Democratic Schooling." Democracy and Education 21, no. 2 (2013): 1–11.

Carter, Edward C. "Jefferson's American Philosophical Society Leadership and Heritage." In *The Most Flattering Incident of My Life: Essays Celebrating the Bicentennial of Thomas Jefferson's American Philosophical Society Presidency*. Philadelphia: Friends of the American Philosophical Society Library, 1997: 9–15.

The Central Gazette (Charlottesville, Va.): "Imported Professors, and Virginia Stump Orators." December 25, 1824.

Chapman, Carleton B. "The Flexner Report by Abraham Flexner." *Daedalus* 104, no. 1 (1974): 105–117.

Chapman, Nathaniel. "American Medicine." *The Philadelphia Journal of Medical and Physical Sciences* 9 (1825): 404–409.

Chinard, Gilbert. "Jefferson and the American Philosophical Society." *Proceedings of the American Philosophical Society* 87, no. 3 (1943): 263–276.

——. "Jefferson's Influence Abroad." *The Mississippi Valley Historical Review* 30, no. 2 (1943): 171–186.

Christian Register and *Boston Observer*, August 20, 1842 (death notice of John Patten Emmet).

Christmas, William A., and James C. Turner. "Varsity Hall: The Infirmary of the University of Virginia." *Journal of American College Health* 57, no. 3 (2008): 349–351.

Clark, Austin H. "Thomas Jefferson and Science." *Washington Academy of Sciences Journal* 33 (1943): 193–203.

Cobbett, William. In "The Rush Light." New York: February 28, 1800: 49. https://archive.org/details/rushlight1718cobb.

Cohen, Mesick. "Wilson Baker Architects and the University of Virginia." *Pavilion X Historic Structure Report*, https://www.officearchitect.virginia.edu/pfds/PavilonX-HSR.pdf>,8.

Cohn, Lawrence H. "Contributions of Thomas Jefferson to American Medicine." *The American Journal of Surgery* 138, no. 2 (1979): 286–292.

Colbourn, H. Trevor. "Thomas Jefferson's Use of the Past." *William and Mary Quarterly* 15, no. 1 (January 1958): 56–70.

Columbian Sentinel, "Something Curious in the Medical Line." March 12, 1799.

Cometti, Elizabeth, ed. *Jefferson's Ideas on a University Library: Letters from the Founder of the University of Virginia to a Boston Bookseller*. Charlottesville: Tracy W. McGregor Library, University of Virginia, 1950.

Commission on Medical Education in Virginia. "Shall the Medical Department of the University of Virginia be Abandoned and Removed to Richmond: The Record of the Case and A Discussion of the Reports." *Alumni News of the University of Virginia*, December 1921 supplement, 52 pages.

Cope, Zachary. "Dr. Charles Thomas Haden (1786–1824), a Friend of Jane Austen." *British Medical Journal* 1 (1966): 974.

——. "Influence of the Society of Apothecaries on Medical Education." *British Medical Journal* 1 (1956): 1–6.

Cordell, Eugene F. "The Importance of the Study of the History of Medicine." *Medical Library and Historical Journal* 2, no, 4 (1904): 268–282.

Corner, George W. "Beginnings of Medical Education in Philadelphia, 1765–1776." *Journal of the American Medical Association* 194 (1965): 719–721.

Creighton, Catherine A. "Pavilion X: A Brief History (1820–1895)." http://juel.iath.virginia.edu/resources

Crispell, Kenneth R. "Beaumont and Dunglison: Who Was Dunglison?" *Transactions of the American Clinical Climatological Assoc.* 92 (1981): 194–198.

C-SPAN Video Library, Attorney General Sessions on Free Speech, September 27, 2017.

Custers, Eugene J.F.M and Olle ten Cate. "The History of Medical Education in Europe and the United States, with Respect to Time and Proficiency." *Academic Medicine* 93, no.3 (2018): S49–S54.

Cutright, Paul Russel. "Jefferson's Instructions to Lewis and Clark." *Bulletin of the Missouri Historical Society* 22 (1965–66): 302–321.

Daniel, Frederick. "Virginian Reminiscences of Jefferson." *Harper's Weekly* 48 (November 19, 1904): 1768.

Davis, John S. "History of the Medical Department of the University of Virginia, 1825–1914." *University of Virginia Alumni Bulletin* 7, no. 3 (July 1914):299–320.

Davison, Wilburt Cornell, and Wiley D. Forbus. "Fourteen distinguished physicians and surgeons; brief sketches of eminent men for whom Duke Hospital wards are named." *Box 53, Wilburt Cornell Davision Papers, Duke University Medical Center Archives*, 1930.

Davy, George Alan. "Argumentation and Unified Structure in Notes on the State of Virginia." *Eighteenth Century Studies* 26(4) (1993): 581–593.

Degrasse, L. "Thomas Jefferson as a Collector of Books." *AB Brookman's W Weekly* 86 (1990): 121–23.

Dewey, Frank L. "Thomas Jefferson's Law Practice: The Norfolk Anti-Inoculation Riots." *The Virginia Magazine of History and Biography* 91 (January 1983): 39–53.

Dilworth, Gwen. "The Destinies of the South Must be Entrusted to Our Keeping: 1850s Secessionist and Pro-Slavery Thoughts at the University of Virginia." https://juel.iath.virginia.edu/node/1061

D'Elia, Donald J. "Jefferson, Rush, and the Limits of Philosophical Friendship," Proc. Am. Phil. Society 73, no. 5 (1973): 333–343.

Doyle, Derek. "James Hamilton, the younger (1767–1839)." *Journal Royal Coll Physicians of Edinburgh*, 42, no.2 (2012): 188.

Dubose, Joseph, and Curtis Tribble. "James Lawrence Cabell, One of the Most Influential of America's Early Surgeons." *The American Surgeon* 81 (2015): 331–335.

Duffy, John. "Sectional Conflict and Medical Education in Louisiana." *Journal of Southern History* 23 (1957): 289–306.

Duffy, Thomas P. "The Flexner Report—100 Years Later." *The Yale Journal of Biology and Medicine* 84, no. 3 (2011):269–76.

Dunn, P. M." William Potts Dewees (1768–1841) of Pennsylvania: Pioneer of Perinatal Medicine in America." *Archives of Diseases of Children and Fetal Neonatal Education*. 75, no. 1 (1996): 69–70.

Eckman, James. "Anglo-American Hostility in American Medical Literature of the Nineteenth Century." *Bulletin of the History of Medicine* 9 (1941): 31–71.

Estes, J. Worth. "George Washington and the Doctors." *Medical Heritage* 1 (January/February 1985): 44–57.

Emmet, Thomas Addis. *A Memoir of John Patten Emmet, M.D.: formerly Professor of Chemistry and Materia Medica in the University of Virginia, with a Brief Outline of the Emmet Family History.* New York: Privately published, 1898. Available at the National Library of Medicine, Bethesda, Md.

Emmet, Thomas Addis. "Memoir of Professor John Patten Emmet." *The Alumni Bulletin of the University of Virginia* 1, no. 4 (1895): 93–101.

Eriksen, Anne. "Cure or Protection? The Meaning of Smallpox Inoculation, ca 1750-1775." *Medical History* 57, no. 4 (2013): 516–536.

Ezell, John S. "A Southern Education for Southerners." *Journal of Southern History* 4 (1951): 303–327.

The Federal Gazette (Baltimore), "Lectures on Preventive Medicine," May 30, 1833.

Finkelman, Paul. "Thomas Jefferson and Antislavery: The Myth Goes On." *The Virginia Magazine of History and Biography* 102, no. 2 (1994): 193–228.

Fitz, R. H. "The Legislative Control of Medical Practice." *Medical Communications of the Massachusetts Medical Society* 16 (1894): 306–307.

Fitzgerald, Faith T. "The Tyranny of Health." *New England Journal of Medicine* 331 (1994): 196–98.

FitzHugh, Slaughter G. "Anatomical Laboratory – Dissecting Hall 1833-1928." [manuscript], 1981, 3, Historical Collections & Services, Claude Moors Health Sciences Library, University of Virginia.

Flexner, Abraham. "The German Side of Medical Education." *Atlantic Monthly* 112 (1913): 655–60.

Forbes, William S. "Addresses Commemorative of James Lawrence Cabell," delivered at the University of Virginia, July 1, 1890 (Charlottesville, Va.: Chronicle and C. M. Brand, Steam Book and Job Printers, 1890), 5–8.

Francavilla, Lisa A. "John Patten Emmet (1796–1842)." *Encyclopedia Virginia, Virginia Foundation for the Humanities* electronic publication (accessed February 4, 2016).

Friedberg, Barbara. "Francis Bacon and the End of Skepticism." *Skeptical Inquirer: The Magazine for Science and Reason* 24, no. 6 (2000)32–36.

Friedenwald, Harry. "The Physician's Aphorisms: A Medieval Hebrew Satire." *Johns Hopkins Hospital Bulletin* 29 (1918): 67–71.

Funderburke, Sarah. "Tucker, George (1775–1861)." in *Encyclopedia Virginia*, February 12, 2012. https://encyclopediavirginia.org/entries/tucker-georg-1775-1861

Furber, Louise. "Smallpox and Vaccination." *American Journal of Nursing* 1 (1904): 257–63.

Fye, Bruce S. "Weir Mitchell, Philadelphia's Lost Physiologist." *Bulletin of the History of Medicine* 57, no. 2 (1983): 188–202.

Ganter, Herbert L. "William Small, Jefferson's Beloved Teacher." *William and Mary Quarterly* 4, no. 4 (1947): 505–11.

Garnett, James M. "The Elective System of the University of Virginia." *Andover Review* (April 1886): 1–17.

Gates, Ernie. "Theatre of the Macabre." *Virginia Magazine* (Spring 2017).

Gemmill, Chalmers L. "The Charlottesville General Hospital, 1861–1865." *Magazine of Albemarle County History* 22 (1963–64):91160.

——. "The Educational Work of Robley Dunglison." *Virginia Medical Monthly* 87 (1960).: 307–309.

Gibson, Robert S. "Medical Education in the Nineteenth Century, Jefferson and Flexner Revisited." In *The Founding of Mr. Jefferson's University*, edited by John A. Ragosta, Peter S. Onuf, and Andrew J. O'Shaughnessy. Charlottesville: University of Virginia Press, 2019: 151–89.

Gittings, John Claxton. "Pediatrics One Hundred Years Ago," *American Journal of Diseases of Children*, (1928): 1–15.

Goode, Gordon Brown. "The Beginnings of American Science: The Third Century: 1782–1886." *Proceedings of the Biological Society of Washington* 4 (1888): 9–94.

——. "The Beginnings of Natural History in America. An Address Delivered at the Sixth Anniversary Meeting of the Biological Society of Washington," 1886: 35–105.

Gray, Lewis C. "History of Agriculture in the Southern United States to 1860." *Carnegie Institute of Washington* 2 (1933): 571–1086.

Greenbaum, Louis S. "A Review of Cabanis: Enlightenment and Medical Philosophy in the French Revolution, by Martin S. Staum," *Eighteenth-Century Studies* 16, no. 3 (1983): 336–340.

——. "Thomas Jefferson, the Paris Hospitals, and the University of Virginia." *Eighteenth-Century Studies* 26, no. 4 (1993): 607–626.

——. "Thomas Jefferson's University of Virginia and the Paris Hospitals on the Eve of the French Revolution." *Medical History* 36, no. 3 (1992): 306–319.

Guinness, Ralph B. "The Purpose of the Lewis and Clark Expedition." *Missouri Valley Historical Review* 20 (1933): 90–100.

Hacker, J. David. "A Census-Based Account of the Civil War Dead." *Civil War History* 57 (2011): 307–48.

Hall, Courtney R. "Jefferson on the Medical Theory and Practice of His Day." *Bulletin of the History of Medicine* 31 (1957): 235–245.

Hall, H. Gaston. "Moliere Satirist of Seventeenth-century French Medicine: Fact and Fantasy." *Proceedings of the Royal Society of Medicine* 70 (1977): 425–31.

Halperin, Edward C. "The Poor, the Black, and the Marginalized as the Source of Cadavers in United States Anatomical Education." *Clinical Anatomy* 20 (2007): 489.

Hamlin, Percy G. "Aesculapius in Charlottesville: Robley Dunglison, M.D." *Virginia Cavalcade* 22 (summer 1972): 14–21.

Hammarsten, James F., W. Tattersall, and J. E. Hammarsten. "Who Discovered Smallpox Vaccination? Edward Jenner or Benjamin Jesty?" *Transactions of the American Clinical and Climatological Assoc.* 90 (1979): 44–55.

Hantman, Jeffrey L., and Gary Dunham. "The Enlightened Archaeologist." *Archaeology* 46. no. 3 (1993): 44–49.

Harley, Earl H. "The Forgotten History of Defunct Black Medical Schools in the 19th and 20th Centuries and the Impact of the Flexner Report." *Journal of the National Medical Association* 98, no. 9 (2006): 1425–29.

Harrison, Fairfax. "A Portrait of Governor Fauquier." *Fauquier Historical Society Bulletin*, no. 4 (1924): 343–350.

Harrison, George Tucker. *Address Commemorative of James L. Cabell.* An address delivered at the University of Virginia, July 1, 1890. Charlottesville, Va.: Chronicle and C. M. Brand, Steam Book and Job Printers, 1890: 9–18.

——. *Memorial Sketch of James Lawrence Cabell, M.A., M.D., L.L.D.* An address delivered at the annual meeting of the Medical Society of Virginia. Roanoke, Va.: September 4, 1889: 1–5.

Hart, Andrew D. "Thomas Jefferson's Influence on the Foundation of Medical Education at the University of Virginia." *Annals of Medical History* 10 (1938): 47–60.

Hartleben, K. Lehmann. "Thomas Jefferson, Archeologist." *American Journal of Archaeology* 47 (1943): 161–163.

Hayes, Kevin J. "The Libraries of Thomas Jefferson." In *A Companion to Thomas Jefferson*, edited by Francis D. Cogliano. Malden, Mass.: Wiley-Blackwell, 2012: 333–348.

Heckscher, Jurretta Jordan. "At All Times His Chosen Companion: Some Notes on What Books Meant to Thomas Jefferson." In *The Founding of Mr. Jefferson's University*, edited by John Ragosta, Peter S. Onuf, and Andrew J. O'Shaughnessy. Charlottesville: University of Virginia Press, 2019: 190-207.

Helo, Ari and Peter Onuf. "Jefferson, Morality, and the Problem of Slavery." *William and Mary Quarterly* 60, no. 3 (2003): 583–614.

Henline, Ruth. "A Study of Notes on the State of Virginia as Evidence of Jefferson's Reaction Against the Theories of the French Naturalists." *Virginia Magazine of*

History and Biography 55 (1947): 233–246.

Hickman, Ellen C. "Robley Dunglison (1798-1869)." *Encyclopedia Virginia, Virginia Foundation for the Humanities* (accessed April 20, 2016).

——. "Avoiding the appearance of dictating to the Assembly: Thomas Jefferson and the Establishment of the University of Virginia." In *The Founding of Mr. Jefferson's University*, edited by John Ragosta, Peter Onuf and Andrew O'Shaughnessy, Charlottesville, University of Virginia Press, 2019: 95–101.

Holcombe, James Philemon. "Is Slavery Consistent with Natural Law?" *Southern Literary Messenger*, December 1858: 1–21.

Holowchak, M. Andrew. "The Diffusion of Light: Jefferson's Philosophy of Education." *Democracy and Education* 21, no. 2 (2012): 1–15.

Hooker, Worthington. "The Present Mental Attitude and Tendencies of the Medical Profession." *New Englander* 10 (1952): 548–68.

Hotez, Peter J. "Vaccine Diplomacy: Historical Perspectives and Future Directions." *PLOS Neglected Tropical Diseases* 8, no. 6 (2014): e2808, 14 pages.

Howard, Thomas, and Alfred Brophy. "Proslavery Thought." In *Educated in Tyranny: Slavery at Thomas Jefferson's University*, edited by Maurie McInnis and Louis Nelson. Charlottesville: University of Virginia Press, 2019: 141–170.

Hulkower, Raphael. "From Sacrilege to Privilege: The Tale of Body Procurement for Anatomical Dissection in the United States." *Einstein Journal of Biology and Medicine*, 27, no. 1 (2011): 23–26.

Hunter, Brook. "The Forgotten Legacy of the Hessian Fly." In *The Economy of Early America: Historical Perspectives & New Directions*, edited by Cathy Matson. University Park, Pa.: Penn State University Press, 2006: 236-62.

Hussain, Azhar, Syed Ali, Madiha Ahmed, and Sheharyar Hussain. "The Antivaccination Movement: A Regression in Modern Medicine." *Cureus* 10, no. 7, 2018: e2919, 8 pages.

Iverson, Ian. "The Enslaved Workers of Pavilion X." http://juel.iath.virginia.edu/resources.

Jacobs, James A. "The Dictionary of Virginia Biography, J. L. Cabell (1813–1889)." *Encyclopedia Virginia, Virginia Foundation for the Humanities* (accessed February 4, 2016).

Jones, Colin, and Michael Sonenscher. "The Social Functions of the Hospital in Eighteenth Century France: The Case of the Hotel-Dieu of Nimes." *French Historical Studies* 13, no. 2 (1983): 172–214.

Jones, Jeanne A., and Chalmers Gemmill. "The Notebook of Robley Dunglison, a Student of Clinical Medicine in Edinburgh." *Journal of the History of Medicine and Allied Sciences* 22, no. 3 (1967): 262–73.

Jones, Kenneth Robert. "The Development of Medical Sects." *Journal of Religion and Health*, 22, no. 4 (1983): 307–21.

Jones, Russel M. "American Doctors in the Parisian Medical World." *Bulletin of the History of Medicine* 47, no. 2 (1973): 40–65.

Jordan, Ervin I. *Charlottesville and the University of Virginia in the Civil War*. Lynchburg, Va.: H. B. Howard, 1988: 45–61.

——. "Charlottesville during the Civil War." *Encyclopedia Virginia, Virginia Foundation for the Humanities* (accessed March 16, 2016).

Kahn, Charles. "History of Smallpox and its Prevention." *American Journal of Diseases of Children* 106 (1963): 597–609.

Kastor, Peter J. "The Lewis and Clark Expedition." *Encyclopedia Virginia, Virginia Foun-*

dation for the Humanities (accessed November 20, 2019).

Kaufman, Martin. "American Medical Education," in *The Education of American Physicians*, edited by Ronald L. Numbers, Berkeley, University of California Press, (1980): 7–28.

Kaufman, M. H. "John Barclay (1758–1826) extra-mural teacher of anatomy in Edinburgh: Honorary Fellow of the Royal College of Surgeons of Edinburgh." *Surgeon*, 4, no.2 (2006): 93–100.

Kelly, Matt. "The Past as Prologue: How UVA Has Risen to Meet Crises Throughout History." *UVA Today*, April 3, 2020.

Kenny, Stephen C. "The Development of Medical Museums in the Antebellum South." Bulletin of the History of Medicine 87 (2013): 32–62.

Kett, Joseph. "Education," In *Thomas Jefferson: A Reference Biography*, edited by M.D. Peterson, New York, Charles Scribner's Sons, (1986): 238.

Keys, Thomas E. "The Colonial Libraries and the Development of Sectional Differences in the Colonies." *The Library Quarterly* 8 (1933): 373–390.

Kilbride, Daniel. "Southern Medical Students in Philadelphia, 1800–1860: Science and Sociability in the 'Republic of Medicine'," *Journal of Southern History* 65, no. 4 (1999): 697–732.

Kluger, Jeffrey. "Too Many Americans Still Mistrust the Covid-19 Vaccines. Here's Why." *Time Magazine*, January 5, 2021.

Koelsch, William A. "Thomas Jefferson, American Geographers, and the Uses of Geography." *Geographical Review* 98 (2008): 260–279.

Kopperman, Paul E. "Venerate the Lancet: Benjamin Rush's Yellow Fever Therapy in Context." *Bulletin of the History of Medicine* 78, no. 3 (2004): 539–574.

Ladlam, David M. "Thomas Jefferson and the American Climate." *Bulletin of the American Meteorological Society* 47 (1966): 974–975.

Larson, Heidi J. "The Biggest Pandemic Risk? Viral Misinformation." *Nature* 562 (2018): 309.

Leavell, Byrd S. "Jeffersonian Ideas Endowed the University of Virginia." *Virginia Medical Monthly* 104 (1977): 91–96.

——. "Thomas Jefferson and Smallpox Vaccination." *Transactions of the American Clinical and Climatological Assoc.* 88 (1977): 119–127.

Lewis, Danny. "The Oldest Chemistry Lab in America?" *Smithsonian Magazine*, SmartNews, October 14, 2015.

Lewis, V. Bradley. "The Politics of Pragmatism," February 7, 2013, available at americamagazine.org/issue/culture/politics-pragmatism.

Littin, Bud. "Citizen Weather Observers." *Weatherwise* 43, no. 5 (1990): 254–259.

Lombardo, Paul A. "The Power of Heredity and the Relevance of Eugenic History." *Genetics in Medicine* 20 (2018): 1305–1311.

London Medical Repository, "Tribute to Robley Dunglison," October 1, 1824.

Longo, Lawrence D. "Obstetrics and Gynecology." In *The Education of American Physicians*, edited by Ronald L. Numbers. Berkeley: University of California Press, 1980: 205–225.

Looney, J. Jefferson. "The Master's Degree: A note to Readers." In *Princetonians: 1791-1794,* edited by J. Jefferson Looney and Ruth L. Woodward. Princeton: Princeton University Press, 1991: 489–490.

——. "From Academy to College to University: The Prehistory of the University of Virginia." In *The Founding of Thomas Jefferson's University*, edited by John A. Ragosta et al, Charlottesville, 2019:1122.

Lucas, Frederic A. "Thomas Jefferson: Paleontologist." *Natural History* 26 (1926): 26.

Lurie, Edward. "Louis Agassiz and the Races of Man." *Isis: a journal of the History of Science Society* 45. no. 3 (1954): 227–242.

Lynchburg Daily Virginian, "Relocating the Medical Department of the University of Virginia to Richmond," an editorial, April 9, 1867.

Malone, Dumas. "Jefferson Goes to School in Williamsburg." *Virginia Quarterly Review* 33 (1957): 481–496.

Mainwaring, Robert D., and Curtis C. Tribble. "The Cardiac Illness of General Robert E. Lee." *Surgery, Gynecology & Obstetrics* 174 (1992): 237–244.

Markel, Howard. "December 14, 1700: The Excruciating Final Hours of President George Washington," *PBS NewsHour*, December 14, 2014.

Martin. Henry A. "Jefferson as a Vaccinator." *North Carolina Medical Journal* 7 (1881): 1–34.

Martin, Russel L. "Jefferson's Cause of Death." *Thomas Jefferson Encyclopedia* (accessed May 1990).

Matson, Emily. "John Staige Davis." *Encyclopedia Virginia, Virginia Foundation for the Humanities* (accessed November 13, 2017).

Matsuura, Jeffrey H. "Thomas Jefferson and the Evolution of a Populist Vision of Intellectual Property Rights and Democratic Values." An address given at the symposium *Technology and Democratic Values in the Early Republic* at the University of Virginia, November 3, 2006. www.archipelago.org/vol10-34/matsuura.htm

Maulitz, Richard. "Channel Crossing: The Lure of French Pathology for English Medical Students, 1816-36." *Bulletin of the History of Medicine* 55 (1981): 475–496.

Mayo, Bernard. "A Peppercorn for Mr. Jefferson." *Virginia Quarterly Review*, 19 (1943): 222–235.

Mayo, Henry W. "Robley Dunglison—1798–1869: First Professor of Medicine in Virginia." *Virginia Medical Monthly* 79 (1952): 708–711.

McCorvey, Thomas Chalmers. "Henry Tutwiler and the Influence of the University of Virginia on Education in Alabama." *Alabama Historical Society*, Montgomery, Ala. (1905): 83-106.

McDaid, Jennifer Davis. "Oriana Russel Moon Andrews (1834–1883)." *Dictionary of Virginia Biography*, Library of Virginia, 2016.

McDaniel, W. B. "A View of 19th Century Medical Historiography in the United States of America," *The Bulletin of the History of Medicine* 33, no. 5 (1959): 415–435.

"Memorial of the Faculty of the University to the Rector and Board of Visitors Touching on the Removal of the Medical Department to Richmond." Special Collections Library, University of Virginia, April 2, 1867.

Miles, Wyndham D. "William James MacNeven and Early Laboratory Instruction in the United States." *Ambix* 17, no. 3 (1970): 143–152.

Miller, August C. "Jefferson as an Agriculturist." *Agricultural History*, 16, no. 2 (1942): 65–78.

Miller, Genevieve. "Smallpox Inoculation in England and America: A Reappraisal." *William and Mary Quarterly* 13, no. 4 (1956): 476–492.

——. "Medical History." In *The Education of American Physicians*, edited by Ronald L. Numbers, Berkeley, University of California, 1980: 290–308.

Miller, Lynn E., and Richard M. Weiss. "Medical Education Reform Efforts and Failures in U.S. Medical Schools, 1870–1910." *Journal of the History of Medicine and Allied Sciences* 63 (2008):348–387.

Minardi, Margot. "The Boston Inoculation Controversy of 1721–1722: An Incident in

the History of Race." *William and Mary Quarterly* 61, no. 1 (2004): 47–76.
Mitchell, Samuel L. "Preface." In *Erasmus Darwin, Zoonomia of Laws of Organic Life*, American edition, New York, 1796: xxii.
Mitchell, Thomas D. "Calomel Considered as a Poison." *New Orleans Medical Journal* 5, no. 1 (1844): 28–35.
Moll, Wilhelm. "History of American Medical Education." *British Journal of Medical Education* 2, issue 3 (1968): 173–181.
——. "Medical Fee Bills." *Virginia Medical Monthly* 93 (1966): 657–664.
——. "University of Virginia's 'Firsts' in the History of Medical Education." *Virginia Medical Monthly* 95 (1968): 158–161.
Moore, John H. "The University of Virginia During the Civil War." *Virginia Cavalcade* 13, no. 3 (Winter 1963–64): 23–32.
Moore, Thomas C., and James A. Shield. "Medical Education at America's First University." *Journal of Medical Education* 44, no. 4 (1969): 241–248.
Morrell, Jack B. "Practical Chemistry in the University of Edinburgh, 1799-1843." *Ambix* 16 (1969): 66–80.
Murray, Jock. "Thomas Jefferson and Medicine." *Journal of Medical Biography* 5 (1997): 146–157.
National Intelligencer. "Regulating Public Markets," October 11, 1802. https://lccn.loc.gov/sn83045242
National Intelligencer. "Health Care for the Poor," November 1, 1802. https://lccn.loc.gov/sn83045242
Neem, Johann N. "Developing Freedom: Thomas Jefferson, the State, and Human Capability." *Studies in American Political Development* 27, no. 1 (2013): 36–50.
New York Times, "Abraham Flexner Is Dead at 92; Revolutionized Medical Schools," September 22, 1959.
——. "The Making of Doctors." June 12, 1910.
——. "Voters in Oregon Allow Doctors to Help the Terminally Ill Die," November 11, 1984.
Neumann, Brian. "UVA Unionists: The University of Virginia's Neglected Alumni." In *Magazine of Albemarle Charlottesville History* 78 (2020): 73–108.
North, Robert. "Benjamin Rush, Md.: Assassin or Beloved Healer?" *Proceedings Baylor Medical Center* 13, no. 1 (2000): 45–49.
Numbers, Ronald L. "William Beaumont and the Ethics of Human Experimentation." *Journal of the History of Biology* 12, no. 1 (1979): 113–135.
O'Brien, Connor Cruise. "Thomas Jefferson: Radical and Racist." *The Atlantic* (October 1, 1996).
Ogden, Emily. "He Blinded Me with Science." *Lapham's Quarterly Online*, August 29, 2018. https://www.laphamsquartertly.org/roundtable/he-blinded-me-science
Oliver, John W. "Thomas Jefferson—Scientist." *The Scientific Monthly* 56, no. 5 (1943): 460–467.
O'Neal, William B. "Financing the Construction of the University of Virginia: Notes and Documents." *Magazine of the Albemarle County History* 23, (1964–1965): 5–34.
Ousager, Jakob, and Helle Johannessen. "Humanities in Undergraduate Medical Education: A Literature Review." *Academic Medicine* 85 (2010): 988–998.
Parshall, Karen Hunger. "Bonnycastle, Charles (12796-184)." in Dictionary of Virginia Biography, available online at Encyclopedia Virginia, https://encyclopediavirginia.org/entries/bonnycastle-charles-1796–1840/.

Parton, James. "College Days of Thomas Jefferson." *Atlantic Monthly* 29, no. 171 (1872): 16–34.

Patten, John S. "A Short Story of Our Library." *Alumni Bulletin of the University of Virginia* 11, (1918): 422–425.

Patton, John S. "The History of Faculty Chairmen of the University of Virginia." *Alumni Bulletin of the University of Virginia*, series 4, no. 4 (1904): 263–273.

Peale, Franklin. "Memorial of the Late Robley Dunglison." Philadelphia: Collins Printer, 1869: 3–19.

Pearson, J. Diane. "Medical Diplomacy and the American Indian: Thomas Jefferson, the Lewis and Clark Expedition, and the Subsequent Effects on American Health and Public Policy." *Wícazo Sa Review* 19, no. 1, 2004: 106–108.

Peden, William. "Some Aspects of Jefferson's Bibliography: A Paper Read before the Bibliographical Society of America." Lexington, Va.: Journalism Laboratory Press, Washington and Lee University, 1941.

——. "Some Notes Concerning Thomas Jefferson's Libraries." *William and Mary Quarterly* 1, no. 3 (1944): 265–272.

Pernick, Martin. "Politics, Parties, and Pestilence: Epidemic Yellow Fever in Philadelphia and the Rise of the First Party System." *William and Mary Quarterly* 29, no. 4 (1997): 559–586.

Peterson, Merrill D. "Thomas Jefferson's Notes on the State of Virginia." In *Studies in Eighteenth Century Culture*, vol. 7, edited by Roseann Runte. Madison, Wis.: University of Wisconsin Press, 1978: 49–62.

Pierre, Joseph. "Antivaxxers and the Plague of Science Denial." *Psychology Today*, February 8, 2019.

Pitts, Grover C. "History of Physiology at the University of Virginia." *The Physiologist* 28, no. 5 (1985): 402–406.

Pritchett, Henry S. "Jefferson's Interest in Science." *Alumni Bulletin of the University of Virginia* 6 (1900): 74–75.

Puzio, Dominic. "The Anatomical Theatre (1825-1939)." *Jefferson's University . . . Early Years,* (June 8, 2015). https://juel.iath.virginia.edu/node/242.

Radbill, Samuel X. "Dr. Robley Dunglison and Jefferson." *Transactions of the American Philosophical Society* 57 (1959): 40–44.

——. "Robley Dunglison: An Eminent Figure in Philadelphia Medicine." *Transactions and Studies of the College of Physicians of Philadelphia* 32, no. 4 (1965): 164–170.

——. "Robley Dunglison, M.D., 1798-1869, American Medical Educator." *Journal of Medical Education* 34, no. 2 (1959): 84–94.

——. "Thomas Jefferson and the Doctors." *Transactions and Studies of the College of Physicians of Philadelphia* 37, no. 2 (1969): 106–114.

Ragosta, John. "Notes on the State of Virginia." *Thomas Jefferson Encyclopedia* (accessed February 22, 2018).

Randolph, Fred J., and Fred L. Francis. "Thomas Jefferson as Meteorologist." *Monthly Weather Review* 23 (1895): 456–458.

Ranlet, Phillip. "The British, Slaves and Smallpox." *The Journal of Negro History* 84 (1999): 217–226.

Reps, John W. "Thomas Jefferson's Checkerboard Towns," *Journal of the Society of Architectural Historians* 20, no. 3 (1961): 108–114.

Reynolds, Terry S. "The Education of Engineers in America before the Morrill Act of 1862." *History of Education Quarterly* 32, no. 4 (1992): 459–482.

Richmond Enquirer, "Calomel, An Old Song," March 2, 1816.

——. "A Friend of the University," May 30, 1845.

——. Obituary and memorial of John Patten Emmet, October 18, 1842.

——. "Typhoid Outbreak at the University," March 10, 1829.

Richmond, I. "Robley Dunglison M.D." *Pennsylvania Medicine* 69 (1966): 76–77.

Richmond Whig, "The College Fusion Question," April 5, 1867

——. "Virginia Medical Education." April 5, 1867.

Riedel, Stefan. "Edward Jenner and the History of Smallpox and Vaccination." *Proceedings Baylor University Medical Center* 18, no. 1 (2005): 21–25.

Ring, Malvin E. "The Dental Health of President John Adams." *New York State Dental Journal* 70, no. 7 (2004): 36–37.

Robb-Smith, Alastair Hamish Tearlock. "Medical Education at Oxford and Cambridge Prior to 1850." In *The Evolution of Medical Education in Britain*, edited by Frederick Noel Lawrence Poynter. London: Pitman Publisher, 1966: 19–52.

Robinson, Daniel N. "Jefferson and Adams on the Mind-Body Problem." *History of Psychology* 6, no. 3 (2003): 228–238.

Roguin, Ariel. "Rene Laennec (1781–1826): The Man behind the Stethoscope." *Clinical Medicine & Research* 4, no. 3 (2006): 230-235.

Rooney, William E. "Thomas Jefferson and the New Orleans Marine Hospital." *Journal of Southern History* 22, no.2 (1956): 167–182.

Rosen, George. "The Philosophy of Ideology and Emergence of Modern Medicine in France." *Bulletin of the History of Medicine* 20 (1946): 328–339.

——. "Political Order and Human Health in Jeffersonian Thought." *Bulletin of the History of Medicine* 26, no. 1 (1952): 32–44.

Rosenfeld, Leonard M. "Physiology at Jefferson Medical College (1842–1982)." *The Physiologist* 27, no. 3 (1984):113–127.

Runk, Benjamin Franklin Dewees. "John Patten Emmet." *Magazine of Albemarle County History* 13 (1953): 54–67.

Rusnock, Andrea. "Catching Smallpox: The Early Spread of Smallpox Vaccination." *Bulletin of the History of Medicine* 83 (2009): 17–36.

Rutkow, Ira. "Joseph Lister and His 1876 Tour of America." *Annals of Surgery* 257, no. 6 (2013):1181–1187.

Saling, E and B. Arabin. "Historical Landmarks of Perinatal Medicine in Obstetrics." *Journal of Perinatal Medicine*, 16, no. 1 (1968): 5–21.

Savitt, Todd L. "Jefferson's Vision of Medical Education and His Quest for a Professor of Medicine." *Virginia Quarterly* 122, no. 4 (1995): 245–251.

----. "The Use of Blacks for Medical Experimentation and Demonstration in the Old South." *The Journal of Southern History* 48, no. 3 (1982): 331–348.

Scherr, Arthur. "An Honest, Intelligent Man: Thomas Jefferson, the Free Black Patrick Henry, and the Founder's Racist Views in His Last Years." *The Virginia Magazine of History and Biography* 127, no. 4 (2019): 300–339.

Schlich, Thomas. "Asepsis and Bacteriology: A Realignment of Surgery and Laboratory Science." *Medical History* 56, no. 3 (2012): 308–334.

Schulman, Gayle M. "Slaves at the University of Virginia." Unpublished paper presented to the African-American Gemology Group of Charlottesville/Albemarle, May 2003, MSS 16138, Albert and Shirley Small Special Collections Library.

Semba, Richard D. "The Ocular Complications of Smallpox and Smallpox Immunization." *Archives of Ophthalmology* 121 (2003): 715–719.

Sherwood, Patricia C., and Joseph M. Lasala. "Education and Architecture: The Evolution of the University of Virginia's Academical Village." In *Thomas Jefferson's*

Academical Village, edited by Richard Guy Wilson. Charlottesville: University of Virginia Press, 1993: 9–45.

Shryock, Richard Harrison. "Empiricism versus Rationalism in American Medicine, 1650–1950." *Proceedings of the American Antiquarian Society* 79 (1969): 99-150.

——. "European Backgrounds of American Medical Education (1600-1900)." *Journal of the American Medical Association* 194 (1965): 709–714.

——. "The Health of the American People." *Proceedings of the American Philosophical Society* 90, no. 4 (1946): 251–258.

——. "The Advent of Modern Medicine in Philadelphia, 1800–1850." *Yale Journal of Biology Medicine* 13 (1941): 715–738.

——. "The Medical Reputation of Benjamin Rush: Contrasts over Two Centuries." *Bulletin of Medical History* 45, no 6 (1971): 507–552.

——. "Nineteenth Century Medicine: Scientific Aspects." *Journal of World History* 3, no. 4 (1957): 881–908.

——. "Public Relations of the Medical Profession in Great Britain and the United States: 1600–1870." In *The Social History of Medicine, Annuals of Medical History* 2 (1930): 308–339.

Shuman, Andrew G, Marc Edelman, and Joseph J. Fins. "Bleeding by the numbers: Rush versus Cobbett." *The Pharos* (autumn 2014): 10–16.

Simpson, George Gaylord. "The Beginnings of Vertebrate Paleontology in North America." *Proceedings of the American Philosophical Society* 80 (1942): 130–188.

Slawson, Robert G. "Medical Training in the United States Prior to the Civil War." *Journal of Evidence-Based Complimentary and Alternative Medicine* 17, no. 1 (2012): 11–27.

Smith, Stephen. "Addresses Commemorative of James L. Cabell." Delivered at the University of Virginia, July 1, 1889, (Charlottesville: Chronicle and C.B. Brand, Stern Book and Job Printers, 1890): 19–40.

Spero, Patrick. "The Other Presidency: Thomas Jefferson and the American Philosophical Society." *Proceedings of the American Philosophical Society* 162, no. 4 (2018): 321–360.

Spillane, John David. "Doctors of 1776: I." *British Medical Journal* 1, no. 6025 (1976): 1571–1574.

Spratt, John G. "Thomas Jefferson: The Scholarly Politician and His Influence on Medicine." *Southern Medical Journal* 69 (1976): 360–366.

The Southern Argus (Norfolk, Virginia), December 3, 1858.

Southern Literary Messenger. "The University: Its Character and Wants." April 1856: 241–269.

——. "Mr. Rives Address." September 9, 1847: 574–576.

Staloff, Darren. "Ideology, Empiricism, and Politics: The Philosophical Exchanges of Thomas Jefferson and John Adams." Paper presented at the 2017 SAR Annual Conference on the American Revolution, Quincy, Mass. (June 9, 2017).

Steele, Brian. "Thomas Jefferson's Gender Frontier." *Journal of American History* 95, no. 1 (2008): 17–42.

Stern, Alexandra M., and Howard Markel. "The History of Vaccines and Immunization: Familiar Patterns, New Challenges." *Health Affairs* 24, no. 3 (2005): 611–621.

Stray, Christopher. "Key, Thomas Hewitt, Latin Scholar (1799–1875)." *Oxford Dictionary of National Biography*, Oxford University Press (2004).

Stricker, Frank. "American Professors in the Progressive Era: Incomes, Aspirations, and Professionalism." *Journal of Interdisciplinary History* 19, no. 2, 1988.

Sturges, Mark. "Founding Farmers: Jefferson, Washington and the Rhetoric of Agricultural Reform." *Early American Literature* 50, no. 3 (2015): 681–709.

Sullivan, Robert B. "Rush, Benjamin." *American National Biography* 19, (1999): 72–75.

Svrluga, Susan. "America's First Chemistry Lab Discovered Accidentally in a Building Designed by Thomas Jefferson." *The Washington Post*, October 13, 2015.

Szmuk, Peter, Tiberiu Ezri, Shmuel Evron, Yehudah Roth, and Jeffrey Katz. "A Brief History of Tracheostomy and Tracheal Intubation, from the Bronze Age to the Space Age." *Intensive Care Medicine* 34 (2008): 222–228.

Tarter, Brent. "Blaetermann, George (1782–1850." in Dictionary of Virginia Biography, available online at Encyclopedia Virginia: https://encyclopediavirginia.org/entries/blaetermann-george-1782-1850/.

Tay, Endrina. "Forming the Body of a Library Based on the 'Illimitable Freedom of the Human Mind.'" In *The Founding of Thomas Jefferson's University*, edited by John Ragosta, Peter S. Onuf, and Andrew J. O'Shaughnessy. Charlottesville: University of Virginia Press, (2019): 208–223.

——. "Jefferson, Thomas and Books." *Encyclopedia Virginia* (2021, February 23). https://encyclopediavirginia.org/entries/jefferson-thomas-and-books.

Taylor, Alan. "The Virtue of an Educated Voter." *American Scholar* 85 (September 6, 2016): 18-27, available at https://theamericanscholar.org/the-virtue-of-an-educated-voter/#.

Thomson, Keith. "The Question of Climatic Stability in America before 1900." *Climate Change* 3 (1981): 227–241.

Thorson, David. Benjamin Rush, *Thomas Jefferson Encyclopedia*, (May 28, 2020)

Thorup, Oscar A. "Thomas Jefferson and Academic Medicine." *The Pharos*, (April 1977): 16–23.

——. "Thomas Jefferson and a Few of His Physician Friends." *Transactions of the American Clinical and Climatological Association* 104 (1992): 138–145.

——. "Thomas Jefferson: Founder of Two Medical Schools." *Transactions of the American Clinical and Climatological Association* 92 (1980): 16–22.

Traill, Thomas S. "Memoir of Dr. Charles Thomas Hope." Transactions of the Royal Society of Edinburgh 16 (1849): 419–434.

Trask, John W. "The United States Marine Hospital, port of Boston: An account of its origin and briefly of its history and of the physicians who have been in charge." Washington, Federal Security Agency, U.S. Public Health Service, 1940: 51–83.

Trent, William P. "The Influence of the University of Virginia upon Southern Life and Thought." In Herbert B. Adams, *Thomas Jefferson and the University of Virginia, 1888*:
150–175.

Turner, W. A. "The College Fusion Question." Broadside, To the Editors of the Richmond Enquirer, 1867.

Tutwiler, Henry. *Address of H. Tutwiler, A.M., L.L.D. of Alabama, Before the Alumni Society of the University of Virginia*. Charlottesville: Charlottesville Chronicle Book and Job Office, 1882: 3–14.

Underwood, E. Ashworth. "Edward Jenner, Benjamin Waterhouse and the Introduction of Vaccination in the United States." *Nature* 163 (1949): 823–828.

Union of Concerned Scientists. *Science and Democracy in the United States: A Rich History*, August 20, 2012. ucsusa.org/resources/science-and-democracy-united-states.

Valley Virginian of Staunton. Editorial on Relocating the Medical Department of the University of Virginia to Richmond. April 24, 1867.

Verner, Coolie. "Mr. Jefferson Makes a Map." *International Journal of the History of Cartography* 14 (1959): 96–108.

von Daacke, Kirt. "Anatomical Theater." In *Educated in Tyranny*, edited by Maurie McInnis and Louis P. Nelson. Charlottesville: University of Virginia Press, 2019: 171–198.

Wagoner, Jennings L. "Honor and Dishonor at Mr. Jefferson's University: The Antebellum Years." *History of Education Quarterly* 26, no. 2 (1986): 155–179.

——. "Mr. Jefferson's Academy: An Educational Interpretation." In *Thomas Jefferson's Military Academy: Founding West Point*, edited by Robert M. McDonald. Charlottesville: University of Virginia Press, 2004: 118–153.

——. "Thomas Jefferson and the Education of a New Nation." Bloomington, Indiana: Phi Beta Kappa Educational Foundation, 1976: 5–41.

——. "Jefferson and Education." *Monticello Monograph Series*, distributed by The University of North Carolina, Chapel Hill, North Carolina (2004): 9–168.

Waite, Frederick C. "American Sectarian Medical Colleges before the Civil War." *Bulletin of the History of Medicine* 19, no. 2 (1946): 1–15.

——. "Grave Robbing in New England." *Bulletin of the Medical Library Association* 33 (1945): 272–294.

Waite, John G., Clay S. Palazzo, and Mathew K. Scheldt. *The Chemical Hearth and the First Chemistry Teaching Laboratories and Lecture Rooms at the University of Virginia, Charlottesville*. John G. Waite Associates, Architects and the University of Virginia, 2017: 7–74.

Wall, L. Lewis. "Thomas Addis Emmet, the Vesicovaginal Fistula, and the Origins of Reconstructive Gynecological Surgery." *International Urogynecology Journal* 13 (2002): 145–155.

Wallace, Henry A. "Keynote Address." *Proceedings of the Association of Land-Grant Colleges and Universities* 51 (1937): 336–346.

Wallenborn, McKenzie. "Thomas Jefferson and the Medicine of His Day." *Medical Alumni News of the University of Virginia* 11, no. 1 (2002): 3–9.

Walterscheid, Edward C. "Thomas Jefferson and the Patient Act of 1793." 40 *Essays in History* 3 (1998): I–VIII. www.stephankinsella.com/2010/06/thomas-jefferson-and-the-patent-act-of-1793/

Warner, John Harley. "Physiology." In *The Education of American Physicians*, edited by Ronald Numbers. Berkeley: University of California, 1980: 48–71.

——. "The Selective Transport of Medical Knowledge: Antebellum American Physicians and Parisian Medical Therapeutics." *Bulletin of the History of Medicine* 59, no. 2 (1985): 213–231.

——. "A Southern Medical Reform: The Meaning of Antebellum Argument for Southern Medical Education." *Bulletin of the History of Medicine* 57, no. 3 (1983): 364–381.

Waterhouse, Benjamin. "Something Curious in the Medical Line." *Columbian Sentinel* (a Boston newspaper), March 12, 1799.

Wehrman, Andrew. "Thomas Jefferson, Inoculation, and the Norfolk Riots," presented at a symposium on *The Spirit of Inquiry in the Age of Jefferson*, American Philosophical Society, 7–8 June 2018.

Weiss, Harry B. "Thomas Jefferson and Economic Entomology." *Journal of Economic Entomology* 37, no. 6 (1944): 836–841.

Weiss, Robin and Jose Esparza. "The Prevention and Eradication of Smallpox." *Philosophical Transactions of the Royal Society London* 370 (2015): 1666.

Welch, William. "Some of the Advantages of the Union of Medical School and University." In *William H. Welch, Papers and Addresses*, vol. 3. Baltimore: Johns Hopkins University Press, 1930.

Wenger, Mark. "Thomas Jefferson, the College of William and Mary, and the University of Virginia." *The Virginia Magazine of History and Biography* 103, no. 3 (1995): 339–374.

Wernau, Julie and Paul Overberg. "Covid-19 Vaccine Hesitancy Present Challenge for Herd-Immunity Push." *Wall Street Journal*, February 3, 2021.

Wertenbaker, Charles Christian. "Early Days of the University." *The Alumni Bulletin of the University of Virginia* 4, no. 1 (May 1897): 21–25.

Wheat, Thomas Adrian. "Medicine in Virginia during the Civil War." *Encyclopedia Virginia, Virginia Foundation for the Humanities* (accessed April 27, 2016).

Whorton, James. "Chemistry", In *The Education of American Physicians*, edited by Ronald L. Numbers, Berkeley, University of California Press, (1980): 72–94.

Williams, Eleri, and A. Neil Turner. "Broadening Our Horizons: Are Medical Humanities an Essential Part of Medical Education?" *Nephrology, Dialysis, Transplantation* 33, (2018): 1511–1513.

Wilson, Douglas L. "The Evolution of Jefferson's Notes on the State of Virginia." *Virginia Magazine of History and Biography* 112 (2004): 98–133.

——. "Jefferson and the Republic of Letters." In *Jeffersonian Legacies*, edited by Peter S. Onuf. Charlottesville: University of Virginia Press, 1993: 50–76.

Wilson, Gayle. "American Philosophical Society." *Monticello Research Report, Thomas Jefferson Encyclopedia* (accessed November 1997).

——. "Jefferson: Advocate of Inoculation." *Monticello Newsletter*, No. 15 (Spring 2004).

____. "Medicine." *Thomas Jefferson Encyclopedia*, (February 2004).

——. "Jefferson Authorizes the Survey of the Coasts." *Monticello Newsletter*, No. 18 (Fall 2007).

Wilson, Richard Guy. "Inspirational Learning. The Architecture of the University of Virginia." *The Journal of Thomas Jefferson's Life and Times* 1, no. 2 (February 2017): 11–21.

Wolfe, Brendan. "Slavery at the University." *Encyclopedia Virginia, Virginia Foundation for the Humanities* (accessed February 2016).

Woods, Mary. "Thomas Jefferson and the University of Virginia: Planning the Academic Village." *Journal of the Society of Architectural Historians* 44, no. 3 (1985): 266–283.

WS. "The Modesty of True Science as Exemplified in the Characters of Newton, Franklin and Humboldt." *The Virginia University Magazine* 4 (October 1859): 93–98.

Woodward, Samuel Bayard. "The Story of Smallpox in Massachusetts." *New England Journal of Medicine* 206, no. 23 (1932): 1181–1191.

Wu, Osmond C., Sunil Manjila, Nima Malakooti and Alan R. Cohen "The remarkable medical lineage of the Monro family: contributions of Alexander primus, secundus, and tertius." *Journal of Neurosurgery* 116, no.6, (2012): 1337–1346.

Yardley, Jonathan. "The Complex Thomas Jefferson in his Time and Place." *The Washington Post*, May 12, 2017.

Young, J. H. "James Hamilton (1767–1839, obstetrician and controversialist." *Medical Hist*ory 7, no.1 (1963): 62-73.

Zechmeister, Gene. "Construction of the University, 1817–1826." *Thomas Jefferson Encyclopedia*, January 2012.

Zirkle, Conway. "The Early History of the Inheritance of Acquired Characters and of

Pangenesis." *Transactions of the American Philosophical Society* 35, no. 2 (1946): 91–151.

Secondary Sources: Dissertations

Atwater, Edward C. "Financial Subsides for American Medical Education before 1940." MA thesis, Johns Hopkins University, 1974.

Carey, John Peter. "Influences on Thomas Jefferson's Theory and Practice of Higher Education." PhD diss., University of Michigan, 1969.

Carlquist-Sagers, Andrea B. "Jefferson's Sensitivities: How Thomas Jefferson's Discussions of Race and Slavery are Influenced by Audience." Undergraduate Honors Capstone Projects. Utah State University, 2020.

Clagett, Martin. "William Small, 1734–1775: Teacher, Mentor and Scientist." PhD thesis, Virginia Commonwealth University, 2002.

Dabney, William M. "Jefferson's Albemarle County, Va., 1727–1819." PhD thesis, University of Virginia, 1951.

Grizzard, Frank E. "Documentary History of the Construction of the Buildings of the University of Virginia, 1817–1828." PhD diss., University of Virginia, August 1996.

Hudson, Robert P. "Patterns of Medical Education in Nineteenth Century America." MA thesis, Johns Hopkins University, 1966.

Neale, Catherine S. "Slaves, Freed People, and the University of Virginia." Undergraduate Honors Thesis, Corcoran Department of History, University of Virginia, April 2006.

Ogden, Emily. "The Science of Error: Mesmerism and American Fiction, 1744–1890." Publically Accessible Penn Dissertations, http://repository.penn.ed/dissertations/296. Pennsylvania State University, 2010.

Peden, William H. "Thomas Jefferson: Book Collector." PhD diss., University of Virginia, 1942.

Rogers, Elizabeth A. "The Foundation and Early History of the Medical School of the University of Virginia. Master of Science thesis, University of Virginia, 1930. Copy in the Virginia Room, University of Virginia Library.

Shawen, Neil McDowell. "The Casting of a Lengthened Shadow: Thomas Jefferson's Role in Determining the Site for a State University in Virginia." EdD diss., George Washington University, 1980.

Smallwood, Mary Lovett. "An Historical Study of Examinations and Grading Systems in Early American Universities." PhD diss., Cambridge: Harvard University Press, 1935.

Smith, Dale C. "The Emergence of Organized Clinical Instruction in Nineteenth-Century Cities of Boston, New York, and Philadelphia." PhD diss., University of Minnesota, 1979.

Wall, Charles C. "Students and Student Life at the University of Virginia: 1825–1861." PhD diss., University of Virginia, 1978.

Wiley, W. H. "Academic Freedom at the University of Virginia: The First Hundred Years from Jefferson through Alderman." Unpublished diss., University of Virginia Library, 1973.

Reading furnishes the mind only with
materials of knowledge;
it is thinking that makes what we read ours.

John Locke, 1706

Index